40.00

ORAL MEDICINE SECRETS

ORAL MEDICINE SECRETS

Stephen T. Sonis, D.M.D., D.M.Sc.
Professor and Chair
Department of Oral Medicine, Infection, and Immunity
Harvard School of Dental Medicine
Brigham and Women's Hospital, and
The Dana-Farber Cancer Institute
Boston, Massachusetts

Robert C. Fazio, D.M.D.
Associate Clinical Professor of Surgery
Yale Medical School
Professor of Biology
University of New Haven
New Haven, Connecticut
Private Practice of Periodontology and Oral Medicine
Norwalk, Connecticut

Leslie Shu-Tung Fang, M.D., Ph.D.
Assistant Professor of Medicine
Harvard Medical School
Physician, Massachusetts General Hospital
Boston, Massachusetts

HANLEY & BELFUS, INC./Philadelphia

Publisher: HANLEY & BELFUS, INC.
               Medical Publishers
               210 South 13th Street
               Philadelphia, PA 19107
               (215) 546-7293; 800-962-1892
               FAX (215) 790-9330
               Web site: http://www.hanleyandbelfus.com

Note to the reader: Although the information in this book has been carefully reviewed for correctness of dosage and indications, neither the author nor the publisher can accept any legal responsibility for any errors or omissions that may be made. Neither the publisher nor the author makes any warranty, expressed or implied, with respect to the material contained herein. Before prescribing any drug, the reader must review the manufacturer's current product information (package inserts) for accepted indications, absolute dosage recommendations, and other information pertinent to the safe and effective use of the product described. This is especially important when drugs are given in combination or as an adjunct to other forms of therapy.

ORAL MEDICINE SECRETS   ISBN 1-56053-419-2

Library of Congress Control Number: 2002107106

Last digit is the print number: 9   8   7   6   5   4   3   2   1

CONTENTS

Contents

PREFACE

Oral medicine has become an important part of dental practice. The population is aging, and with better medical management, patients with many significant chronic diseases are living longer. The amount and number of medications being consumed have skyrocketed. Patients take drugs to manage diseases, modulate symptoms, and prevent new pathology. With an emphasis on medical cost-containment, patients who, in the past, were hospitalized are now treated on an ambulatory basis. The bottom line for us is that there are a lot of patients with systemic disease who will regularly seek dental care, and these patients expect that the dentist will be able to deliver sophisticated treatment despite any underlying pathology. Dental management of medically compromised patients has thus become a routine part of dental practice.

Furthermore, many patients are affected by the lumps, bumps, blisters, ulcers, and white lesions that affect the mouth. Although most of these are benign, many represent diseases that affect morbidity and mortality.

All three of us have taught oral medicine to dentists, physicians, residents, and students. We like the subject and we like to teach. The question and answer format of this book is not dissimilar to the dialogue that takes place between student and teacher on rounds or at seminars. While this book should not replace the many excellent texts in oral medicine and oral pathology on your bookshelf, we think that we have captured the key elements of oral medicine in a very pragmatic format.

We would like to thank Bill Lamsback and Linda Belfus at Hanley & Belfus for their advice, assistance, and patience.

Stephen Sonis
Robert Fazio
Leslie Fang

1. PATIENT ASSESSMENT

Stephen T. Sonis, D.M.D., D.M.Sc.

1. What are the major objectives of pretreatment patient evaluation?
- Establishing the diagnosis
- Determination of pre-existing medical conditions that could affect the oral treatment plan.
- Discovery of concomitant disease
- Management of medical emergencies
- Patient management

2. Give some examples of concomitant disease that can be discovered by a thorough pretreatment evaluation.

Hypertension, diabetes mellitus, coagulopathies, and some infectious diseases are a few examples of undiagnosed illnesses that can be discovered by a thorough pretreatment evaluation.

3. What does the pretreatment evaluation have to do with patient management?

The pretreatment evaluation is generally the first interaction between the provider and the patient. Consequently, it affords the provider the opportunity to evaluate the patient's demeanor and state of mind. If a patient is overly anxious during the first visit, this might suggest the need for increased stress management for subsequent visits.

4. What are the five basic categories of information to be obtained in the course of every formal history?
- Identification of the reason the patient has come to see you (chief complaint).
- Description of the circumstances and history surrounding the onset, development, and course of the chief complaint (history of the present illness).
- Documentation of past diseases or conditions (past medical history).
- Investigation of possible genetic, social, or environmental factors influencing the chief complaint (e.g., family health, personal and social history).
- Summary of additional symptoms or diseases by organ system (review of systems).

5. Does the patient need to be the only source of the history?

Of course not. The history may be obtained from a variety of sources, including family members or friends, a referring physician, or even an old medical record. If the history is obtained from someone other than the patient, it is advisable to obtain identifying information in case the individual needs to be recontacted. It is always important to evaluate the reliability of the source of information, and if it is in question, to solicit additional input.

6. What information should be included in the history of the present illness?
- Location of the problem
- Duration of the problem
- Progression of the condition
- Character of the disease
- Effect of the condition on function
- Effects of previous treatment

7. How is the past medical history usually obtained?

Typically, patients complete a medical history form. These can be purchased from a variety of sources, such as the American Dental Association or commercial printers, or the practitioner can customize them. The form must include space for demographic information and may include billing and insurance information as well. Both the patient and the person reviewing the history should sign the completed form. It is critical to supplement the written form with a verbal review of the medical history because patients may misinterpret questions, omit critical information, or provide erroneous information.

8. The medical history is usually divided into two parts: a history of past illnesses and a review of systems. What four pieces of information constitute the past illnesses?
1. Hospitalizations
2. Medications
3. Allergies
4. Diseases

9. Which diseases should the patient be specifically queried about?
- Diseases or conditions that put the patient at risk for subacute bacterial endocarditis.
- Diseases or conditions that indicate existing artherosclerotic disease.
- Pulmonary diseases that may compromise function or result in acute problems.
- Gastrointestinal and hepatic diseases that may have oral manifestations, be infectious, or affect drug metabolism.
- Endocrine disorders that may require alterations in patient management, predispose the patient to medical emergencies, or affect the course of dental disease.
- Neurologic conditions such as headaches, strokes, or seizures.
- Hematologic conditions that may influence the patient's risk of infection, affect hemostasis, or result in oral lesions.
- Psychiatric diseases and substance abuse problems.
- Infections that may have oral manifestations or influence the course of patient management.

10. What is the review of systems? How does it differ from querying the patient about specific diseases?
Unlike the identification of specific diseases, the review of systems actually entails asking the patient about symptoms associated with specific organ systems. Comprehensively, it evaluates the patient from head to toe. Practically, its use is usually driven by the patient's chief complaint. For example, if the patient complained of a swollen gland and the clinician was concerned about the possibility of lymphoma, the patient might be queried about fevers, night sweats, and weight loss. Similarly, if the patient complained of multiple recurrent periodontal abscesses and the clinician was considering a diagnosis of diabetes mellitus, the patient might be asked about polyuria, polydipsia, and weight loss.

11. What are the four methods of observation that are used as part of a physical examination?
- Inspection
- Palpation
- Percussion
- Auscultation

12. What does the pulse measure?
The pulse is a peripheral measurement of heart rate and rhythm.

13. How is the radial pulse taken? How about the carotid pulse?
The radial pulse is taken by having the patient rotate the hand to the palms-up position. The pulse can be felt by resting the fingers just above the wrist and behind the thumb. The carotid pulse can be palpated by placing the fingers just anterior to the sternocleidomastoid muscle at the level of the thyroid cartilage.

14. How do you actually determine the heart rate and rhythm when taking a patient's pulse?
The first thing to measure is the patient's heart rate. With the fingers in place, you will be able to feel the pulse. Count the number of beats for one full minute. The normal rate is about 72 bpm for a patient at rest (normal range is about 60 to 100 bpm). Once you have finished getting the rate, take note of the rhythm to be sure that its consistent and regular.

USE OF THE CLINICAL LABORATORY IN DENTAL PRACTICE

15. What are the most common indications for laboratory studies in dental practice?
The number of laboratory tests typically used by dentists is relatively small. In general these include examinations to diagnose or rule out anemia, neutropenia, leukemia, diabetes mellitus, coagulopathies, and infectious diseases such as human immunodeficiency virus (HIV) infection or hepatitis. Laboratory culture studies may be important for the diagnosis of certain bacteriologic, viral, or fungal infections.

16. If you practice in a hospital, getting laboratory tests is not difficult, but what if you're in a private, community setting?
Getting laboratory tests done for a patient is actually straightforward no matter where you practice. Two types of laboratories are anxious for your business: hospital laboratories or commercial laboratories. If you write to the Pathology Department of your community hospital, they will be happy to send you requisition slips. When you have a patient who needs a test, simply complete the slip by checking off the appropriate test and send the patient and slip to the hospital. Once there, a phlebotomist will draw the patient's blood and the test will be executed. Commercial laboratories provide a similar service, and may also offer to go to the patient's home to collect the sample.

If you do not have any formal requisition slips, you can write the test you want done on a prescription form and send it to the hospital with the patient.

Remember that the laboratories want your business and will generally be very accommodating.

17. You have a patient taking coumadin who is coming in for an extraction. You want to check the patient's prothrombin time the day of the procedure. What is the best way to get this information?
Almost all laboratory tests of interest to dentists are automated and therefore the turn-around time is pretty rapid. Nonetheless, if you want a result as soon as it's available, indicate that on the requisition by writing STAT, and ask the technician to call you as soon as the result is available.

18. A complete blood count (CBC) is one of the most common tests requested. If you order a CBC, what information will you get? How much does a CBC cost?
Historically, a CBC was composed of hemoglobin, hematocrit, white blood cell count and differential white blood cell count. With automation, red blood cell counts and parameters are included as is platelet number. CBCs thus provide a lot of information. The charge for a CBC varies widely from $35 to $70.

19. What are "normal" values for the following laboratory tests:
  - White blood cell count   (WBC) 4500 to 10,000 cells/mm^3
  - Hemoglobin (Hgb) males = 14 – 18 g/dl; females = 12 – 16 g/dl
  - Hematocrit (Hct) males = 40 – 54%; females = 37 – 47%
  - Differential white blood cell count
    - Neutrophils 50–70%
    - Lymphocytes 30–40%
    - Monocytes 3–7%
    - Eosinophils 0–5%
    - Basophils 0–1%

20. What is neutrophilia and what causes it?
Neutrophilia is an increase in the absolute neutrophil count above 7500 cells/mm^3. It can be caused by any of the following:
  - Physiologic causes–exercise or stress
  - Infections–acute localized or systemic bacterial infections primarily but also as a consequence of fungal or certain viral infections

- Inflammation caused by burns, surgery, and tissue injury, such as myocardial or pulmonary infarction
- Metabolic disorders such as diabetic ketoacidosis, uremia, and eclampsia
- Acute hemorrhage
- Acute hemolysis
- Myeloproliferative diseases may result in abnormal neutrophils; an example is myelocytic leukemia
- Iatrogenic causes are mostly due to drugs such as epinephrine, lithium or steroids
- Malignant tumors
- Hereditary neutrophilia

21. What is neutropenia? What causes it?

Neutropenia is a decrease in the absolute neutrophil number to less than 1500 cells/mm^3. The four major causes of neutropenia are
- Drugs
- Certain infections
- Hematologic diseases
- Autoimmune disorders

22. Name some drugs that can cause neutropenia.

- Cancer chemotherapy agents such as cyclophosphamide and 5-fluorouracil
- AZT (azidothymidine)
- Phenothiazines
- Sulfonamides
- Phenytoin

23. What are the major causes of eosinophilia?

- Parasitic infections
- Allergic diseases
- Skin diseases
- Drug reactions
- Certain malignancies (e.g., Hodgkin's disease, chronic myelogenous leukemia)
- Collagen vascular disorders
- Radiation therapy

24. What are the major causes of lymphocytosis?

- Certain acute infections such as mononucleosis, infectious hepatitis, and cytomegalovirus infection
- Endocrine disorders such as thyrotoxicosis and adrenal insufficiency
- Certain chronic infections such as tuberculosis and syphilis
- Hematologic diseases such as some lymphomas and leukemias
- Recovery from acute infections

25. What is a normal platelet count?

The normal range for a platelet count is between 150,000 and 450,000 cells/μl.

26. What is thrombocytopenia? What are the most likely causes of thrombocytopenia in a dental patient?

Thrombocytopenia is a decrease in the platelet count below normal. The most likely causes of thrombocytopenia in a dental patient are
- Drug induced - cancer chemotherapy drugs, alcohol, estrogens
- HIV infection
- Autoimmune disorders such as systemic lupus erythematosus
- Viral infections such as infectious mononucleosis
- Leukemia

27. What does the prothrombin time measure?

Prothrombin time measures the extrinsic (factor VII) and common (factors V and X, prothrombin, fibrinogen) pathways of coagulation.

28. How is the prothrombin time expressed?

Historically the prothrombin time was expressed in seconds. However, because values varied from laboratory to laboratory a new unit called the International Normalized Ratio or INR was introduced. The INR is based on the ratio of a patient's prothrombin time divided by a reference control.

2. ATHEROSCLEROSIS

Robert C. Fazio, D.M.D., and Leslie S.T. Fang, M.D., Ph.D.

1. What is atherosclerosis?
Atherosclerosis is a disease of unknown origin that is caused by the accumulation of an abnormal amount of lipids on the walls of the arteries, with resultant plaque formation. The disease can affect any vessel and represents the most common pathophysiologic cause of cardiovascular (angina, myocardial infarction, and risks of cardiac arrhythmias), cerebrovascular (transient ischemic attack and stroke), and peripheral vascular disease.

2. What are the consequences of atherosclerosis?
• Vascular thrombosis (clots)
• Embolism (traveling clots)
• Aneurysms (weakened and dilated vascular wall)

3. What is the mechanism for the development of these complications?
These atherosclerotic plaques encroach upon the vascular lumen. As the vessel narrows, blood and oxygen supply to the distal tissue becomes compromised and ischemic injury ensues. These atherosclerotic plaques can act as seeding areas for thrombosis or clots, with resultant infarction of the area supplied. Thrombosis may also produce circulating blood clots, or emboli, which can cause infarctions in other parts of the body. Atheromatous changes of the vascular wall can also result in weakening of the area and create a bulge, or aneurysm, that can rupture and cause hemorrhage.

4. Which vessels are affected by atherosclerosis?
Virtually all vessels, large or small, can be affected by atherosclerosis. The most important vessels affected are the coronary arteries. Other important vessels affected include those supplying the brain and peripheral circulation.

5. What are the consequences of atherosclerotic involvement of the coronary vessels ?
Disease in the coronary vessels results in an imbalance of limited myocardial oxygen supply and excessive oxygen demand. This can lead to the development of angina, myocardial infarction, arrhythmia, or sudden death. Most men and women above the age of 50 in the United States have moderately advanced coronary atherosclerosis, even though they have no symptoms. After a variable presymptomatic period, various clinical manifestations of atherosclerotic heart disease may appear.

6. What are the consequences of atherosclerotic involvement of the cerebral vessels?
Atherosclerotic changes of vessels supplying the brain can lead to transient ischemic attacks or strokes as a result of compromised blood flow to the brain.

7. What are the consequences of atherosclerotic involvement of the peripheral circulation?
Atherosclerosis involving the vessels supplying the extremities can result in muscular cramping or intermittent claudication. Further compromises of the vessels can result in ischemic or gangrenous changes to the digits.

8. What are the implications of atherosclerosis for the dentist?
For the dentist, it is important to identify patients who may be at high risk for atherosclerosis. Although these patients may be asymptomatic at the time of presentation, symptoms can develop while they are under the care of the dentist and complicate dental management. These patients are the most likely to develop cardiac and cerebrovascular complications during the

stresses of dental procedures. It is therefore important to identify patients who are likely to be at risk for atherosclerosis.

9. What are the risk factors contributing to atherosclerosis?
The population at risk includes men above the age of 50 and postmenopausal women.

Some factors are definitely associated with the development of atherosclerotic coronary artery disease, cerebrovascular disease and peripheral vascular disease. These include hypertension, cigarette smoking and elevated blood cholesterol levels, particularly low-density lipoprotein levels.

Other risk factors, such as diabetes mellitus, genetic factors, postmenopausal state, family history, and the use of contraceptive pills, are thought to be important, but their association with atherosclerosis has not been convincingly demonstrated.

10. What should be the dental approach to the management of patients with risk factors for atherosclerosis?
Before the dentist undertakes a complex dental treatment plan, a patient with multiple risk factors for atherosclerosis should have had a medical evaluation within the past 18 months. The evaluation should include a physical examination and an electrocardiogram to rule out clinically silent atherosclerotic disease. Patients with risk factors who have not had a recent medical evaluation can have nonsurgical dental procedures and simple surgical procedures carried out using normal dental operating procedures. More advanced surgical procedures that would involve long operative time or extensive soft-tissue and bone trauma should be deferred until after medical evaluation.

3. HYPERTENSION

Robert C. Fazio, D.M.D., and Leslie S.T. Fang, M.D., Ph.D.

1. What is hypertension?

Hypertension is the abnormal elevation of the resting arterial systolic blood pressure above 140 mm Hg and/or the elevation of the diastolic blood pressure above 90 mm Hg.

2. What is the prevalence of hypertension?

The National Health and Nutrition Examination Survey (NHANES III) revealed that about 50,000,000 Americans have hypertension. One in four American adults has hypertension.

3. What is the significance of hypertension?

Hypertension accelerates atherosclerosis. Epidemiologic studies have demonstrated that untreated hypertension is associated with increased morbidity and mortality from cerebrovascular disease, peripheral vascular disease, renal disease and cardiovascular disease. Studies have also shown that control of hypertension would prevent cerebrovascular accidents, congestive heart failure and, to a lesser extent, coronary atherosclerosis. Hypertension was listed as a primary or contributing cause of death in about 210,000 of more than 2,000,000 U.S. deaths in 1997 in NHANES III.

4. What causes hypertension?

Of the patients with hypertension, 90% have no definable cause and are therefore categorized as having essential hypertension (primary or idiopathic hypertension). The remaining 10% of patients have secondary hypertension, which is most often the result of renal disease, renovascular disease, or adrenal diseases such as Cushing's disease, primary aldosteronism, or pheochromocytoma. Whereas some forms of secondary hypertension can be cured surgically, most patients with primary or essential hypertension require long-term use of medications.

5. Describe the medical approach to evaluating patients with hypertension.

The primary goal of the medical evaluation is to identify that small percentage of patients with secondary hypertension in the hope of being able to cure the disease. If the evaluation is negative, the patient will, in all likelihood, need long-term medical therapy.

Not all patients require elaborate evaluation for secondary hypertension, since the majority of patients have essential hypertension. Patients requiring more focused evaluation include those who develop hypertension either at a very young age (younger than age 30) or at a late age (older than age 70). Young patients with hypertension are more likely to have renovascular disease as a result of renal artery hyperplasia or adrenal diseases. Patients who develop hypertension for the first time at age 70 or older often have renovascular disease as a result of atherosclerotic disease of the renal artery.

6. What is the goal of blood pressure treatment?

According to the Sixth Report of the Joint National Committee on Prevention, Evaluation and Treatment of High Blood Pressure (JNC VI), the target blood pressure should be tailored according to the health of the patient.

- For individuals with no diabetes or renal disease, the blood pressure goal should be <140/90 mm Hg.
- For individuals with diabetes, the blood pressure goal is <130/85 mm Hg.
- For individuals with renal disease, the blood pressure goal is <130/85 mm Hg.
- For individuals with proteinuria higher than 1 g/24 hr, the blood pressure goal should be <125/75 mm Hg.

7. What is the status of treating blood pressure in the United States?

About one in four patients in the US has hypertension. Of those, 46.4% are not treated. Of the patients treated, the hypertension of 49% is not adequately controlled.

8. What is the strategy in the management of patients with hypertension?

The goal is to be able to control the blood pressure with either a single drug or combinations of drugs. In general, medications are started at a low dose, which is increased according to the level of blood pressure control. The goal is to be able to attain a balance of effective drugs with minimal side effects.

9. Describe the classes of drugs usually used for the management of patients with hypertension.

Patients with mild hypertension are usually managed with a single drug. A number of drugs are regarded as reasonable first-line medications for the management of hypertension.

Diuretics are still used frequently but are less popular because of concerns over side effects, which range from volume depletion, hypokalemia, and hyperuricemia to a mild degree of hyperlipidemia.

Beta-blockers are also reasonable first-line drugs but may create problems with bradycardia, bronchospasm, and increased serum lipid levels.

Converting enzyme inhibitors are now used as first-line medications with increasing frequency. These drugs are effective, but a small proportion of patients may develop cough from this class of medication.

Calcium channel blockers are effective agents with few side effects. However, some patients may develop peripheral edema. There are also increasing concerns about adverse cardiovascular sequelae from these drugs.

Other drugs are less likely to be used as first-line drugs. These include alpha-blockers and angiotensin II receptor blockers. All these drugs are effective antihypertensive agents, but they have variable side effect profiles. Alpha blockers such as hydralazine, prasozin, terazosin, and doxazosin can cause postural hypotension. Alpha-blockers such as methyldopa can cause orthostatic hypotension, impotence, and drowsiness and are seldom prescribed. Clonidine is a centrally acting alpha blocker that is quite effective in the control of blood pressure but can cause xerostomia. More importantly, clonidine cannot be withdrawn abruptly because severe rebound hypertension can result. Angiotensin II receptor blockers belong to an exceedingly effective new class of antihypertensive agents with very few side effects and will undoubtedly gain increasing acceptance over the next few years.

Patients with moderate hypertension often require a combination of drugs to obtain adequate control. Not infrequently, diuretics are added to drugs such as converting enzyme inhibitors, calcium channel blockers, angiotensin II receptor blockers, or beta-blockers to augment their effectiveness. Other effective combinations include the use of vasodilators together with beta-blockers and the use of converting enzyme inhibitors or angiotensin II receptor blockers with calcium channel blockers.

There are a number of other antihypertensive agents available but these are less frequently used because of their side effect profiles.

10. What are the diuretics commonly prescribed for hypertension?

Thiazide diuretics are mild diuretics and are often the first-line drug of choice. Drugs in this class include

GENERIC NAME	BRAND NAME
Hydrochlorothiazide	HydroDIURIL
	Esidrix
Chlorothiazide	Diuril

Some thiazide diuretics are long-acting and are therefore more potent diuretics. Drugs in this category include

GENERIC NAME	BRAND NAME
Chlorthalidone	Hygroton
	Thalitone
	Uridon
Metolazone	Zaroxolyn
	Mykrox
	Diulo
Benzthiazide	Exna
	Hydrex
Cyclothiazide	Anhydron
Hydroflumethiazide	Diucardin
	Saluron
Methylclothiazide	Aquatensen
	Duretic
	Enduron
Polythiazide	Renese
Quinethazone	Hydromox
Trichlormethiazide	Naqua
	Metahydrin
	Trichlorox

The most potent diuretics are the loop diuretics, including

GENERIC NAME	BRAND NAME
Furosemide	Lasix
	Furoside
	Myrosemide
	Uritol
Ethacrynic acid	Edecrin
Bumetanide	Bumex
Torsemide	Demadex

Some diuretics are potassium-sparing:

GENERIC NAME	BRAND NAME
Amiloride	Midamor
Spironolactone	Aldactone
Triamterene	Dyrenium

Because of concerns over hypokalemia, some combination of drugs are used to protect against potassium wasting. These include

GENERIC NAME	BRAND NAME
Amiloride + hydrochlorothiazide	Moduretic
Spironolactone + hydrochlorothiazide	Aldactazide
	Spirozole
Triamterene + hydrochlorothiazide	Dyazide

11. What are the commonly prescribed beta-blockers?

Beta-blockers are designed to decrease sympathetic nervous system activity. These drugs are useful in treating hypertension, angina, and congestive heart failure. Because they slow down the heart rate, they are also effective antiarrhythmics. Beta-blockers can be subdivided into cardioselective and nonselective types. Cardioselective beta-blockers act on beta-1 receptors and block beta receptor sites in the cardiovascular system. Non–selective beta-blockers block both beta-1 and beta-2 receptors.

Commonly prescribed non–selective beta-blockers include

GENERIC NAME	BRAND NAME
Carteolol	Cartol
Nadolol	Corgard
Oxyprenolol	Trasicor
Penbutolol	Levatol
Pindolol	Visken
Propranolol	Inderal Detensol
Sotalol	Betapace Sotocor
Timolol	Blocadren

Commonly prescribed cardioselective beta blockers include

GENERIC NAME	BRAND NAME
Acebutolol	Monitan Sectral
Atenolol	Tenormin
Betaxolol	Kerlone
Bisoprolol	Zebeta
Esmolol	Brevibloc
Metoprolol	Lopressor Betalol Durules Toprol XL

12. What are the commonly prescribed angiotensin converting enzyme (ACE) inhibitors?

ACE inhibitors are drugs that inhibit the conversion of angiotensin I to angiotensin II. This class of drugs is effective agents for reduction of blood pressure and for afterload reduction in congestive heart failure.

Drugs in this class include

GENERIC NAME	BRAND NAME
Benazepril	Lotensin
Captopril	Capoten
Enalapril	Vasotec
Fosinopril	Monopril

(Cont'd. on next page)

GENERIC NAME	BRAND NAME
Lisinopril	Zestril, Prinivil
Moexipril	Univasc
Perindopril	Aceon
Quinapril	Accupril
Ramipril	Altace
Trandolapril	Mavik

13. What are the commonly prescribed calcium channel blockers?

Calcium channel blockers are commonly prescribed antihypertensive, antianginal, and anti-arrhythmic drugs.

Drugs in this category include

GENERIC NAME	BRAND NAME
Bepridil	Bepadin
Diltiazem	Cardiazem
	Cardiazem CD
	Cardiazem SR
	Covera SR
	Dilacor XR
Felodipine	Renedil
Flunarazine	Sibelium
Isradipine	DynaCirc
Nicardipine	Cardene
Nifedipine	Adalat
	Procardia
Nimodipine	Nimotop
Nisoldipine	Sular
Verapamil	Calan
	Calan SR
	Isoptin
	Verelan

14. What are the commonly prescribed angiotensin II receptor blockers?

Angiotensin II receptor blockers are drugs that block the angiotensin II receptor. They are effective agents for reduction of blood pressure and for afterload reduction in congestive heart failure.

Drugs in this class include

GENERIC NAME	BRAND NAME
Candesartan	Atacand
Eprosartan	Treveten
Irbesartan	Avapro
Losartan	Cozaar
Telmisartan	Micardis
Valsartan	Diovan

15. Name the commonly prescribed alpha-blockers.

Alpha-blockers are effective antihypertensive agents that act on the sympathethic nervous system.

GENERIC NAME	BRAND NAME
Phenoxybenzamine	Dibenzyline
Phentolamine	Regitine
Prazosin	Minipress
Doxazosin	Cardura
Terazosin	Hytrin

16. List the common centrally acting antihypertensive agents.

GENERIC NAME	BRAND NAME
Clonidine	Catapress
	Catapres TTS
Guanabenz	Wytensin
Guanfacine	Tenex
Methyldopa	Aldomet

17. What are the side effects of the antihypertensive drugs?

Different antihypertensive agents have different side effects. The choice of an antihypertensive agent is therefore a careful balancing act between attaining ideal blood pressure control and minimizing side effects. Some of the side effects may have significant dental implications, e.g., problems with gingival hyperplasia with calcium channel blockers and problems with xerostomia with clonidine (Catapres) (discussed in greater detail later on). Nonselective beta-blockers and alpha-blockers may influence the choice of vasconstrictors.

18. What is the role of the dentist in the detection of hypertension?

Dentists should play a major role in the detection of hypertension because they routinely see patients for multiple visits and semiannual checkups. Severity of blood pressure elevation is in part dependent on the blood pressure measured and in part on the presence of symptoms. of Guidelines exist for the clinical status of blood pressure. Monitoring a patient's blood pressure is an easy task and an important aspect of comprehensive dental-medical care.

19. How can hypertension complicate dental therapy?

Poorly controlled hypertension may lead to acutely elevated blood pressure during stressful situations and precipitate angina, congestive heart failure, or, rarely, a cerebrovascular event such as stroke or hemorrhage.

20. How should a patient with hypertension be evaluated by the dentist?

A dentist can assess the severity of a patient's hypertension by means of a medical history and a blood pressure determination. Patients often record a history of hypertension in the dentist's medical questionnaire. The dentist should then determine the time of the diagnosis, past and present treatment and complications. Most important, the dentist should ask about the types and dosages of current medications and especially note recent changes in regimen.

A list of the patient's medications can provide some idea of the severity of the patient's hypertension and can alert the dentist to the possible side effects that may complicate dental therapy.

21. How should a dentist approach a patient with hypertension?

The control of anxiety is an important therapeutic adjunct in the management of the hypertensive dental patient. Patient rapport is therefore crucial. As the difficulty of the dental procedures increases, so does the patient's anxiety level. It is therefore important to monitor the patient's blood pressure throughout complicated procedures.

22. How should a dentist manage a patient with controlled or mild hypertension (140–159/ 90–99 mm Hg)?

The patient with controlled or mild hypertension can tolerate all nonsurgical and simple surgical procedures using normal operative protocol. Complex periodontal and oral surgery may require the use of various sedation techniques, including N_2O/O_2 inhalation analgesia or additional augmentation with oral sedatives or anxiolytics such as diazepam. Patients who receive oral premedication must be accompanied to the dental visit by an adult. Shorter appointment with the goal of reducing stress to the patient are preferred. Longer appointments, when necessary, may be accomplished with the use of adjunctive sedation techniques.

23. How should a dentist manage a patient with moderate hypertension (160–169/100–109 mm Hg)?

The patient with undiagnosed moderate hypertension should be referred to a physician for management. No complex elective dentistry should be considered. If the dentist elects to use a local anesthetic with epinephrine, the amount used should be limited to 2 Carpules of local anesthetic containing 1:100,000 epinephrine (4 Carpules of 1:200,000). In the case of local anesthetic with levonordefrin, the dentist should limit the total amount used to 2 Carpules of local anesthetic containing 1:20,000 levonordefrin. Treatment of an advanced case of dental pathology might proceed through phase I therapy, including oral hygiene instruction, scaling, root planing, and simple operative dentistry. However, complex procedures should be deferred until the blood pressure is under better control. Similarly, for shorter appointments, N_2O/O_2 inhalation analgesia and oral anxiolytics and sedatives may be appropriate for managing a dental emergency. Intravenous sedation should be deferred until blood pressure control is attained.

The patient with diagnosed, treated but still moderate hypertension should be referred to a physician for a review of the medical management and possibly more aggressive medical therapy.

Patients with moderate hypertension can undergo nonsurgical procedures using normal operating methods. In advanced crown and bridge and all simple surgical procedures, adjunctive sedation techniques should be used. Intermediate and advanced surgical procedures should be performed in the office for a patient with moderate hypertension only with aggressive monitoring of the patient's vital signs and only after all therapeutic options to control the blood pressure have been exhausted. Vigorous bleeding may occur during dentosurgical procedures in patients with poorly controlled hypertension.

24. How should a dentist manage a patient with severe hypertension (>170/>100 mm Hg)?

The patient with severe hypertension should receive dental examination only and be referred to a physician for further medical management prior to receiving additional dental care. Palliative care is mandated and a controlled, monitored environment is necessary for dental emergencies. Use of vasoconstrictors is contraindicated.

25. How should a dentist manage a patient with malignant hypertension (severe hypertension associated with central nervous system symptoms such as blurring of vision, headache, or changes in mental status)?

Malignant hypertension is a medical emergency and the patient should immediately be referred to a physician for acute intervention.

26. What special consideration should be given to the patient taking calcium channel blockers?

Calcium channel blockers carry significant risks for gingival hyperplasia. Although the *Physicians' Desk Reference* lists the frequency of gingival hyperplasia at 0.5 to 1%, the actual prevalence is considerably greater. About 30–40% of patients on nifedipine (Procardia, Adalat) develop clinically significant gingival hyperplasia. Most of the other calcium channel blockers carry a 10–20% risk. The discrepancy appears to revolve around the clinical definition of gingival hyperplasia. The drug company reports gingival hyperplasia as a complication only when ½–¾ of the clinical crown is covered. In clinical practice, concerns about gingival hyperplasia are raised at a much lower threshold.

The risk of developing gingival hyperplasia does not appear to be dose-related but rather patient-specific. A patient is either a reactor or a non-reactor to calcium channel blockers, and the effect is independent of the dose administered. Severity of the gingival hyperplasia is dependent on the quality of the patient's oral hygiene, the frequency of dental prophylaxis, and the presence of crowded teeth and defective restorations.

27. How should we manage patients who develop gingival hyperplasia on calcium channel blockers?

Phase I hygiene therapy, including oral hygiene instruction, scaling, root planing, and curettage, should be completed. The correction of defective restorations and caries is essential. The frequency of dental prophylaxis should be increased.

If these conservative means are inadequate for the control of gingival hyperplasia, consultation with the patient's physician should be undertaken in order to assess the possibility of discontinuing the calcium channel blocker. Only then should surgical excision be considered.

28. What should the discussion with the patient's physician center around when confronted with significant and refractory gingival hyperplasia in a patient on a calcium channel blocker?

a. The frequency of occurrence of gingival hyperplasia on the particular calcium channel blocker
b. The possibility of using alternate agents in the management of the patient
c. The fact that some calcium channel blockers are less likely to induce gingival hyperplasia: nifedipine appears to be the major offender, and isradipine appears to be the least, damaging with the remainder of the calcium channel blockers somewhere in-between.

29. What special consideration should be given to patients on clonidine?

Clonidine is a drug that can cause significant xerostomia. Patients on clonidine should be placed on an antixerostomia protocol.

30. What is an antixerostomia protocol?

The dentist should see these patients on a more frequent recall program. A patient who might normally be seen twice a year may be seen three to four times a year.

The patient should be advised of the increased caries risk. Dietary counseling to avoid simple sugars and multiple meals should be given. Salivary stimulation with sucrose-free lemon drops is recommended. In cases in which significant xerostomia exists, salivary replacement with artificial saliva or mouth moisturizers (e.g., Xero-lube, Oralube, Salivart) is often indicated. If necessary, pilocarpine HCl, 5 mg tid, may be prescribed.

31. Is there any other protocol that the dentist should recommend for the patient on clonidine?

The dentist should strongly recommend the fluoride protocol. At a minimum, 1.1% pH neutral sodium fluoride gel (Fluorident) should be applied topically daily. Full oral hygiene measures (brushing, flossing, and use of the water pik) should be implemented. The patient should then rebrush the teeth using the fluoride gel and be instructed to spit out the excess but not to rinse out. Additional food or drink before going to bed should be avoided.

32. What is the approach to the patient on clonidine who has a significant history of caries?

The dentist should strongly consider the fabrication of custom fluoride trays for this patient. This would permit a 7-minute application with significantly increased contact time between the fluoride gel and the dentition.

33. Why is it not desirable to use an acidulated phosphate fluoride gel in the patient on clonidine who has a significant history of caries?

Acidulated phosphate fluoride gels have an acidic pH that can etch porcelain restorations and compromise the aesthetics of the dentition. Frequent use of these gels can cause gingival and mucosal irritation.

34. What special consideration should be given to patients on non-selective beta-blockers?

Beta-blockers, particularly the non–selective beta-blockers such as propranolol (Inderal), nadolol (Corgard), and timolol (Blocadren), can interact with epinephrine in the commonly used local anesthetics by potentiating the effect of epinephrine. This can result in a hypertensive reaction with significant cardiovascular consequences.

Levonordefrin is an alternative vasoconstrictor without potential drug-drug interactions with beta blockers. Local anesthetic preparations utilizing levonordefrin (e.g., 2% mepivacaine with 1:20,000 levonordefrin) as the vasoconstrictor are probably the preferred agents to use in these patients.

35. What special consideration should be given to patients taking alpha-blockers?

Alpha-blockers theoretically have the potential to interact with epinephrine, resulting in the "epinephrine reversal effect."

36. What is the epinephrine reversal effect?

Alpha-blockers can reverse the epinephrine effect. Instead of prolonging the anesthetic effect, epinephrine, in the presence of alpha-blockers, may actually shorten the anesthetic effect. Rather than enhancing hemostasis, epinephrine, in the presence of alpha-blockers, may induce vasodilatation and bleeding.

37. How does epinephrine reversal effect occurs?

The vasculature has alpha- and beta-receptors. Alpha-receptors are responsible for vasoconstriction and beta-receptors are responsible for vasodilatation. Epinephrine has a dominant alpha effect, but it also has a lesser beta-2 effect. When alpha-receptors are given alone, vasoconstriction dominates. In the presence of alpha-blockers, the beta-2 effect of epinephrine is unmasked, resulting in vasodilatation.

38. Does this epinephrine reversal effect occur with use of the vasoconstrictor levonordefrin?

No, levonordefrin does not have a beta-2 effect. For patients on alpha-blockers, the preferred anesthetic when vasoconstriction is desired is a preparation using levonordefrin (e.g., 2% mepivacaine with 1:20,000 levonordefrin).

4. ANGINA PECTORIS

Robert C. Fazio, D.M.D., and Leslie S.T. Fang, M.D., Ph.D.

1. What is angina pectoris?

Angina pectoris is a form of symptomatic ischemic heart disease. When there is a transient myocardial oxygen demand in excess of the available oxygen delivery for the coronary arteries, the patient exhibits a symptom complex with chest pain.

2. Why is angina an important issue for the dentist?

A stressful dental procedure can precipitate an acute attack of angina. This requires emergency intervention. Prolonged angina can result in a life-threatening myocardial infarction.

The presence of angina is indicative of significant coronary artery disease and should alert the dentist to judicious use of vasoconstrictors in local anesthetics.

3. What is the cause of angina pectoris?

In the majority of cases, atherosclerotic changes of the coronary vessels can result in lack of blood supply to the myocardium. Less frequently, angina can result from excess oxygen demand, limited oxygen-carrying capacity of the blood (e.g., anemia) or inadequate perfusion of the coronary arteries due to hypotension or coronary vessel spasm.

4. What is the clinical manifestation of angina pectoris?

A classic case of angina is precipitated by emotional stress or physical exertion and is relieved by rest. Typically, the patient complains of a compression of the chest in the retrosternal area. The pain is often described as a heavy sensation over the precordial area and can radiate to the left shoulder and arm or to the jaw. It is usually of brief duration, lasting 3 to 5 minutes if the precipitating factor is removed.

5. What should the dentist do if an episode of angina occurs in the dental chair?

1. Stop the dental procedure
2. Place the patient in a supine position
3. Administer sublingual nitroglycerin
4. Administer oxygen
5. Monitor serial blood pressure and heart rate
6. If angina is not relieved after 5 minutes, give a second sublingual nitroglycerin and transfer the patient to a medical facility. (A protracted bout of angina can result in life-threatening myocardial infarction.)

6. How are the symptoms of angina pectoris and myocardial infarction different?

The pain associated with myocardial infarction is usually more severe and more protracted. Myocardial infarction is usually the result of an occlusion of the coronary vessel. Whereas angina is reversible, myocardial infarction results in actual tissue damage.

7. What does the medical evaluation of the patient with angina consist of?

The diagnosis of angina is usually made on the basis of the history. During an attack, the electrocardiogram may show ischemic changes in the area affected. However, cardiovascular examinations between attacks are usually unrevealing, and the resting electrocardiogram may show only nonspecific changes.

If the diagnosis remains in doubt after the initial evaluation, an exercise stress test may be performed to demonstrate ischemic changes. The stress test is often done with the use of a radionuclide injection in order to enhance the sensitivity of the test. Thallium-201 and MIBI (sestamibi) are the agents most commonly used.

19

If there is sufficient clinical indication, the patient may have to undergo an arteriogram to further define the anatomy of the coronary vessels. The physician could thus be able to assess the need for further intervention. If the anatomy is appropriate, at the time of the angiography angioplasty and placement of stents can be performed to correct the stenosis. If the anatomy is not amenable to angioplastic intervention, the patient would qualify for coronary artery bypass graft.

8. How is angina managed medically?

Medical management of angina pectoris includes a modification of the patient's lifestyle as well as the use of medications.

The patient is encouraged to lose weight, discontinue smoking, reduce anxiety and tension, and avoid situations that provoke stress.

For immediate relief of chest pain, nitroglycerin, a short-acting nitrate, is prescribed in doses ranging from 0.3 to 0.6 mg given sublingually. Nitrates can also be given prophylactically in anticipation of increased physical activity or stress.

Long-acting nitrates such as isosorbide dinitrate (Isordil, Imdur) or nitropatch can be prescribed to prevent anginal attacks. Beta-blockers (e.g., propranolol, atenolol, metoprolol) are also often prescribed because they can reduce myocardial oxygen demand. Calcium channel blockers are sometimes prescribed because they can cause dilatation of the coronary arteries and enhance blood flow to the myocardium. However, there is some concern that calcium channel blockers may be associated with adverse cardiovascular events in ways that as yet are unclear.

9. What is unstable angina?

Occasionally, a patient may experience a change in the pattern of angina. With an increase of the frequency and severity of the pain or with the appearance of angina at rest, the patient is said to have unstable angina. In a significant fraction of patients with unstable angina, the condition progresses to myocardial infarction within a short time. These patients therefore must be treated aggressively.

10. How is angina treated by interventional means?

When appropriate, the patient with angina may have to undergo coronary angiography. For lesions amenable to this procedure, the patient may have percutaneous transluminal coronary angioplasty with the use of a balloon-tipped catheter to dilate the coronary vessel, with or without placement of a stent. The procedure has considerably less risk of morbidity than coronary surgery, but the dilated vessel may restenose in months or years. This would necessitate a repeat procedure by coronary artery bypass graft.

11. How should the dentist approach a patient with a recent angioplasty?

A patient with a recent angioplasty still has an unstable coronary situation. Complex elective dental procedures should be deferred for 6 months.

In a dental emergency, the most simple treatment plan consistent with a stable outcome should be utilized. Emergency surgical care should be performed in a controlled, monitored setting.

12. Should a patient with a coronary stent be given antibiotic dental prophylaxis?

Currently, 90–95% of patients who undergo coronary angioplasty also have placement of an intracoronary stent. Although conclusive data are currently lacking, it is prudent to use antibiotic prophylaxis for 6 months following stent placement. Dental prophylaxis is not necessary thereafter.

13. Who should have coronary artery bypass surgery?

Coronary artery bypass surgery is more invasive but is more effective in alleviating anginal symptoms. Coronary artery bypass surgery is usually reserved for patients with intractable angina despite maximal medical therapy and those whose lesions are not amenable to angioplasty. Patients with high-grade obstruction of the left main coronary artery (this group has a high mortality rate when managed medically) should be treated with coronary artery bypass surgery.

14. What are the guidelines for use of local anesthetics with vasoconstrictors in the patient with angina?

If the dentist elects to use a local anesthetic with epinephrine, the amount used should be limited to 2 Carpules of local anesthetic containing 1:100,000 epinephrine (4 Carpules of 1:200,000). In the case of the use of local anesthetic with levonordefrin, the dentist should limit the amount used to 2 Carpules of local anesthetic with 1:20,000 levonordefrin (mepivacaine with levonordefrin).

15. How should the dentist approach the patient with angina on beta-blockade?

Beta-blockers, particularly the non–selective beta-blockers such as propranolol (Inderal), nadolol (Corgard), and timolol (Blocadren), can interact with epinephrine in the commonly used local anesthetics by potentiating the effect of epinephrine. This can result in a hypertensive reaction with significant cardiovascular consequences.

Levonordefrin is an alternative vasoconstrictor without potential drug-drug interactions with beta-blockers. Local anesthetic preparations utilizing levonordefrin (e.g., 2% mepivacaine with 1:20,000 levonordefrin) as the vasoconstrictor are probably the preferred agents to use in these patients.

16. How should the dentist approach the patient with angina on calcium channel blockers?

Calcium channel blockers carry significant risks for gingival hyperplasia. Although the *Physicians' Desk Reference* lists the frequency of gingival hyperplasia at 0.5 to 1%, the actual prevalence is considerably greater. About 30–40% of patients on nifedipine (Procardia, Adalat) develop clinically significant gingival hyperplasia. Most of the other calcium channel blockers carry a 10–20% risk. The discrepancy appears to revolve around the clinical definition of gingival hyperplasia. The drug company reports gingival hyperplasia as a complication only when $\frac{1}{2}$ to $\frac{3}{4}$ of the clinical crown is covered. In clinical practice, concerns about gingival hyperplasia are raised at a much lower clinical level.

The risk of development of gingival hyperplasia does not appear to be dose related but rather patient-specific. A patient is either a reactor or a nonreactor to calcium channel blockers, and the effect is independent of the dose administered. The severity of the gingival hyperplasia depends on the quality of the oral hygiene, the frequency of dental prophylaxis, and the presence of crowded teeth and defective restorations.

17. How should we manage patients on calcium channel blockers who develop gingival hyperplasia?

Phase I hygiene therapy, including oral hygiene instruction, scaling, root planing, and curettage, should be completed. The correction of defective restorations and caries is essential. The frequency of dental prophylaxis should be increased.

If these conservative means are inadequate for the control of gingival hyperplasia, consultation with the patient's physician should be undertaken in order to assess the possibility of discontinuing the offending calcium channel blocker. Only then should surgical excision be considered.

18. What should the discussion with the patient's physician center around when the dentist is confronted with significant and refractory gingival hyperplasia in a patient on a calcium channel blocker?

- The frequency of gingival hyperplasia experienced by the patient on the calcium channel blocker
- The possibility of using alternate agents in the management of the patient with angina
- The fact that some calcium channel blockers may be less prone to inducing gingival hyperplasia: nifedipine appears to be the major offender, and isradipine (DynaCirc) appears to cause the least gingival hyperplasia, with the remainder of the calcium channel blockers somewhere in between

19. What are the guidelines for the use of prophylactic nitroglycerin prior to dental procedures?

If the patient has a relatively stable pattern of angina occurring less than once a week, no prophylaxis is necessary.

If the patient has frequent angina, nitroglycerin prophylaxis is probably warranted.

In either instance, the dentist should have access to nitroglycerin in his or her practice.

20. How should the dentist approach a patient with a history of unstable angina?

These patients are not candidates for complex elective dental procedures. Palliative measures are indicated. When needed, complex dental procedures should be managed in a controlled, monitored setting. The use of vasoconstrictors is contraindicated.

5. MYOCARDIAL INFARCTION

Robert C. Fazio, D.M.D., and Leslie S.T. Fang, M.D., Ph.D.

1. What is myocardial infarction?

Myocardial infarction is the result of prolonged ischemic injury to the heart. The most common reason for having a myocardial infarction is progressive coronary artery disease secondary to atherosclerosis.

2. What are the symptoms of myocardial infarction?

The patient usually has severe chest pain in the substernal or left precordial area. The pain can radiate to the left arm or the jaw and may be associated with shortness of breath, palpitations, nausea or vomiting. The pain is often similar to that of angina but is more protracted and prolonged.

3. What are the complications of myocardial infarction?

The complications include arrhythmias and congestive heart failure. Complications depend upon the extent of the myocardial infarction. Patients with a small infarct usually recover with minimal morbidity. Patients with large areas of injury are more likely to suffer heart failure and life-threatening arrhythmias.

4. What are the concerns for the dentist managing a patient who has had a myocardial infarction?

The main concern is the aggravation of cardiac ischemia or precipitation of arrhythmia during the dental procedure. This risk is more likely to occur the closer in time the dental procedure is to the myocardial infarction. This risk is also increased with increasing complexity of the dental procedure and with the use of vasoconstrictors in local anesthetics.

5. How common is the history of myocardial infarction in the dental population?

In one prospective study, 1.3% of patients above age 30 and 10% of patients above age 40 undergoing noncardiac surgery gave a history of a previous myocardial infarction.

6. What is the most important factor in assessing a patient with a history of myocardial infarction?

The amount of time that has elapsed from the episode of myocardial infarction is the most important factor to consider. Other considerations include the size of the infarct and complications such as arrhythmias and congestive heart failure.

7. What is the clinical significance of a recent myocardial infarction?

A recent myocardial infarction is perhaps the most important risk factor to consider for patients with cardiac diseases prior to any surgical procedure. There is an increased likelihood of arrhythmia during anesthesia and stress as well as possible myocardial suppression secondary to general anesthesia.

8. How should risks in a patient with a history of myocardial infarction be stratified?

- Highest risk during the first 6 months after a myocardial infarction
- Moderate risk during the 6–12-month period after a myocardial infarction
- Lowest risk after 12 months

9. What are the risks of surgical intervention in patients with a recent myocardial infarction?

Reports have indicated that the first 6 months after a myocardial infarction is the period of highest risk for a recurrence. Major surgery during this period carried a 50% risk of recurrent myocardial infarction, with an extremely high mortality rate. More recent studies have placed the incidence at 18–22%, undoubtedly the result of improved anesthestic and surgical techniques and better perioperative monitoring of patients.

After the 6-month period, the incidence of perioperative myocardial infarction decreases progressively. After the first 12 months, the incidence stabilizes at approximately 5%.

It is important to point out that the data available are derived from patients undergoing major surgical procedures, and it is difficult to extrapolate these data to dental stress. Nevertheless, it is best to err on the side of safety in these instances to avoid unnecessary morbidity.

10. What are the other factors that would contribute to the risk of a patient with a history of myocardial infarction requiring dental intervention?

The dental management of the patient with a previous myocardial infarction depends on the severity and course of the myocardial infarction. A patient with a small uncomplicated myocardial infarction is less likely to have problems than a patient with a large complicated myocardial infarction. Patients with arrhythmias and congestive heart failure are much more likely have acute problems. Similarly, a patient with a history of multiple myocardial infarctions is at higher risk than a patient with a single myocardial infarction.

11. How should the dentist approach patients who have had myocardial infarctions within the past 6 months?

Because of the high risk of recurrent myocardial infarction and arrhythmia in these patients, dentistry should be limited to palliative treatment only. Emergency dental care should be delivered in a controlled, monitored environment. The use of vasoconstrictors in local anesthetics is relatively contraindicated.

Good patient-dentist communication, stress reduction, and monitoring are essential for the safe management of the postinfarction patient.

12. How should the dentist approach patients who have had myocardial infarctions 6-12 months previously?

Nonsurgical and simple surgical procedures should be carried out with judicious use of local anesthetics. Lidocaine, 2%, with 1:100,000 lidocaine, and 2% mepivacaine with 1:20,000 levonordefrin, should be limited to 2 Carpules for each appointment. Complex elective procedures, both restorative and surgical, are still relatively contraindicated. Care should be taken to minimize stress. Longer procedures should be divided into several shorter ones, and adjunctive sedation techniques should be strongly considered.

13. How should the dentist approach patients who have had their most recent myocardial infarctions more than a year ago?

It is important to remember that these patients still have significant coronary artery disease despite their stability during the past year. They can, however, more readily tolerate complex procedures than patients with more recent myocardial infarctions. If the patient has had a complicated myocardial infarction with residual sequelae such as arrhythmia and congestive heart failure, the dental plan should be substantively altered. For example, simple removable partial denture fabrication would be preferred over complex periodontal fixed prostheses. Again, limiting vasoconstrictors to 2 Carpules of conventional local anesthetics with 1:100,000 epinephrine or 1:20,000 levonordefrin or equivalent is still recommended.

6. CONGESTIVE HEART FAILURE

Robert C. Fazio, D.M.D., and Leslie S.T. Fang, M.D., Ph.D.

1. What is congestive heart failure?

Congestive heart failure is the result of the inability of the heart to deliver an adequate supply of oxygenated blood to meet the metabolic demands of the body.

2. Why should the dentist be attuned to issues around the patient with congestive heart failure?

Congestive heart failure indicates significant cardiac dysfunction. Dental procedures in patients with congestive heart failure are associated with increased risk of arrhythmia, angina, and precipitation of heart failure.

The medications used to manage the patient with congestive heart failure can also complicate dental management of the patient.

3. What are the signs and symptoms of congestive heart failure?

Patients with congestive heart failure often complain of shortness of breath or dyspnea, particularly on exertion. Shortness of breath can cause the patient to awaken at night (paroxysmal nocturnal dyspnea) and is often worse when the patient lies flat (orthopnea). Patients often have to sleep on several pillows. Dyspnea is the result of pulmonary congestion caused by compromised left ventricular function.

Patients may also have symptoms associated with failure of the right ventricle. This results in swelling and fluid accumulation in the ankles (peripheral edema) and in the abdomen (ascites). Passive congestion of the liver from elevated right-sided pressure can cause right upper abdominal discomfort.

4. What are the causes of heart failure?

Heart failure can result any time there is an imbalance between the metabolic demands of the body and the ability of the heart to deliver oxygenated blood to the body.

The most common cause of heart failure is poor myocardial function as a result of ischemic heart disease. Coronary artery disease with myocardial infarction can result in significant compromises in myocardial function. Another common cause of congestive heart failure is long-standing hypertension. Increased resistance to cardiac output compromises the diastolic function of the heart. Cardiomyopathy secondary to coronary artery disease and uncontrolled and persistent hypertension account for a significant percentage of the identifiable causes of congestive heart failure.

Poor myocardial function can also result from infiltrative diseases of the heart (e.g., amyloidosis), metabolic disorders (e.g., hypothyroidism) and pharmacologic agents with a negative inotropy (e.g., beta-blockers).

Increased vascular resistance results not only from hypertension, but also from aortic stenosis or coarctation of the aorta.

An increase in the volume of blood that the heart must pump greatly increases the workload of the heart and can result in compromised cardiac performance. Valvular insufficiency (e.g., aortic or mitral regurgitation), atrial or ventricular septal defects and fluid retention states (e.g., renal failure).

Less commonly, increased metabolic demand can precipitate heart failure (e.g., severe anemia or thyrotoxicosis).

5. How is congestive heart failure managed medically?

- Correction of factors that can precipitate or aggravate congestive heart failure: control of hypertension, management of ischemic heart disease, and correction of anemia, thyrotoxicosis, and valvular dysfunction

- Salt and fluid restriction
- Use of diuretics
- Use of digoxin
- Use of afterload reducing agents: angiotensin converting enzyme inhibitors, angiotensin II receptor blockers, and vasodilators
- Use of beta blockers

6. What are the diuretics used in the management of congestive heart failure?

Thiazide diuretics are mild diuretics and are often the first-line drug of choice. Drugs in this class include

GENERIC NAME	BRAND NAME
Hydrochlorothiazide	HydroDIURIL
	Esidrix
Chlorothiazide	Diuril

Some thiazide diuretics are long-acting and are therefore more potent diuretics. Drugs in this category include

GENERIC NAME	BRAND NAME
Chlorthalidone	Hygroton
	Thalitone
	Uridon
Metolazone	Zaroxolyn
	Mykrox
	Diulo
Benzthiazide	Exna
	Hydrex
Cyclothiazide	Anhydron
Hydroflumethiazide	Diucardin
	Saluron
Methylclothiazide	Aquatensen
	Duretic
	Enduron
Polythiadine	Renese
Quinethazone	Hydromox
Trichlormethiazide	Naqua
	Metahydrin
	Trichlorox

The most potent diuretics are the loop diuretics, including

GENERIC NAME	BRAND NAME
Furosemide	Lasix
	Furoside
	Myrosemide
	Uritol
Ethacrynic acid	Edecrin
Bumetanide	Bumex
Torsemide	Demadex

Because of concerns about hypokalemia, some combination of drugs are used to protect against potassium wasting. These include

GENERIC NAME	BRAND NAME
Amiloride + hydrochlorothiazide	Modiuretic
Spironolactone + hydrochlorothiazide	Aldactazide
	Spirozole
Triamterene + hydrochlorothiazide	Dyazide

7. What are angiotensin converting enzyme (ACE) inhibitors?

ACE inhibitors are drugs that inhibit the conversion of angiotensin I to angiotensin II. These drugs are effective agents for reduction of blood pressure and for afterload reduction in congestive heart failure. Drugs in this class include

GENERIC NAME	BRAND NAME
Benazepril	Lotensin
Captopril	Capoten
Enalapril	Vasotec
Fosinopril	Monopril
Lisinopril	Zestril, Prinivil
Moexipril	Univasc
Perindopril	Aceon
Quinapril	Accupril
Ramipril	Altace
Trandolapril	Mavik

8. What are angiotensin II receptor blockers?

Angiotensin II receptor blockers are drugs that block the angiotensin II receptor. They are effective agents for reduction of blood pressure and for afterload reduction in congestive heart failure. Drugs in this class include

GENERIC NAME	BRAND NAME
Candesartan	Atacand
Eprosartan	Treveten
Irbesartan	Avapro
Losartan	Cozaar
Telmisartan	Micardis
Valsartan	Diovan

9. What are vasodilators?

Vasodilators work directly on the peripheral vasculature to decrease arterial and venous tone. Drugs in this class include

GENERIC NAME	BRAND NAME
Hydralazine	Apresoline
Minoxidil	Loniten

10. How should the dentist approach a patient with a history of congestive heart failure?

The dentist should adjust the dental treatment plan according to the severity and complexity of the patient's congestive heart failure.

11. How should a dentist approach a patient with a history of mild congestive heart failure?

Patients with a history of mild congestive heart failure who are asymptomatic on medical therapy are at low risk for complications during dental therapy. Nonetheless, most of these patients have coronary artery disease and the use of vasoconstrictors should be limited. If the dentist elects to use a local anesthetic with epinephrine, the amount used should be limited to 2 Carpules of local anesthetic containing 1:100,000 epinephrine (4 Carpules of 1:200, 000). In the case of local anesthetic with levonordefrin, the dentist should limit the amount used to 2 Carpules of local anesthetic containing 1:20,000 levonordefrin.

12. How should a dentist approach a patient with a history of moderate congestive heart failure?

Patients with moderately severe heart failure have intermittent symptoms despite medical therapy. These patients can go into congestive heart failure with stress. It is therefore important to modify the treatment plans. Nonsurgical and simple surgical procedures should be carried out with judicious use of local anesthetics. Lidocaine, 2%, with 1:100,000 lidocaine, and 2% mepivacaine with 1:20,000 levonordefrin, should be limited to 2 Carpules for each appointment. Complex elective procedures, both restorative and surgical, are still relatively contraindicated. Care should be taken to minimize stress. Longer procedures should be divided into several shorter ones, and adjunctive sedation techniques should be strongly considered.

13. How should a dentist approach a patient with a history of severe congestive heart failure?

Patients with severe heart failure have symptoms in spite of escalating doses of medications. They are usually on high doses of potent diuretics such as furosemide (Lasix), ethacrynic acid (Edecrin) or bumetanide (Bumex). They are also on significant doses of afterload reducing agents such as angiotensin converting enzyme inhibitors, angiotensin II receptor blockers, or vasodilators.

The dentist should consider substantive changes in the dental treatment plan. Advanced periodontal surgery and complex fixed prosthetics are generally contraindicated. Palliative care, including possible extraction of questionable teeth and removable prosthetic management, may be indicated.

A controlled monitored facility should be utilized for extensive surgical care.

Vasoconstrictors should be avoided in these unstable patients.

14. What are the complications of diuretic therapy that the dentist should be aware of?

- Diuretics can cause dehydration and hypovolumia, which can result in orthostatic hypotension in the dental chair.
- Diuretics can cause hypokalemia, which in turn can produce arrhythmia; the latter can complicate dental management.

To avoid orthostasis, patients should be instructed not to stand up from a sitting or lying position too abruptly.

15. What are the complications of afterload reducing agents?

The angiotensin converting enzyme inhibitors and angiotensin II receptor blockers are relatively free of significant side effects.

Vasodilators can cause orthostatic hypotension. To avoid orthostasis, patients should be instructed not to stand up from a sitting or lying position too abruptly.

7. ARRHYTHMIAS

Robert C. Fazio, D.M.D., and Leslie S.T. Fang, M.D., Ph.D.

1. What is arrhythmia?

A disturbance of the normal rhythm of the heart is called an arrhythmia. The abnormality may arise from disturbances in either the atria or the ventricles. The arrhythmia may be completely asymptomatic, detected only by routine examination and electrocardiograms, or the patient may have symptoms ranging from palpitations to syncope.

2. Why is arrhythmia of concern to the dentist?

Anxiety experienced during dental therapy may exacerbate arrhythmia. Significant arrhythmias increase the risk of angina, myocardial infarction, transient ischemic attacks, cerebrovascular accidents, and sudden death.

3. How are arrhythmias classified?

Arrhythmias can be separated into abnormal rhythm arising either from the atrium (atrial arrhythmias) or from the ventricles (ventricular arrhythmias). In general ventricular arrhythmias are of more concern than atrial arrhythmias. However, both atrial and ventricular arrhythmias can result in symptoms.

4. What are the common atrial arrhythmias?

The most common atrial arrhythmia is sinus tachycardia. Other atrial arrhythmias include atrial premature contractions, paroxysmal atrial tachycardia, atrial flutter, and atrial fibrillation.

5. What is sinus tachycardia?

Normal pulse rate should be regular and between 60 and 100 bpm. In response to stress, exercise, excitement, or anxiety, the pulse rate may exceed 100 bpm. This rapid rhythm is called sinus tachycardia. It is seldom associated with symptoms and does not require therapy. Sinus tachycardia can be seen in association with the stresses of dentistry.

6. What are atrial premature contractions?

Patients with atrial premature contractions have an impulse coming from the atrium prematurely and may notice an occasional "skipped beat." Atrial premature contractions are the most common cause of an irregular pulse. They do not normally require treatment.

7. What are the common atrial tachycardias?

Patients with paroxysmal atrial tachycardia, atrial flutter, or atrial fibrillation have heart rates of 120 to 180 bpm. Healthy patients should be able to tolerate such rates, although they may complain of palpitations, dizziness or light-headedness. In patients with underlying heart disease, however, such arrhythmias can precipitate hypotension, angina, congestive heart failure, or syncope.

8. What are the common drugs used to treat atrial tachycardias?

Digoxin, beta blockers such as propranolol (Inderal), sotalol, and amiodarone are the most frequently prescribed medications. Patients with atrial fibrillation are also given anticoagulants such as warfarin because of symptoms of systemic emboli associated with this arrhythmia. Systemic embolization is particularly significant in patients with concurrent mitral stenosis.

9. Name the common ventricular arrhythmias.

The most common ventricular arrhythmia is the ventricular premature contraction. The patient may be asymptomatic or may notice only an occasional "skipping" or "fluttering sensation in the chest." Ventricular premature contractions (PVCs) can occur in normal individuals.

Electrocardiographic evaluation usually reveals fewer than five premature contractions per minute from a single focus in the heart. Such contractions are benign and do not warrant medical intervention. However, frequent ventricular contractions arising from several foci (multifocal PVCs) are more significant because they can degenerate into life-threatening ventricular tachycardia or ventricular fibrillation. Symptomatic patients with significant ventricular arrhythmias are therefore treated medically on a chronic basis.

10. What is ventricular tachycardia?

Clusters of three or more consecutive PVCs at a rate of about 150 bpm produce a rhythm known as ventricular tachycardia. Patients with long runs of ventricular tachycardia often have significant hemodynamic compromise. It is a life-threatening rhythm that frequently degenerates into ventricular fibrillation and is a medical emergency necessitating hospitalization.

11. Define ventricular fibrillation.

Ventricular fibrillation is a totally chaotic ventricular rhythm that is hemodynamically compromising. It may revert spontaneously but often requires cardioversion. Most of the out-of-hospital "sudden death" is caused by ventricular fibrillation.

12. What is the common therapeutic intervention for ventricular arrhythmia?

Patients with significant ventricular arrhythmias are usually on one or more antiarrhythmics including beta-blockers, sotalol, or amiodarone. In patients with significant ventricular tachycardia or ventricular fibrillation, an automatic implanted cardiac defibrillator (AICD) is often placed surgically. This device allows for detection of the tachyarrhythmia and immediate automatic defibrillation. This has significantly altered the mortality of patients with severe ventricular arrhythmias.

13. What is bradycardia or bradyarrhythmia?

A pulse rate of less than 60 bpm in an adult is called bradycardia.

14. What is the most common bradyarrhythmia?

Sinus bradycardia is the most common bradyarrhythmia. Sinus bradycardia is a resting heart rate of less than 60 bpm with no associated pathology. Electrocardiographic evaluation reveals that the electrical impulse originates normally from the sinus node. Sinus bradycardia may be normal in young and physically active people, such as athletes. Other patients may have sinus bradycardia because of conditions that slow the discharge rate of the sinus node. Increased vagal tone, medications with parasympathetic effects (e.g. digoxin and phenothiazines), and medications that suppress the excitability of the heart (beta-blockers, sotalol) can cause bradycardia.

15. How is sinus bradycardia treated?

In young patients with no symptoms, sinus bradycardia requires no treatment. In patients with bradycardia related to medications, modification of the drug regimen is indicated only if symptoms of bradycardia result.

16. What is sick sinus syndrome?

Some patients have diseases affecting the sinus node and present with inappropriate sinus responses. These patients are usually elderly and may have symptoms of palpitations, light-headedness, or syncope. An electrocardiogram may reveal abnormalities ranging from sinus bradycardia to sinus arrest. There may also be episodic supraventricular tachycardias such as atrial flutter, atrial fibrillation, or paroxysmal atrial tachycardia.

17. How is sick sinus syndrome treated?

Patients without symptoms do not require therapy. Patients with symptoms from tachycardia require medications such as beta-blockers, sotalol, or amiodarone for rate control. Patients with symptomatic bradycardia, either because of sick sinus syndrome or because of the medications needed to treat the bradycardia, require placement of a permanent pacemaker.

18. What is complete heart block?

Degenerative, inflammatory, and infiltrative diseases affecting the atrioventricular node or the conduction system can result in heart block and bradyarrhythmia. Drugs can also block conduction through the atrioventricular node. The most common culprit is excessive digoxin, which can produce bradycardia in patients with atrial fibrillation.

19. What is the treatment of complete heart block?

In most patients with complete heart block, bradycardia causes light-headedness, dizziness, or syncope (Stokes-Adams attacks). These patients need placement of a permanent pacemaker.

20. In general, how does a dentist assess risk?

The highest risk patient is the one with no known arrhythmia who has symptoms or who on examination has a pulse higher than 100 bpm or less than 60 bpm, or who has an irregular pulse. No dental treatment is indicated, and the patient must be referred to a physician for evaluation.

21. Is a patient with a known arrhythmia at risk?

A patient at minimal risk is one with an atrial arrhythmia or infrequent unifocal PVC that do not require medication. An asymptomatic young active patient with sinus bradycardia is also at negligible risk.

Patients at moderate risk are those with atrial arrhythmias on chronic medication who have no symptoms. Patients with cardiac pacemakers are also at moderate risk.

Patients at significant risk are those with ventricular arrhythmias on chronic medication who have no symptoms.

22. List the dental management issues for patients with arrhythmias.
- Determine whether the arrhythmia is well controlled
- Minimize stress to the patient +/– sedation techniques
- Minimize the use of vasoconstrictors
- Consider hospitalization for more stressful procedures for patients with more severe arrhythmias
- Consider less complex dental treatment plans for patients in the higher risk categories

23. How does a dentist determine whether an arrhythmia is well controlled?

The dentist should first determine whether the patient is symptomatic and should inquire if the patient's medical regimen has recently been changed. The dentist also should know if the patient has had a recent physical examination and electrocardiogram. If there are any concerns, a physician consultation is advised.

24. What should the consulting physician be asked?

The dentist needs to know how well the patient will tolerate the dental procedure and needs to be assured that the patient's arrhythmia is clinically stable. It is important to determine if the patient can tolerate a 1- or 2-hour appointment.

If vasoconstrictors are needed, advise the physician that you plan on using less than 2.0 Carpules of 2% lidocaine with 1:100,000 epinephrine, or 2% mepivacaine with 1:20,000 levonordefrin or an equivalent such as 4.0 Carpules of prilocaine with 1:200,000 epinephrine.

25. If the physician is concerned about the dental stress, what are the dentist's options ?

The dentist can suggest that the most difficult procedures be done in the hospital setting, where closer monitoring is available.

Alternately, the dentist can divide large procedures into multiple small ones requiring less time and less anesthetic. The dentist can also simplify the overall treatment plan.

Finally, the dentist can consider the use of sedation techniques such as N_2O/O_2 or oral anti-anxiety medications.

8. BACTERIAL ENDOCARDITIS

Robert C. Fazio, D.M.D., and Leslie S.T. Fang, M.D., Ph.D.

1. What is bacterial endocarditis?

Bacterial endocarditis is a serious infection of the heart valves or the endothelial surfaces of the heart. In recent decades the mortality rate has been 7–10%. Considerable progress in medical and surgical intervention has reduced the mortality rate for bacterial endocarditis to about 3%. Because dental manipulation is the leading identifiable cause of transient bacteremia that can result in infectious endocarditis, it is important for the dentist to understand the pathogenesis of the disease, to be able to identify the population at risk, and to be able to administer appropriate prophylactic antibiotic therapy.

2. How does a patient get bacterial endocarditis?

• The susceptible patient has a pre-existing cardiac defect.
• Transient bacteremia from some source occurs.
• The organisms of that bacteremia implant at the site of the cardiac defect.
• Bacteria proliferate at the site of the implantation.

3. What is the significance of an underlying cardiac abnormality in the development of bacterial endocarditis?

Bacterial endocarditis results from bacterial implantation and proliferation at the site of a cardiac abnormality. In the absence of such cardiac defect, the risk of bacterial endocarditis is infinitely small. The nature of the cardiac lesion also dictates the risk for endocarditis.

4. What are the most common cardiac abnormalities associated with bacterial endocarditis?

• Damaged heart valves as a sequela of rheumatic fever
• Damaged heart valves as a result of previous bacterial endocarditis
• Acquired valvular lesions such as calcific aortic stenosis in the aging population
• Roughened cardiac surfaces as a result of a jet-stream effect from blood crossing congenital cardiac lesions (such as mitral valve prolapse or ventricular septal defect)
• Prosthetic heart valves

5. How common a condition is bacterial endocarditis?

Bacterial endocarditis is rare in the general population. (approximately 2–5 cases per 100,000 patient years). The incidence increases substantially in those patients with a pre-existing cardiac defect. The risk of bacterial endocarditis is dependent on the nature of the underlying cardiac defect. For the patient with congenital bicuspid aortic valve, the prevalence is approximately 20 cases per 100,000 patient years. For the patient with a ventricular septal defect, the risk of bacterial endocarditis increases to approximately 220 cases per 100,000 patient years. The risk for infection for a patient with a previous bout of bacterial endocarditis is approximately 700–1000 per 100,000 patient years.

6. Why is this condition so important to the dentist?

The organism most commonly associated with bacterial endocarditis is *Streptococcus viridans*, a common oral organism. Dental manipulations have repeatedly been implicated as the source of transient bacteremia that leads to bacterial endocarditis.

7. What species is the most common pathogen in bacterial endocarditis?

Streptococcus sanguis and *S. mitis* are the two most common organisms. Other organisms include *S. salivarius* and *S. mutans*.

8. What percentage of patients with bacterial endocarditis have *S. viridans* as the infecting organism?

The current estimate is that 30–40% of patients with bacterial endocarditis have *S. viridans* as the underlying cause. In the earlier decades of the 20th century, the incidence of this organism was even higher. In 1968 DeMoor and associates studied 500 patients suspected of having bacterial endocarditis and isolated *S. sanguis* from the blood of 208 patients and *S. mutans* from 35 patients. Serotyping the organisms, they found remarkable similarities between the blood isolates of these strains, those of *S. viridans,* and those of strains previously isolated from the dental plaque of the same patients. These early studies suggested that the oral cavity is an important source of organisms causing bacterial endocarditis.

9. Are there other organisms in the oral cavity that produce bacterial endocarditis?

A number of other organisms normally found in the oral cavity account for a significant proportion of the causative agents of bacterial endocarditis: alpha-hemolytic streptococci, enterococci (*Streptococcus faecalis*), pneumococci, staphylococci, and group A streptococci. In addition, some organisms associated with rapidly progressive periodontitis are implicated in some cases. These have included *Actinobacillus actinomycetemcomitans* and *Eikenella corrodens*. These latter two organisms are members of the HACEK group of organisms found increasingly to be causative agents in patients with bacterial endocarditis (see question 73).

10. Is bacterial endocarditis a serious illness?

Overall, there is about a 3% mortality rate for patients who develop bacterial endocarditis. The mortality is depends in part on the underlying cardiac defect and its propensity for infection. Moreover, the morbidity of the disease is profound because of the many clinical complications from bacterial endocarditis.

11. What are the clinical consequences of bacterial endocarditis?

The clinical consequences of bacterial endocarditis may be grouped into three major categories.

1. Local bacterial proliferation may damage valvular function, resulting in valvular insufficiency and, ultimately, congestive heart failure. The infection may cause the development of an abscess of the myocardium, with subsequent disruption of the normal conduction pathways of the heart. The resultant arrhythmia can be life-threatening.

2. Pieces of infected valvular vegetation may break off and travel through the patient's body through the bloodstream. These infectious emboli may lodge in a number of organs and produce infection there as well. Among the organs most commonly targeted by such emboli are the brain, kidney, and spleen.

3. Antibodies directed against the bacteria may bind to circulating bacterial antigens to form immune complexes. Deposition of these complexes may produce arthritis or glomerulonephritis or both by the activation of complement and other biologically active substances.

12. How should the dentist assess a patient for risk of endocarditis?

• The risk of endocarditis depends primarily upon the pre-existing underlying cardiac condition.
• The dental health and hygiene of the patient also contribute to the relative risk. Patients with active periodontal disease and patients with periapical infection are more likely to have transient bacteremia both in the absence of dental procedures and during dental manipulation. The likelihood of transient bacteremia from the oral cavity is related directly to the degree of oral inflammation and infection.
• The likelihood of transient bacteremia is also related to the degree of soft-tissue trauma. The greater the soft-tissue trauma, the greater the risk of bacteremia (i.e., extractions versus prophylaxis).

13. How is risk assessed based upon the underlying cardiac defect?

The American Heart Association SBE Prophylaxis Committee regards several pre-existing cardiac conditions as high-risk lesions. Patients with these lesions are more likely to develop bacterial

endocarditis and are likely to have significant morbidity and mortality if bacterial endocarditis does occur. The high-risk patients include patients with the following conditions:
- Prosthetic cardiac valves
- A history of previous bacterial endocarditis
- Complex cyanotic congenital disease (e.g., single cardiac ventricle states, transposition of the great arteries, tetralogy of Fallot)
- Surgically constructed systemic pulmonary shunts or conduits

14. What is the prevalence of bacterial endocarditis in these patients?
These patients are at significantly increased risk for development of bacterial endocarditis. For example, patients who have prosthetic cardiac valves or patients who have a previous history of bacterial endocarditis have a prevalence of between 300 and 700 cases of bacterial endocarditis per 100,000 patient years. The general population, on the other hand, has a prevalence of 2 to 5 cases of bacterial endocarditis per 100,000 patient years.

15. Who are the patients at moderate risk for the development of bacterial endocarditis?
- Those with mitral valve prolapse with valvular regurgitation and/or thickened leaflets and hypertrophic cardiomyopathy.
- Those with congenital cardiac malformations such as uncorrected patent ductus arteriosus, ventricular septal defect, coarctation of the aorta, and bicuspid aortic valve.
- Those with acquired valvular disease such as rheumatic heart disease with carditis and calcific aortic stenosis in the aging population

16. What is the prevalence of bacterial endocarditis in patients at moderate risk?
A patient with ventricular septal defect has a 220 per 100,000 patient year risk for the development of bacterial endocarditis. Patients with pulmonary stenosis have a 20 per 100,000 patient year risk. Patients with congenital heart disease in all categories have 120 per 100,000 patient year risk. Patients with mitral valve prolapse with regurgitation have a 50 per 100,000 patient year risk. In contrast, the general population has a 2 to 5 cases per 100,000 patient year risk for the development of bacterial endocarditis.

17. Which patients are at negligible risk?
The American Heart Association defines a group of patients with negligible risk for the development of bacterial endocarditis, although these patients have some cardiac issues. Patients in this category include:
- Patients who have had surgical repair of atrial septal defect, ventricular septal defect or patent ductus arteriosus without residual complications beyond 6 months from the surgical date.
- Patients who have had mitral valve prolapse without valvular regurgitation. Unlike the patient with mitral valve prolapse with regurgitation, which carries a 5 per 100,000 patient year risk for the development of bacterial endocarditis, mitral valve prolapse without regurgitation carries approximately a 5 per 100,000 patient year risk. The latter prevalence is nearly coincident with that in the general population. Therefore, antibiotic prophylaxis is not recommended for these patients.
- Patients with isolated atrial septal defect of the secundum type.
- Patients with previous rheumatic fever without valvular dysfunction.
- Patients with functional or innocent heart murmurs.
- Patients with cardiac pacemakers.
- Patients with implanted defibrillators.

18. What is the difference between the secundum type and the primum type of atrial septal defect? Why is dental prophylaxis recommended for one and not the other?
Atrial septal defect of the secundum type is the most common atrial septal defect. The defect is located high in the atrial septum away from the valves. There is virtually no pressure gradient

across the atrial defect, and there is no jet-stream effect created by this lesion. There is therefore minimal turbulent blood flow and minimal risk for a roughened endothelial surface. Dental prophylaxis is therefore not necessary.

Atrial septal defect of the primum type is usually a larger defect located low in the septum with a position closer to the valves. This lesion is often seen in patients with trisomy 21 (Down's syndrome). It is accompanied by turbulence and a jet-stream effect. The endothelial surface has a roughened surface and creates a situation where fibrin clot can form. These patients should therefore receive dental prophylaxis.

19. Why is it that not every patient with a history of rheumatic fever requires prophylaxis?

Only 50% of patients who have had rheumatic fever actually have had the carditis and valvular disease associated with rheumatic fever. Only those patients with permanently damaged valves require antibiotic prophylaxis. Those without carditis do not have roughened endothelial surfaces and do not require antibiotic prophylaxis.

20. Why does a patient with previous coronary artery bypass graft surgery not need dental prophylaxis?

Coronary artery bypass surgery is the placement of a vessel often taken from the leg and sewn into the aorta and the coronary vessel to bypass an occluded area of the artery. Once the suture lines from the vascular surgery heal, there is no turbulent blood flow over a damaged site. Therefore, there is no platelet fibrin clot susceptible to transient bacteremia, and dental prophylaxis is not necessary.

21. Why do patients with surgically repaired atrial septal defects, ventricular septal defects, or patent ductus arteriosus not need bacterial endocarditis prophylaxis?

When atrial septal defects, ventricular septal defects, or patent ductus arteriosus are surgically corrected, there is no longer turbulent blood flow and no nidus for bacterial implantation even if there is transient bacteremia. It is therefore reasonable to use dental prophylaxis during the first 6 months after surgery when suture lines and grafts are being endothelialized. Prophylaxis is not necessary thereafter.

22. Are many of these defects being repaired via transcatheter insertion of prosthetic devices rather than by surgical repair?

Septal occluders and vascular coils are placed via catherization procedures. The issue of dental prophylaxis remains the same. Patients should receive dental prophylaxis for the 6 months following surgery; it is not necessary thereafter.

23. What is an innocent or functional murmur?

Innocent or functional murmurs are usually found in children. The murmurs are usually heard during periods when there is a hyperdynamic circulatory state (e.g., high fevers). During these periods, the discrepancy in the size of the heart valve and the developing heart muscle may result in "innocent murmurs" or "flow murmurs." These murmurs usually disappear with the maturation and growth of the individual and are often absent when the circulatory tree is no longer in a hyperdynamic state. Not infrequently, the murmur was present during childhood and is gone in adult life.

24. How about flow or innocent murmurs present in the adult population?

Flow or innocent murmurs in the adult population are more difficult to evaluate. A persistent murmur in an adult may be innocent if it is of no functional significance, but this does not necessarily mean that dental prophylaxis is not necessary. The exact valvular pathology should be defined prior to labeling a murmur innocent with no requirement for dental prophylaxis. These murmurs are often evaluated by studies such as echocardiography, which identify the source of the murmur and verify that the heart is structurally normal. Echocardiography may, however, detect mitral valve prolapse with regurgitation or thickened leaflets that will require prophylaxis.

25. Are there any murmurs in the adult population that the dentist can assume are innocent based on the interview with the patient alone?

Generally, a patient who reports a murmur detected in childhood but not in adulthood can be assumed to have a truly innocent murmur and does not require prophylaxis. Similarly, a patient who reports a murmur only heard during pregnancy may have a flow murmur during a hyperdynamic state. Patients who are pregnant often have cardiac output that is two to three times the cardiac output of a nonpregnant patient. These high-flow states can result in turbulent blood flow that makes a noise heard on auscultation as a murmur or flow murmur. The murmur resolves after the delivery, when the cardiovascular system returns to a normal state. These patients indeed have functional murmur and do not require prophylaxis.

26. Has the American Heart Association changed its recommendation on dental prophylaxis for patients with mitral valve prolapse?

Previously, the American Heart Association recommended dental prophylaxis for all patients with mitral valve prolapse. Epidemiologic data, however, revealed that only patients with mitral valve prolapse and regurgitation and/or thickened leaflets have an increased risk for bacterial endocarditis (nearly 10 times the risk of the general population). On the other hand, patients with mitral valve prolapse but no regurgitation or thickened leaflets are at no increased risk for development of bacterial endocarditis. Therefore, no prophylaxis is recommended for these patients.

27. What if the patient with mitral valve prolapse is not sure if he or she has thickened mitral valve or regurgitation? What should the dentist do?

If the patient does not know whether he or she has thickened mitral valve leaflet or regurgitation and an emergent procedure is needed, antibiotic prophylaxis should be given until further evaluation of the mitral valve can take place. Typically, the patient's physician would have an echocardiographic report that will clarify the situation. Future need for prophylaxis is dictated by the echocardiographic findings.

28. What if the physician reports that the murmur is innocent and no prophylaxis is required and no studies are indicated?

The dentist can proceed with all procedures without antibiotic prophylaxis. A formal correspondence between the dentist and the physician is recommended. The correspondence should record the consultation and indicate that the patient is believed not to be at risk for bacterial endocarditis.

29. What should the dentist do with regard to dental prophylaxis in a patient with a history of rheumatic fever in whom cardiac involvement is uncertain?

If a patient with a history of rheumatic fever is not sure whether he or she has a murmur, the dentist should assume that there is a murmur and cover any risk prophylactically. Consultation with the physician with regard to future dental prophylaxis is mandated.

30. Why is there no need for prophylaxis for patients with cardiac pacemakers and implanted defibrillators? What should the dentist do if the patient's physician recommends prophylaxis nevertheless?

Normally, the wires from the pacemaker and the implanted defibrillators are endothelialized within a few weeks after placement and prophylaxis is not necessary.

However, there are data in the medical literature to suggest that transient bacteremia (e.g., after dental manipulation) can seed the subdermal pouch where the pacemaker or the defibrillator is implanted. Therefore, some cardiologists recommend prophylaxis, not so much to prevent bacterial endocarditis but to prevent skin infection at the subdermal pouch.

Specific physicians, for a variety of reasons, may recommend prophylaxis for specific patients in spite of the American Heart Association's recommendations. It is important to note that the American Heart Association's recommendations are guidelines only. The clinical judgment of the individual physician and dentist may call for over-riding the recommendations. However, the rationale for deviation from the recommendations should be carefully documented.

31. What dental procedures would place the patient at risk for bacterial endocarditis?
The American Heart Association has recommended that any dental procedure that causes "significant bleeding" places the patient with an underlying cardiac defect at risk for bacterial endocarditis and mandates prophylaxis.

32. What procedures are these?
• All dental extractions; all periodontal procedures including surgery, scaling, and root planing; probing alone; or recall maintenance
• Dental implant placement and reimplantation of avulsed teeth
• Endodontic instrumentation or surgery beyond the apex
• Subgingival placement of antibiotic fibers or strips
• Initial placement of orthodontic bands but not brackets
• Intraligamentary local anesthetic injections
• Prophylactic cleaning of teeth or implants where bleeding is anticipated

33. How is significant bleeding defined?
Previous American Heart Association recommendations indicated that "any bleeding" merited consideration for prophylaxis. The Committee's recommendation has been tempered to recommend prophylaxis in instances where "significant bleeding" is anticipated. Unfortunately, no precise definition of significant bleeding is offered, and it is left to the dentist's discretion to gauge whether significant bleeding is likely to occur with any given procedure. Since the American Heart Association's recommendations delineate probing of the gingiva as an at risk procedure, it can be assumed that virtually any bleeding should be considered significant. Clearly, the clinician should not lose sight of the fact that the risk of bacteremia is far greater following the extraction of a tooth compared with the probing of the periodontium around the tooth. The clinician is also reminded of the variability of bleeding on probing based on the presence of periodontal disease, inflammation, infection, and pocket depth.

34. Is dental instrumentation the major cause of bacterial endocarditis?
No; the predominant source of oral bacteremia with resultant bacterial endocarditis is "spontaneous bacteremia" induced by the patient when he or she is chewing food or carrying out oral hygiene measures. In patients with poor periodontal health, spontaneous bacteremia occurs frequently.

35. How often are dental procedures implicated as the cause of endocarditis?
In order to separate bacteremia caused by dental intervention from spontaneous bacteremia, it is important to understand the course of clinical disease in a patient with bacterial endocarditis.
In patients with streptococcal endocarditis, 85% are symptomatic within 2 weeks after the introduction of bacteria into the susceptible host. The disease then progresses slowly, but most patients require hospitalization in approximately 2 months. Therefore, dental procedures within 30 to 90 days of the diagnosis of streptococcal endocarditis may be implicated as the cause of the endocarditis. On the other hand, if no dental interventions have been done within 30 to 90 days of the diagnosis, it is more likely that the condition has been brought on by other causes of transient bacteremia.

36. How many patients with bacterial endocarditis have historically seen the dentist within 90 days of contracting the disease?
CE Cherubin, in the *American Journal of Medicine*, 1971, and several others suggest that approximately 15 percent of patients with bacterial endocarditis have seen a dentist in the previous 90 days.

37. How often is bacterial endocarditis the result of bacteremia induced by a dental procedure?

WE Guntheroth, in the *American Journal of Cardiology*, 1984, and R Bayliss, in the *British Journal*, 1983, estimated that 4% or less of all subacute bacterial endocarditis cases are the result of bacteremia induced by dental procedures.

38. Based on the literature, what is the association between dental manipulation and bacterial endocarditis?

Oral bacteria cause approximately 40% of cases of bacterial endocarditis. Approximately 15% of patients with bacterial endocarditis have seen the dentist within 90 days. Studies suggest that the cases of bacterial endocarditis directly attributable to specific dental manipulation represent only approximately 4% or less of all reported cases. Therefore, most cases (approximately 96%) are actually caused by bacteremia induced by nondental procedures.

39. Are there any population based case control studies?

Strom and coworkers in *Annals of Internal Medicine*, volume 129, 1998, published an article entitled "Dental and Cardiac Risk Factors for Infective Endocarditis."

A population case-controlled study of 54 hospitals in the Philadelphia, Pennsylvania, area attempted to quantitate the risk for endocarditis from dental treatment. In this hospital population, 273 cases of bacterial endocarditis were isolated. These cases were compared with a case-control group without bacterial endocarditis from the same area, which was matched for age, sex, and other parameters.

The study concluded that dental therapy was virtually identical in the two groups. However, pre-existing cardiac lesions were significantly more common in the group who developed endocarditis (38% versus 6%).

The authors concluded that there was a strong correlation between the presence of a cardiac valvular abnormality and the risk for development of bacterial endocarditis. However, whether the patient had had dental interventions was not significant. The study ultimately questions the value of dental prophylaxis.

40. Are there other studies questioning the effectiveness of dental prophylaxis?

In a similar population based study in the Netherlands, Van Der Meer and colleagues reported similar results, again questioning the wisdom of dental prophylaxis.

41. Should these data impact the dentist's opinion with regard to dental prophylaxis?

As data accumulate, the American Heart Association has been simplifying antibiotic prophylaxis, and current recommendations call for relatively simple single-dose therapy in the majority of instances. Until the American Heart Association publishes new guidelines, those delineated in the *Annals of Internal Medicine*, November, 1997, should be adhered to. The dentist, however, should anticipate that future recommendations may suggest that many patients currently needing prophylaxis would no longer require it.

However, it is hard to see how prophylaxis can be withheld from the high risk group of patients and those with prosthetic valves. In addition, those with a prior history of bacterial endocarditis would probably always be recommended to receive dental prophylaxis.

In patients with other pre-existing cardiac abnormalities, it is likely that dental prophylaxis would be recommended only in instances where high-grade bacteremia (significant bleeding) is anticipated.

One recent set of recommendations editorialized by an author of previous guidelines suggests the possibility of limiting prophylactic antibiotic use to those patients at high risk for infection who are undergoing high-risk procedures (for example, patients with prosthetic valves, patients with a history of previous bacterial endocarditis, and patients having extractions, oral surgery, or other gingival surgery).

42. How effective is antibiotic prophylaxis in preventing bacterial endocarditis?

The data available are equivocal and largely presumptive. There have been published reports of patients acquiring bacterial endocarditis in the face of appropriate antibiotic prophylaxis. What is unclear is whether the antibiotic prophylaxis failed to suppress the bacteremia at the time of the dental manipulation or if the bacterial endocarditis was caused by other incidental bacteremia, perhaps induced by the patient (spontaneous bacteremia).

In the Stromm study, 37 of 273 patients diagnosed as having bacterial endocarditis had an underlying cardiac abnormality, and their bacterial endocarditis was caused by dental flora and dental therapy within the preceding 90 days. Of the 37, 27 patients had the appropriate American Heart Association–approved antibiotic prophylaxis.

43. If a patient is edentulous, is there a risk of bacteremia from an oral source?

There are case reports of bacterial endocarditis as a result of bacteremia from a denture sore. Therefore, patients with a history of pre-existing cardiac defects should be monitored closely when fitted for a new full denture. Efforts should be made to avoid abrasion-induced denture sores in these patients.

44. For a patient undergoing general dentistry and prosthetics, is prophylaxis recommended?

The current recommendations suggest that dental prophylaxis is necessary only in instances in which significant bleeding is anticipated. Since significant bleeding is generally not encountered in routine general dentistry and prosthetics, antibiotic prophylaxis is generally not necessary.

45. What are the recommended regimens for antibiotic prophylaxis?

The basic choices are generally 2 g of amoxicillin po 1 hour before the appointment or clindamycin 600 mg po 1 hour prior to the appointment. Amoxicillin is typically prescribed in 500-mg capsules times four. Clindamycin can be prescribed as 150-mg tablets times four or 300-mg tablets times two.

46. What is the need for follow-up antibiotics (second dose)?

The American Heart Association has dropped its recommendation for a second dose. This is based on the consideration that most bacteremia occurs within the first 15 minutes of the procedure. The currently recommended oral doses give coverage between 6 and 14 hours post therapy.

47. Has the amoxicillin dose been reduced in the most recent set of recommendations?

Yes, the 1990 recommendation was for 3 g (3000 mg of amoxicillin) preoperatively. Subsequent studies have demonstrated that the 2-g dose provided therapeutic levels of the drug for 6–12 hours. The new guidelines call for 2 g of amoxicillin. The advantage of the 2-g dose is to diminish the risk of gastrointestinal side effects of the higher dose.

48. Can I use penicillin VK?

Amoxicillin is recommended because it is better absorbed from the gastrointestinal tract and provides higher and more sustained serum levels.

49. How about the former erythromycin regimens?

For a number of reasons, erythromycin regimens have been eliminated. The drug required administration 2 hours rather than 1 hour prior to the appointment. The different preparations of erythromycin, erythromycin stereate, delayed released capsules erythromycin, enteric-coated erythromycin, and erythromycin ethyl succinate, all had variable pharmacokinetics, making dosing difficult and leading to significant confusion.

50. Are any of the macrolides recommended?

Azithromycin (Zithromax), 500 mg 1 hour before the appointment, or clarithromycin (Biaxin), 500 mg 1 hour before the appointment, is recommended by the American Heart Association.

51. Are there any other acceptable regimens?

Cephalexin (Keflex), 2 g, or cefadroxil (Duricef), 2 g, can be used 1 hour before the appointment.

52. Can I use cephalexin or cefadroxil in patients with penicillin allergy?

Unfortunately, 5–8% of patients who are allergic to penicillin are also allergic to cephalosporins. Since dentistry is generally conducted in an outpatient setting, it is recommended that cephalosporins not be used when the patient has a history of penicillin allergy.

53. Are there intramuscular or intravenous options?

Yes, 2 g of ampicillin IM or IV, 600 mg of clindamycin IV or 1 g of cefazolin (Ancef) IM or IV within 30 minutes of the procedure are parenteral preparations recommended by the American Heart Association.

54. What is the status of the vancomycin recommendation for the penicillin-allergic patient?

Vancomycin is no longer recommended by the American Heart Association. Although vancomycin is an effective drug, overprescription of this drug would remove the agent as a last line of defense against penicillin-resistant *Staphylococcus* species. It is feared that the overuse of vancomycin in the nonemergent prophylaxis setting may increase the development of resistant strains.

55. What are the major dental management considerations for patients who require dental prophylaxis?

There are three primary issues:
1. The timing of the appointment when multiple visits are necessary.
2. Potential changes in treatment plan based on the underlying cardiac condition.
3. An aggressive prevention protocol.

56. What is the appropriate spacing of appointments?

The American Heart Association recommends that for patients requiring multiple visits, a time interval of between 9 and 14 days elapse between appointments. The concern is relative to the development of strains resistant to the prophylactic drug. If procedures are done within a shorter time interval, theoretically amoxicillin-resistant bacteria can emerge. With a 9- to 14-day interval, the oral flora will recolonize, reducing the likelihood that a resistant strain will be present at the time of the dental intervention.

57. How should the dentist do this on a practical basis?

If the patient needs two visits only, a 9-day interval seems reasonable. If, on the other hand, the patient requires more than two visits, a 14-day interval between visits would probably be preferable in order to minimize the emergence of resistant organisms.

58. What if the dentist cannot adhere to this interval?

There are times when optimal dental intervention precludes such a long waiting period between visits. For example, a patient who had acute endodontic treatment developed recurrent symptoms in 4 days. In this setting, it is recommended that the dentist prescribe a different medication than the one initially prescribed. For patients who received amoxicillin initially, clindamycin, azithromycin, or clarithromycin can be used. For penicillin-allergic patients who received clindamycin, azithromycin, or clarithromycin can be used.

59. What should the dentist do if the patient is already taking amoxicillin for other conditions?

Amoxicillin should be continued, and dental prophylaxis should be carried out using clindamycin, azithromycin, or clarithromycin. This rule would apply to the patient who has finished a course of amoxicillin within the past 9–14 days. These patients should have clindamycin, azithromycin, or clarithromycin for dental prophylaxis because they may have amoxicillin-resistant organisms in the oral cavity.

60. What if the dentist is unaware of this until the patient appears at the office and has already taken his or her normal prophylactic amoxicillin dose?

There is obviously concern that there may be resistant organisms in the oral cavity that are not adequately covered by the amoxicillin prophylaxis. It would therefore be reasonable to add clindamycin, 600 mg, at the time of the visit and proceed with the planned procedure.

61. What if the patient has forgotten to take his or her premedication?

The American Heart Association guidelines do not specify a recommendation in this setting. Previously, the consensus was for the drug to be given in the dental office and the dental procedure delayed for an hour in order to ensure maximum blood levels of the antibiotic at the time of anticipated clinical bleeding.

In the most recent 1997 guidelines, the American Heart Association suggested that in the setting of unanticipated bleeding, effective prophylaxis is possible if the patient is medicated anytime up to 2 hours from the time of the induced bacteremia. That same study by Berney and colleagues in the *Journal of Infectious Diseases*, 1990, suggested that, if the patient is medicated 4 hours after the unanticipated bleeding, there is no prophylactic benefit.

Based on these data, some dentists may elect to give antibiotic prophylaxis chairside just prior to the dental procedure.

Until the American Heart Association discusses this specific clinical situation, caution is advised.

62. What is the conservative approach to the patient who has forgotten to take the premedication?

The most conservative approach would be to reschedule the patient for a time when the premedication has been taken 1 hour before the procedure.

63. What is a practical solution to dental prophylaxis for a patient who has forgotten to take the premedication?

On the basis of the Berney data suggesting that antibiotics have been shown to be effective for up to 2 hours after a dental procedure, the dentist may elect to medicate the patient chairside and proceed with the planned procedure.

64. When would chairside antibiotic prophylaxis not be appropriate?

Patients at high risk for development of bacterial endocarditis who are to undergo procedures that can result in significant clinical bleeding are poor candidates for chairside prophylaxis.

65. What is the role of a prevention protocol?

Antiseptic mouth rinses applied immediately prior to dental procedures may reduce the bacteremia load for that patient. Chlorhexidene or povidone-iodine gentle oral rinsing with 15 ml of the solution for 30 seconds prior to the dental treatment is recommended.

66. Should the dentist recommend water piks, electric toothbrushes and other electrically powered dental hygiene aids?

Package inserts on water piks and electric toothbrushes specifically caution against the use of these products if the patient has a heart murmur. The American Heart Association, on the other hand, notes that home use devices pose far less risk of bacteremia in a healthy mouth than does ongoing oral inflammation. The American Heart Association does list water piks and electric-powered toothbrushes as recommended dental aids.

67. When would these agents be appropriate?

A clinician might avoid recommending electric oral hygiene devices in the early part of periodontal treatment when the patient has significant oral inflammation and uncontrolled disease. Once ideal soft tissue health is attained, it is probably appropriate to recommend these devices.

68. Should the dentist change the treatment plan for patients at risk for bacterial endo-carditis?

Many dentists opt to retain teeth with deep residual pockets that often demonstrate clinical purulence. The dentist must be cognizant of the fact that when manipulated at home by the patient during oral hygiene procedures, these teeth are more likely to yield a clinically significant bacteremia than teeth with good periodontal health. A more aggressive extraction strategy for highly questionable teeth should be undertaken in patients with cardiac defects at high risk for endocarditis. More aggressive treatment of asymptomatic periapical lesions should also be considered.

69. What is the HACEK group of organisms?

The HACEK group of pathogens are organisms that are found increasingly in patients diagnosed as having bacterial endocarditis. This group of organisms includes *Haemophilus influenzae*, *Actinobacillus actinomycetemcomitans*, *Cardiobacterium hominis*, *Eikenella corrodens*, and *Kingella kingae*. Two of the four, *A. actinomycetemcomitans* and *E. corrodens*, are bacteria that have been isolated in aggressive periodontal lesions.

70. What are the recommendations for patients undergoing cardiac surgery?

A preoperative dental evaluation is recommended by the American Heart Association for patients who will be undergoing cardiac surgery. The goal of the dental evaluation is to be able to reduce the likelihood of bacteremia from an oral source postoperatively. Acutely infected teeth must be treated or extracted. Poorly controlled periodontal disease should be controlled aggressively with scaling, root planing and, if tolerated, curettage. When in doubt, selective extraction of teeth of questionable health should be considered.

It is important to stress that the level of aggressiveness in extraction should be governed by the cardiac surgical procedures being undertaken. Many reparative cardiac procedures do not modify the patient's long term risk for infective endocarditis. In patients with coronary artery bypass grafts, closure of ventricular septal defect or patent ductus arteriosus there is little risk for bacterial endocarditis following cardiac surgery. On the other hand, patients who receive prosthetic valves have a markedly higher risk for bacterial endocarditis. It is therefore important to recognize the varying risks for patients and temper the therapeutic plans accordingly.

71. What are the recommendations for the patient having noncoronary artery vascular grafts (e.g., correction of aortic defects)?

The American Heart Association recommends prophylaxis 6 months following the placement of these grafts. Generally, it is not recommended after the 6-month interval. However, some vascular surgeons may suggest to the dentist that antibiotic prophylaxis is necessary for specific individuals.

72. Are there specific recommendations for patients with heart transplants?

The cardiologist is generally concerned about an increased risk of acquired valvular dysfunction, especially during episodes of rejection for patients with heart transplants. In addition, a significant amount of immunosuppression is necessary in such patients. Most transplant physicians, therefore, would recommend oral prophylactic antibiotics prior to any dental therapy that would cause significant bleeding.

73. Vascular stents are commonly being used to treat coronary artery disease. Do these stents require antibiotic prophylaxis prior to dental visits?

A vascular stent placed in the coronary artery will epithelialize soon after the placement. Therefore, there is no chance for platelet fibrin clot to form in the stent after the epithelialization. Generally, patients with vascular stents are not recommended for antibiotic prophylaxis. However, in the immediate postoperative period, the stent is a foreign body in the bloodstream and theoretically can become infected. Therefore, the cardiologist may prefer dental prophylaxis for up to as long as 6 months after stent placement.

74. When should the dentist be concerned that dental manipulation might have caused bacteremia and bacterial endocarditis?

Most cases of bacterial endocarditis related to dental procedures produce symptoms after a short incubation period. The symptoms usually begin within a few weeks after the procedure. A patient who complains of constitutional symptoms with persistent fever, chills, malaise, and other nonspecific findings of distress should be referred to the physician for evaluation. It is always desirable to maintain a good line of communication with the physician with regard to your concerns.

75. What is the single most important recommendation for the patient with a cardiac defect that places him or her at risk for bacterial endocarditis?

It is critical that these patients have the best oral hygiene possible. The dentist should design a program to improve poor gingival health. Patients who have underlying cardiac defects that place them at risk for bacterial endocarditis should be advised that inadequate oral hygiene, unhealthy gingiva and periodontium, and untreated endodontic problems or soft-tissue infection markedly increase the risk for bacterial endocarditis, a potentially life-threatening disease. A strict prevention protocol should be maintained for all such patients. The cornerstone of a successful therapeutic plan is based upon the patient's understanding of the risks.

76. Are there any specific recommendations for the way consultation with physicians should be carried out?

The dentist should understand that the best result from a consultation is obtained when specific information is asked for. Unfortunately, a physician may not be as familiar with the latest American Heart Association recommended regimens as the dentist. One study in 1989 demonstrated that only 27% of physicians and 39% of dentists could identify the correct antibiotic regimen for various patients at risk for bacterial endocarditis. (CL Nelson, and coworkers, *Journal of the American Dental Association*, 1989).

77. What kind of information should the dentist specifically seek during a physician consultation?

For information that will help in the management of a patient with a heart murmur, a typical conversation would be: "Does this murmur place the patient at risk for bacterial endocarditis? If so, I would like to use the American Heart Association's recommended medications for prophylaxis." Such a question specifically asks the physician whether the underlying cardiac defect places the patient at risk for bacterial endocarditis, and this specific point would not be lost in the fine details of the cardiac examination. Second, it suggests that the dentist would prefer to follow the American Heart Association recommendations with which the physician should be familiar. It also precludes the physician's suggesting a regimen that may be outdated. It is not unreasonable for the dentist to suggest that he or she will fax or send a letter to the physician confirming the consultation and the recommendations.

9. MANAGEMENT OF THE CARDIAC SURGERY PATIENT

Robert C. Fazio, D.M.D., and Leslie S.T. Fang, M.D., Ph.D.

DENTAL CONSIDERATION FOR PATIENTS ABOUT TO UNDERGO CARDIAC SURGERY

1. What is the role of the dentist in the management of patients who are about to undergo cardiac surgery?

The dentist may be consulted for an evaluation of the oral health of a patient who is scheduled to undergo cardiac surgery. A number of cardiac surgical procedures can increase the patient's risk of developing bacterial endocarditis. Because the oral cavity is a major source of transient bacteremia that can result in bacterial endocarditis, the oral health of the patient should be optimized preoperatively whenever feasible.

2. List the common cardiac surgical procedures.

Coronary artery bypass grafts, heart valve replacement, and the repair of congenital cardiovascular defects such as atrial septal defects, ventricular septal defects, tetralogy of Fallot, transposition of the great vessels, and coarctation of the aorta.

3. Describe the role of the dentist in the evaluation of the patient prior to planned cardiac surgery.

The dental evaluation should be directed primarily at the risk of developing bacterial endocarditis after cardiac surgery. Patients who are at high risk for developing endocarditis postoperatively should have aggressive preoperative intervention to minimize the risk. Different cardiac surgical procedures place the patients at varying risk for the development of postoperative bacterial endocarditis and require different dental therapeutic intervention

4. Which patients are at low risk for developing bacterial endocarditis postoperatively?

Patients who have undergone coronary artery bypass procedures or successful repair of an atrial septal defect, a ventricular septal defect, or patent ductus arteriosus are at low risk for the development of bacterial endocarditis beyond the immediate postoperative period. These patients do not require special intervention preoperatively.

5. Which patients are at risk for developing bacterial endocarditis postoperatively?

Patients requiring valvular replacement, either with a prosthetic or a homograft, are at risk for the development of bacterial endocarditis postoperatively. Patients who are to undergo repair of complicated congenital lesions such as transposition of the great vessels, tetralogy of Fallot, or coarctation of the aorta are also at risk for developing bacterial endocarditis postoperatively.

6. What should be the dental approach to the patients who are at risk for developing bacterial endocarditis postoperatively?

The primary goal is to eliminate infection quickly before the cardiac surgical procedure in order to minimize the risk of postoperative bacterial endocarditis. In addition to the extraction of acutely infected teeth, any tooth with a questionable prognosis because of pulpal or periodontal disease should be extracted.

7. List the dental considerations for patients undergoing cardiac transplant.

• Patients are often quite unstable, and dental therapy has to be tailored according to the clinical situations.

- Patients are under a considerable amount of immunosuppressive therapy after the procedure and are at high risk for infection.
- Teeth with slight to moderate caries should be excavated and restored.
- Teeth with deep caries, pulpal exposure, or near-pulpal exposure should be extracted
- Teeth with moderate to severe periodontal disease should be extracted.
- The dentist should understand that time constraints may alter the therapeutic approach to these patients, many of whom may require urgent cardiac transplant.
- The dentist should try to minimize stress to the patient. Whenever feasible, lengthy procedures should be spread over shorter appointments. Adjunctive sedation techniques should be considered when appropriate.
- In general, the use of epinephrine should be minimized in patients with significant underlying cardiac disease, especially if arrhythmia is a concern.

8. What precautions should the dentist take in addressing these patients preoperatively?
- The dentist should remember that patients with significant valvular disease and congenital cardiac anomalies often need antibiotic prophylaxis prior to any dental procedures
- The dentist should understand that time constraints may alter the therapeutic approach to these patients, many of whom may require urgent cardiac surgical procedures.
- The dentist should try to minimize stress to the patient. Whenever feasible, lengthy procedures should be spread over shorter appointments. Adjunctive sedation techniques should be considered when appropriate.
- In general, the use of epinephrine should be minimized in patients with significant underlying cardiac disease, especially if arrhythmia is a concern.

9. Describe the general guidelines to the management of the patients who are at risk for the development of bacterial endocarditis after cardiac surgery.
- Teeth with slight to moderate caries should be excavated and restored
- Teeth with deep caries, pulpal exposure, or near-pulpal exposure should be extracted
- Teeth with moderate to severe periodontal disease should be extracted

DENTAL CONSIDERATION FOR THE PATIENT WHO HAS UNDERGONE CARDIAC SURGERY

10. What are the dental considerations for any patient who has undergone cardiac surgery?
Patients who have undergone cardiac surgery should not have elective dental procedures done within the first 3 months after surgery. Patients are often still recovering from surgery and are not ideally suited to undergoing elective procedures.

11. What are the dental considerations for a patient who has undergone coronary artery bypass graft?
Patients who have undergone coronary artery bypass graft should not have elective dental procedures done within the first 3 months after surgery. Patients are often still recovering from surgery and are not ideally suited to undergoing elective procedures. Beyond the first 3 months, there is no need for dental prophylaxis in these patients.

12. What are the dental considerations for a patient who has undergone valvular replacement?
- Patients who have undergone valvular replacement should not have elective dental procedures done within the first 3 months after surgery when they are still clinically unstable.
- Many patients will be on anticoagulation therapy after valvular replacement. In general, patients with prosthetic valves require lifelong anticoagulation therapy. Patients with porcine valve and valvular reconstruction often need anticoagulation therapy only within the first 3 months after surgery and do not require anticoagulation thereafter. It is important to know the anticoagulation status of the patient and manage him or her accordingly.

- All patients who have undergone valvular replacement or reconstruction are at high risk for the development of bacterial endocarditis and should have antibiotic prophylaxis.
- Patients should be instructed about the need for aggressive oral hygiene and placed on frequent maintenance recall schedules.

13. What are the dental considerations for a patient who has undergone surgery for congenital anomalies?
- Patients who have undergone surgery for congenital anomalies of the heart should not have elective dental procedures done within the first 3 months after surgery when they are still clinically unstable.
- Antibiotic prophylaxis should be considered for patients who have had repair of tetralogy of Fallot, coarctation of the aorta, or transposition of the great vessels.
- Patients should be instructed about the need for aggressive oral hygiene and placed on frequent maintenance recall schedules.
- Antibiotic prophylaxis is not necessary for patients who have had successful primary repair of an atrial septal defect, ventricular septal defect, or patent ductus arteriosus.

14. What are the dental considerations for a patient who has undergone cardiac transplant?
- Patients who have undergone cardiac transplant should not have elective dental procedures done within the first 3 to 6 months after surgery because of their clinical instability and the amount of immunosuppressive therapy they are often administered.
- Antibiotic prophylaxis is recommended.
- Aggressive treatment of dental infection is recommended.
- Patients should be instructed about the need for aggressive oral hygiene and placed on frequent maintenance recall schedules.
- Cyclosporine therapy, particularly in higher doses, can cause gingival hyperplasia. Patients with gingival hyperplasia should have rigorous oral hygiene and recall prophylaxis and surgical gingivectomy in some circumstances.

10. DIABETES MELLITUS

Robert C. Fazio, D.M.D., and Leslie S.T. Fang, M.D., Ph.D.

1. What is diabetes mellitus?

Diabetes mellitus is an absolute or relative insulin insufficiency caused either by a low output of insulin from the pancreas or by unresponsiveness of peripheral tissues to insulin.

2. What is the clinical relevance of diabetes mellitus?

Diabetes mellitus is the sixth leading cause of death in the United States. It is one of the most costly illnesses, and diabetic complications such as blindness, renal failure, and limb amputation contribute significantly to the cost.

3. What is the clinical relevance of diabetes mellitus for dentistry?

There is a strong correlation between diabetes and the risk of chronic periodontitis.

4. How is this correlation substantiated?

Grossi and coworkers (*Journal of Periodontology*, 1994) showed that only two positive answers on the medical questionnaire are positively correlated with the risk for periodontitis. The presence of diabetes mellitus and/or a heavy smoking habit strongly impact the development of periodontitis.

5. Are there correlations between diabetic complications and dental pathology?

Rylander and coworkers (*Journal of Clinical Periodontology*) reported an association between retinopathy and nephropathy and the development of gingivitis.

Glavind and colleagues (*Journal of Periodontology*, 1968) noted that the presence of retinopathy was associated with greater loss of periodontal attachment.

6. What is the implication of these findings for the dentist?

The dentist should be particularly diligent in the diagnosis and prevention of periodontal disease for those patients with diabetes mellitus and related complications.

7. What is the worldwide prevalence of diabetes mellitus?

Currently, approximately 130 million people around the world have diabetes. Projections by the International Diabetes Institute suggest that this figure will rise to more than 220 million by the year 2010.

8. What is the prevalence of diabetes mellitus in the United States?

Diabetes now affects 1 in 15 white adults in the United States. The prevalence is considerably higher in the elderly and in certain ethnic groups such as blacks, Native Americans, Asian Indians and Pima Indians.

9. What is the impact of diabetes mellitus on the dental practice?

An average dental practice of 1000 patients should expect to have 50–200 patients with diabetes mellitus. Diabetes mellitus affects 17 people per 1000 between the ages of 25 and 44 and 79 people per 1000 over the age of 65.

10. How often would the dentist see a diabetic patient?

Of the overall patient population in the average dental office, 7% are diabetic. The projected prevalence over the next decade as the "baby boomer" population ages is 10%. Currently, 18% of the elderly population are diabetic.

11. Why do many dentists feel that they are seeing fewer diabetics in their practice?
Estimates are that one of every two diabetics do not know they have diabetes mellitus.

12. What is the current classification of diabetes?
Diabetes mellitus is now classified according to etiology.
  a. Patients with type 1 diabetes mellitus have either an autoimmune or an idiopathic disease in which the pancreatic beta-cells are destroyed, usually leading to absolute insulin deficiency.
  b. Patients with type 2 diabetes mellitus may have insulin resistance with relative insulin deficiency, a secretory defect with or without insulin resistance, or an increase in glucose production by the liver. In developed countries, approximately 90% of patients with type 2 diabetes mellitus are obese.

13. What is the importance of this new classification?
The new classification defines diabetes mellitus by its cause. This classification would allow for more rational therapeutic strategies. Correct classification would allow for tailoring of therapy for the patient.

14. What is the distribution between types 1 and 2 diabetes mellitus?
Type 2 diabetes mellitus is the most common kind; in the United States, 85–90% of patients with diabetes mellitus have type 2.

15. What are the symptoms of diabetes mellitus?
Many patients with diabetes mellitus have no symptoms, and the diagnosis is made because of abnormal blood glucose levels detected on a routine screening.
Some patients may develop polydipsia, polyuria, polyphagia, and weight loss.
In patients with severe insulin deficiency, development of ketoacidosis may cause nausea, vomiting, lethargy, confusion, and coma.

16. How might an undiagnosed diabetic with no symptoms appear to the dentist?
The patient might appear with aggressive periodontitis out of proportion to age or local factors or both. In other words, the dentist may diagnose significant periodontitis but recognize that the patient seems too young for that level of disease or lacks an appropriate amount of plaque and calculus to justify such periodontal destruction.

17. What is the differential diagnosis of periodontitis that appears out of proportion to age or local factors or both?
The two most common diagnoses are rapidly destructive periodontitis associated with an aggressive microbiota or undiagnosed diabetes mellitus.

18. What other clinical findings suggest this differential diagnosis?
A patient with periodontitis and a poor response to treatment should be evaluated for diabetes mellitus. The patient might have undergone scaling, root planing, and curettage but continues to demonstrate signs of active disease with poor tissue tone and ongoing purulence and exudation. These patients should be suspected of having undiagnosed diabetes mellitus.

19. How would a consideration of this differential diagnosis affect treatment plans?
Besides conventional dental therapy, a patient with diabetes mellitus requires concurrent medical management of the disease to allow for ideal healing. Left untreated, the diabetes will increase the risk of progressive periodontal disease later on.
The patient with rapidly progressive periodontitis usually responds to conventional periodontal therapy if adjunctive antibiotic therapy is utilized. The choice of an appropriate antibiotic is usually determined by culture and sensitivity data.
The dentist, therefore, is choosing between a medical referral or subgingival flora bacterial testing.

20. Are there any clues that would lead the dentist to one diagnosis over another?

Reviewing the family history may be helpful. Children of known diabetics are 2.5 times more likely to develop diabetes mellitus in their lifetimes. In the United States, obesity is also correlated with the development of type 2 diabetes mellitus.

21. How about the undiagnosed patient presenting with polydipsia, polyuria, polyphagia, and weight loss?

These classic symptoms demand medical referral regardless of the periodontal status.

22. How is diabetes mellitus diagnosed?

The diagnosis of diabetes mellitus may occasionally be made during a routine test on an asymptomatic patient by the demonstration of an elevated blood glucose levels (hyperglycemia) or glucose in the urine (glycosuria).

Symptomatic patients with polyphia, polydipsia, polyuria and weight loss may have the diagnosis of diabetes mellitus confirmed by blood tests.

Patients with a fasting plasma glucose level higher than 120 or a random plasma glucose of greater than 200 have diabetes mellitus.

23. Does the dentist have options for screening patients for diabetes mellitus?

There are three options:
a. Referral to the physician's office.
b. Referral to a commercial laboratory for blood sugar determination.
c. The use of a glucometer test in the dental office.

24. What are the advantages and disadvantages of referral to the physician?

The referral to the patient's physician places the patient in the hands of the professional who will treat him or her if the blood tests confirm the diagnosis. The disadvantage is that the dentist needs to consult with the physician to explain and confirm his suspicions. The physician will probably do a clinical examination of the patient, resulting in a longer time to schedule planned procedures and an inconvenience to the patient.

25. What are the pros and cons of referring a patient to a commercial laboratory?

The dentist can use forms from the local commercial laboratory or write a prescription for a fasting blood glucose test. Often the laboratories have walk-in hours that should be convenient for the patient and they will fax the results to the referring dentist. The test is, therefore, reasonably easy to execute at minimal cost. If the test is positive for diabetes mellitus, the patient must be referred to the physician for further evaluation and management.

26. Is it advisable to have a glucometer in the dental office?

This is probably the best approach. The dentist with a glucometer in the office can test the patient immediately for a random blood glucose level. The dentist can also instruct the patient not to eat or drink after midnight before his or her next dental visit and obtain a fasting blood glucose measurement at that visit. If the fasting blood glucose level is above 120, the patient should be referred to the physician for further management. If the results are within normal limits (fasting glucose 80–110), the dentist can reassure the patient. The test is both inexpensive and convenient

27. What is a glucometer?

A glucometer is a small (approximately 4" × 3") machine used to screen blood glucose levels. It is designed for use of patients at home and is easy to operate. Commercially available glucometers cost less than $100 and can be obtained in any pharmacy.

28. What is the best overall strategy in approaching a patient suspected having diabetes mellitus on clinical grounds?
- Advise the patient of your concern about a possible diagnosis of diabetes mellitus.
- Reassure the patient that a screening procedure can be done in the dental office without requiring a separate visit with the patient's physician.
- Reassure the patient that you do not need to draw blood from the veins but can get the sample from a simple finger stick.
- A positive result demands referral to the physician. A negative result reassures the patient of the absence of the disease and directs the dentist to consider the diagnosis of rapidly progressive periodontitis with its therapeutic implications.

29. What are the complications of diabetes mellitus?
In addition to the metabolic complications of diabetes, patients may develop vascular, cardiovascular, renal, and neurologic complications.
- Large vessel complications of diabetes mellitus include peripheral vascular disease, coronary artery disease, and cerebrovascular disease.
- Small vessel complications lead to diabetic retinopathy and diabetic kidney disease.
- Neurologic complications include peripheral neuropathy with prominent sensory losses.
- Autonomic insufficiency is seen in patients with severe disease and can result in postural hypotension, sexual impotence, and abnormality in gastrointestinal motility.
- Diabetics are more prone to infections in general and periodontitis specifically because of compromised host responses.

30. Does control of diabetes affect the risk for periodontitis?
The glucose hypothesis states that sustained hyperglycemia is correlated with the occurrence of all diabetic complications, including periodontitis. Managan and associates noted that patients with "uncontrolled" diabetes mellitus have a 2- to 4-fold risk of periodontitis when compared with patients with "controlled" diabetes mellitus.

31. How is adequacy of diabetic control assessed?
The patient should have a reasonable feel about the adequacy of diabetic control by readings obtained on home monitoring using a glucometer. Hemoglobin A_{1C} (glycosylated hemoglobin) is also an important test that can show the degree of blood glucose control over a 2-month period. This blood test is usually done in the physician's office.

32. How does a diabetic patient use a glucometer?
Diabetics are taught to do home monitoring of blood glucose with a glucometer. The glucometer is a small hand held machine measuring approximately $4" \times 3"$. The machine and all its supplies are available in any pharmacy at minimal cost. The glucometer is intended for home monitoring and is reasonably easy to learn to operate. The patient obtains a drop of blood by finger stick with a disposable small lancet. The drop of blood is placed on a small disposable strip that is inserted into the glucometer. Within a few seconds, the glucometer display shows the blood glucose measurement. Not infrequently, the patient performs multiple measurements during the course of the day to guide titration of his or her insulin therapy.

33. What is Hemoglobin A_{1C}?
Hemoglobin A_{1C} (HbA_{1C}) is an important gauge of adequacy of control. It is a blood test done in the physician's office. HbA_{1C} reflects the proportion of the hemoglobin that is glycosylated. Normal patients usually have about 5% of their hemoglobin glycosylated. The goal is to attain a HbA_{1C} level less than 7% (usually obtained with preprandial blood glucose levels of 70–120 mg/dl).

Glycosylated hemoglobin indicates mean glucose levels over approximately a 60-day period. Physicians periodically repeat the test to assess long-term control of the diabetic and to make long-term therapeutic decisions. The following table demonstrates the correlations between

HbA_{1C} results and level of control. An HbA_{1C} greater than 9% indicates that the patient has a mean glucose level higher than 200 mg/dl. An HbA_{1C} less than 7% is equivalent to a mean glucose level of less than 140 mg/dl.

Hemoglobin A1C Level as an Indicator of Adequacy of Control of Diabetes Mellitus

HbA_{1C}	LEVEL OF CONTROL
<7%	Good
7–9%	Fair
>9%	Poor

34. Why is HbA_{1C} important to the dentist?

All diabetics are monitored by serial HbA_{1C} by their physicians. Since the risk of progressive periodontitis is closely correlated with sustained hypoglycemia, HbA_{1C} is a simple assessment of that risk. A dentist anticipating a treatment plan may downgrade the prognosis of specific teeth based on HbA_{1C} values that suggest poor diabetic control (HbA_{1C} of greater than 9%).

35. How might HbA_{1C} levels affect dental plans?

When treated, a patient with a certain level of periodontal disease might be a candidate for a fixed prosthesis or a complex perioprosthetic fixed treatment plan. This same patient with poorly controlled diabetes mellitus and therefore a downgraded abutment prognosis may now be a candidate for a less sophisticated prosthetic treatment plan that does not strictly rely on specific abutments (i.e., a simple removable prosthesis).

36. How is diabetes mellitus diagnosed?

The diagnosis of diabetes mellitus may occasionally be made during a routine test on an asymptomatic patient by the demonstration of an elevated blood glucose levels (hyperglycemia) or high amounts of glucose in the urine (glycosuria).

Symptomatic patients with polyphagia, polydipsia, polyuria, and weight loss may have the diagnosis of diabetes mellitus confirmed by blood tests.

Patients with fasting plasma glucose levels higher than 120 mg/dl or a random plasma glucose of higher than 200 mg/dl have diabetes mellitus.

37. How is type 1 diabetes mellitus treated?

Patients with type 1 diabetes mellitus are treated with insulin.

38. How is type 2 diabetes mellitus treated?

Patients with type 2 diabetes mellitus should be treated with oral hypoglycemic agents. With time, oral hypoglycemic agents may not be sufficient and insulin may have to be added.

39. What are the different preparations of insulin commonly used?

Although there are many different preparations of insulin, the most commonly used insulin are NPH Insulin and regular insulin. NPH is an intermediate-acting insulin, whereas regular insulin is a short-acting insulin. Not infrequently, synthetic human insulin is the preparation of choice. In most patients, a mixture of NPH and regular insulin preparations is used to optimize control.

Commonly Used Insulin Preparations

	EFFECT BEGINS (HR)	MAXIMAL ACTION (HR)	DURATION (HR)
Short–Acting Regular	½	4–6	6–8
Intermediate–Acting NPH	3	8–12	18–24

40. What are the commonly prescribed oral hypoglycemics?

Five different classes of oral antidiabetic agents are available (see table).

- Sulfonylureas act to enhance insulin secretion. Chronic administration of sulfonylureas also decreases insulin resistance.
- Metformin acts on intestinal absorption of glucose, decreases insulin resistance, and also enhances anaerobic glycolysis.
- Glitazones act primarily to decrease insulin resistance.
- Glucosidase inhibitors acts to decreases intestinal absorption of glucose.
- Repaglinide act to stimulate pancreatic secretion of insulin.

The United Kingdom Prospective Diabetes Study indicated that many patients with diabetes mellitus eventually require a combination of oral antidiabetic agents. If the patient's target is not reached within 2 to 3 months, the next level of antidiabetic agent should be introduced.

Commonly Prescribed Oral Hypoglycemic Agents

Sulfonylureas: First Generation:	Metformin (Glucophage)
• Acetohexamide (Dymelor)	
• Chlorpropamide (Diabinese)	Glitazones
• Tolazamide (Tolinase)	• Rosaglitazone (Avandia)
• Tolbutamide (Orinase)	• Pioglitazone (Actos)
Sulfonylureas: Second Generation:	Glucosidase inhibitors
• Glimepiride (Amaryl)	• Acarbose (Precose)
• Glipizide (Glucotrol)	
• Glyburide (DiaBeta; Micronase)	Repaglinide (Prandin)

41. Which are the commonly prescribed sulfonylureas?

First-generation sulfonylureas: these have been available in the United States for the treatment of type 2 diabetes mellitus for over 20 years. They are

- Acetohexamide (Dymelor)
- Chlorpropamide (Diabinese)
- Tolazamide (Tolinase)
- Tolbutamide (Orinase)

Second-generation sulfonylureas: these have been available since 1984 and tend to produce fewer side effects and interact less frequently with other drugs.

- Glimepiride (Amaryl)
- Glipizide (Glucotrol)
- Glyburide (DiaBeta; Micronase)

42. What is the role of metformin?

The United Kingdom Prospective Diabetes Study suggests that metformin (Glucophage) should be the first oral antidiabetic agent used. The actions of metformin include delayed glucose absorption, inhibition of gluconeogenesis, and slight increased peripheral glucose uptake. It is the drug of choice for patients who are overweight. Lactic acidosis is a rare but serious side effect and is most likely to occur in those with renal or hepatic disease.

43. Which are the commonly prescribed glitazones?

Glitazones improve insulin action by reducing insulin resistance.

- Rosaglitazone (Avandia)
- Pioglitazone (Actos)

44. Which are the commonly prescribed glucosidase inhibitors?

Acarbose (Precose) lowers postprandial blood glucose levels.

45. What is repaglinide?

Repaglinide (Prandin) is a rapid and short-acting agent that stimulates pancreatic insulin release. Repaglinide has to be taken about 30 minutes before each meal.

46. What is the strategy for the use of oral antidiabetic agents?

The United Kingdom Prospective Diabetes Study indicated that many patients with diabetes mellitus eventually require a combination of oral antidiabetic agents. A single oral antidiabetic agent should be used and gradually increased to the maximal dose. If the patient's target is not reached within 2 to 3 months, the next level of antidiabetic agent should be introduced. Although the majority of patients with type 2 diabetes mellitus can be controlled with a combination of oral antidiabetic agents, insulin may be necessary in the later phases of the disease.

47. How do patients' drug regimens affect the dentist?

Major dental procedures, most often surgical but some advanced prosthetic procedures, may compromise the ability of the patient to maintain a normal oral caloric intake. If the dentist is sure that there will be a significant drop in oral intake, a consultation with the physician is indicated. The dental management issue is to consider a short-term discontinuation of the medication until normal caloric intake resumes.

48. How should the dentist manage insulin therapy in the out-patient setting?

1. A mid-morning dental appointment should be scheduled.
2. A normal breakfast should be consumed by the patient.
3. Insulin doses should be tailored to the procedures proposed.
   a. Patients who are expected to resume normal oral intake immediately after the procedure can take their normal dose of insulin.
   b. Patients who are expected to have some delay in the resumption of oral intake following the procedure should take one half their normal morning insulin dose. This must be confirmed by consultation with the physician.
4. Resume normal diet following the procedure as soon as possible.

49. How would you manage insulin therapy in the in-patient setting?

1. Schedule early morning surgery.
2. No oral intake after midnight.
3. A fasting blood glucose level should be obtained on the morning of the surgery.
4. Begin intravenous infusion of D_5W at 100 ml/hr on the morning of the surgery.
5. Administer half the normal dose of insulin.
6. Maintain the intravenous fluid infusion until oral intake is resumed.
7. Use a sliding scale of insulin administration based on blood glucose determinations in order to optimize blood glucose control.
8. Blood glucose determinations should be made at 3 PM and at 11 PM.
9. Resume oral intake as soon as possible.
10. The patient should be on a normal insulin regimen 1 to 2 days after surgery and can usually be discharged and followed as an outpatient.

50. What is a "sliding scale" for supplemental insulin therapy for the in-hospital patient?

The physician prescribes supplemental insulin based on specific blood glucose levels typically performed at 3 PM and 11 PM after an early morning surgery. An example would be

BLOOD GLUCOSE	INSULIN DOSE
>250 mg/dl	8 U Regular
200–250 mg/dl	6 U Regular
<200 mg/dl	No additional insulin

51. What is hypoglycemia?

Hypoglycemia is the most serious complication of therapy. It usually occurs as a result of excessive insulin or hypoglycemic agents. Inadequate oral intake may aggravate the situation. The clinical signs and symptoms of hypoglycemia include weakness, nervousness, tremulousness, palpitations, and excessive sweating. The patient's sensorium may progress from confusion and agitation to seizures and coma.

52. How can the dentist minimize the risk of hypoglycemia?

All patients with diabetes mellitus should have their food intake reviewed for the day of the appointment. Before a dental procedure, a patient who has not had food intake within 2 hours should have some orange juice or a soft drink prior to the appointment. The dental management issue is that the dentist would prefer to have the glucose level higher during the procedure rather than lower; symptoms are more likely to occur at the lower level.

53. What are the early symptoms of hypoglycemia?

The weakness, nervousness, tremulousness, palpitations, and excessive sweating appear very much like the effect of inadvertent uptake of vasoconstrictor from local anesthetic injections. If the dentist has given the patient oral glucose before the appointment, the symptoms are much less likely to be the result of hypoglycemia.

54. What is the importance of hypoglycemia to the dentist?

Because of the serious potential sequelae of hypoglycemia, (seizure and coma), the condition should be recognized and promptly treated. As noted, the treatment of hypoglycemia includes the administration of sugar in the form of candy or glucose solutions such as orange juice. However, lethargic patients who are unable to take oral fluids must be treated with the intravenous administration of concentrated glucose solutions such as 50% dextrose in water ($D_{50}W$); these solutions must be part of the dental emergency kit. Many dentists are uncomfortable administering intravenous medication. This points out the crucial role of prevention (e.g., diet history and preappointment oral glucose administration). Usually, patients respond within 1–3 minutes of the administration of glucose.

55. Are there certain patients at greater risk of hypoglycemia than others?

Patients who have had a recent history of hypoglycemic events are at greater risk. The dentist should ask the patient if he or she has had to take dietary sugar between meals based on symptoms and if they regularly carry sugar products for these events?

Another problem is that many patients mistakenly believe that they should have an empty stomach for dental visits. Patients with diabetes mellitus should specifically receive the opposite advice. They should be sure to have had oral intake just before outpatient appointments.

56. What are the implications of diabetes mellitus for the dental practice?

About 5% of dental patients have diabetes. These patients require careful dental evaluation.
- The dentist should know the type of diabetes the patient has.
- The dentist should know the form of treatment the patient is on.
- The dentist should modify the treatment plan to accommodate the needs of the diabetic patient.
- The dentist should be able to recognize the signs and symptoms of hypoglycemia.
- The dentist should be able to treat hypoglycemia.
- The dentist should be mindful of infectious complications in the diabetic patient.

57. What is the dental evaluation of patients with diabetes mellitus?

The dental evaluation of a patient known to have diabetes should include the determination of the form of diabetes (type 1 versus type 2), the therapy being employed, the adequacy of diabetic control, (HbA_{1C}), and the presence of neurologic, vascular, renal, or infectious complications.

58. Why is the information about the type of diabetes important to the dentist?

Type 1 patients are on insulin and are usually young patients with more labile diabetes. They tend to have a higher predisposition for ketoacidosis, and oral infections can significantly affect the adequacy of diabetic control in these patients.

Type 2 patients tend to be on oral hypoglycemic agents. Although they are less prone to ketosis, they tend to have more cardiovascular complications and may need their dental care plan altered because of their comorbid conditions.

59. Which is a greater risk to the dentist, ketoacidosis or hypoglycemia?

Hypoglycemia is by far the most common potential emergency in the dental office. Relative excess insulin can be acute with changes in diet.

Ketoacidosis, the result of too little insulin, develops over time and is not precipitated by the stress of the dental visit. The addition of orange juice or a soft drink in the office just before the appointment will not induce ketoacidosis. It will only prevent a hypoglycemic event.

60. What are the general guidelines for the dental management of patients with diabetes mellitus?

- The primary goal should be to avoid untoward metabolic imbalances during the period of dental therapy.
- Patients should be carefully instructed about their diet and their medications during the course of therapy so as to minimize problems related especially to hypoglycemia.
- The dentist should attempt to minimize stress.
- The dentist should aggressively address the risk of infection.

61. What should the dentist instruct patients about their diet on the day of the dental procedure?

- A diabetic patient should be scheduled for a mid-morning appointment.
- The patient should be instructed to have a normal breakfast. This minimizes the likelihood of the occurrence of hypoglycemia during the dental procedure.
- Attention should be paid to the length of the dental sessions. If a session runs into normal mealtime, arrangements should be made to allow interruptions for appropriate snacks (e.g., orange juice).
- Some patients may have limited ability to chew after certain dental procedures. These patients should be instructed to have soft foods or liquids (e.g., powdered instant breakfast drinks, milk shakes, soups, or scrambled eggs) to maintain their blood glucose at a reasonable level.

62. What are the appropriate instructions to patients on oral hypoglycemic agents?

Patients generally should be instructed to take their normal dose of oral hypoglycemic agents before all outpatient dental procedures. For some advanced surgical procedures, when postoperative oral intake will definitely be compromised, the dentist may want to decrease oral medications the day of the procedure in order to avoid hypoglycemia later in the day. This must be done in consultation with the physician. Most often, the longer procedure should be divided into shorter ones to ensure adequate postoperative oral intake.

63. What are the appropriate instructions to the patients on insulin?

- Modification of insulin therapy must be considered for patients with diabetes who have their meal timing altered or are about to undergo stressful dental procedures.
- When necessary, the patient may be instructed to take half the normal morning insulin amount and to have a normal breakfast.
- The patient can often be given the other half of the insulin dose when a normal diet is resumed after the dental procedure.
- These modifications should ensure that hypoglycemia does not occur.
- Instructions must be given in consultation with the physician.

64. How should the dentist minimize stress for the diabetic patient?
- Whenever feasible, lengthy procedures should be spread out over several shorter appointments.
- Adjunctive sedation techniques should be considered when appropriate.

65. How should the dentist minimize the risk of infection?
Diabetic patients are at increased risk of developing dental and other infections, a risk that can be minimized by preventive and therapeutic measures.
- The patient with diabetes should have aggressive preventive dental services, including frequent recall examinations, oral hygiene instructions, prophylaxis, and treatment of periodontal disease.
- The patient should also be considered for antibiotic prophylaxis following surgical procedures, endodontic therapy, and subgingival scaling in the presence of suppurative periodontitis.
- Antibiotics are important in the treatment of all acute infections.

66. What are the oral findings in the diabetic patient?
- Periodontal disease is the most consistent finding in patients with poorly controlled diabetes mellitus. Approximately 75% of these patients have periodontal disease, with increased alveolar bone resorption and inflammatory gingival changes.
- Diabetics whose disease is under good control also have a higher incidence and greater severity of periodontal disease.
- Diabetics may demonstrate xerostomia and recurrent abscesses.
- Enamel hypoplasia and hypocalcification can result in an increased frequency of caries.
- The oral flora is often altered by colonization with *Candida albicans*, hemolytic streptococci, and staphylococci.
- Abnormal eruption patterns may be noted in children with diabetes. Advanced eruption may be seen before the age of 10, whereas delayed eruption occurs after the age of 10.

11. ADRENAL DISORDERS

Robert C. Fazio, D.M.D., and Leslie S.T. Fang, M.D., Ph.D.

1. What are the adrenal glands?

Adrenal glands are small, multifunctional endocrine organs located above the kidneys. Each gland is divided into an inner zone called the adrenal medulla and an outer zone called the adrenal cortex.

2. What are the hormonal functions of the adrenal glands?

The adrenal medulla produces the catecholamines epinephrine and norepinephrine, which play an integral role in the maintenance of blood pressure, the control of myocardial contractility and excitability, and the regulation of body metabolism. '

The adrenal cortex produces three different hormones:
- Glucocorticoids: help regulate carbohydrate, protein and fat metabolism and are important in the suppression of inflammation
- Mineralocorticoids: help maintain sodium and potassium balance
- Sex hormones: play a secondary role in sexual maturation

3. What disorders are associated with hyperfunction of the adrenal medulla?

Tumors called pheochromocytomas, affecting the adrenal medulla, can lead to hypersecretion of epinephrine and norepinephrine. Patients with this tumor experience episodic hypertension, headaches, flushing, sweating, and palpitations.

4. How can pheochromocytomas be diagnosed?

Pheochromocytomas are diagnosed by determination of serum concentrations of epinephrine and norepinephrine or by the detection of elevated levels of metabolites of catecholamines such as vanillylmandelic acid (VMA) or metanephrines in the urine

5. What disorders are associated with hyperfunction of the adrenal cortex?

The adrenal cortex secretes three classes of hormones. Diseases of the hypothalamus, pituitary gland, or adrenal cortex can all result in hypersecretion of these hormones.

Glucocorticoids: Patients with glucocorticoid hypersecretion have Cushing's syndrome, which results in characteristic changes in body hiatus including moon facies, truncal obesity, muscular wasting, and hirsutism. They are often hypertensive because of fluid retention. Long-term glucocorticoid excess can result in decreased collagen production, a tendency to bruise easily, poor wound healing, and osteoporosis. Patients with Cushing's syndrome are often at increased risk for infection. Laboratory studies may reveal increased blood glucose levels because of interference with carbohydrate metabolism, and examination of the peripheral blood smear may demonstrate slight decreases in eosinophil and lymphocyte counts. The diagnosis is made on the basis of elevated plasma cortisol or urinary 17-hydroxycorticosteroids and 17-ketosteroids. Patients suspected of having adrenal tumors can have the diagnosis confirmed by imaging studies such as adrenal ultrasound, computed tomographic (CT) scan or magnetic resonance imaging (MRI). Occasionally, the adrenal hyperfunction is a result of a tumor in the pituitary of the hypothalamus. These patients have Cushing's disease and would have elevated serum adrenocorticotrophic hormone levels. The diagnosis can be confirmed by tomography of the sella, cranial CT, or cranial MRI.

Mineralocorticoids: Hypersecretion of mineralocorticoids can be the result of a tumor or bilateral hyperplasia of the adrenals. Patients with hypersecretion of mineralocorticoids have low serum potassium levels, fluid retention, mild hypertension, and possibly symptoms of muscle weakness and transient paresthesia. Diagnosis can be confirmed by the finding of an elevated serum aldosterone level. Radiographic evaluation may include the use of ultrasonography, CT scan, MRI, or arteriography.

Sex hormones: Hypersecretion of sex hormones can result from tumors of the adrenals. Excessive sex hormone production can produce masculinization in females and in prepubertal boys. Diagnosis can be confirmed by an elevated serum testosterone level. Radiographic evaluation may include the use of ultrasonography, CT scan, MRI or arteriography.

6. How are patients with hyperfunction of the adrenal cortex managed medically?

Adrenal adenoma and adrenal carcinoma are usually treated by surgical excision. Bilateral adrenal hyperplasia may require bilateral adrenalectomy. Patients with an adenoma causing hyperaldosteronism are usually treated surgically; patients with bilateral hyperplasia and aldosterone hypersecretion may sometimes be managed medically. Patients with adrenogenital syndrome may be managed either medically or surgically. Surgical approach requires bilateral adrenalectomy.

7. What are disorders of hypofunction of the adrenal glands?

Chronic loss of adrenal function is called Addison's disease. The most common cause is the autoimmune destruction of the adrenal gland, which accounts for over half of all cases of adrenal hypofunction. Tubecular, fungal, and (rarely) viral diseases can also destroy the adrenal glands and result in chronic adrenal insufficiency. Acute adrenal insufficiency can occur as a result of bilateral adrenalectomy or overwhelming sepsis causing bilateral adrenal hemorrhage (Waterhouse-Friderichsen syndrome). Occasionally, hyposecretion is a result of pituitary insufficiency.

8. What are the symptoms of adrenal insufficiency and why is adrenal insufficiency important to the dentist?

Patients with decreased adrenal gland hormone production experience weakness, weight loss, orthostatic hypotension, nausea, and vomiting. Patients with severe adrenal insufficiency cannot increase steroid production in response to stress and in extreme situations may have cardiovascular collapse. It is important that an adrenally insufficient patient have adequate steroid replacement, since the stress of surgery can precipitate adrenal crisis.

9. What are the signs of adrenal insufficiency?

Patients with adrenal insufficiency are hyperpigmented. This is most noticeable on the buccal and labial mucosae, although other areas such as the gingival may be involved. The hyperpigmentation is a result of hypersecretion of ACTH, which can stimulate melanocytes to produce pigment.

10. How is adrenal insufficiency diagnosed?

Adrenal insufficiency can be suspected on routine blood testing. Patients with adrenal insufficiency often have hyperkalemia as a result of inadequate mineralocorticoid secretion. They may also be hypoglycemic as a result of inadequate corticosteroid secretion. The diagnosis can be confirmed on the basis of serum cortisol determination, which would be inappropriately low. An ACTH stimulation test can also be performed to examine the response of the adrenal gland to an exogenously administered dose of ACTH. Normal patients have a doubling of the serum cortisol level after a dose of ACTH. An inadequate response suggests adrenal gland hypofunction.

11. How are patients with adrenal insufficiency managed?

Patients with Addison's disease are managed by steroid supplements. While there are many preparations available, prednisone is the most common preparation used to replace glucocorticoid insufficiency. Steroid dosages ought to be as low as possible to avoid side effects. The usual daily maintenance dose of prednisone is 10 to 15 mg. Patients with mineralocorticoid deficiency may require supplementation with fluorocortisone. Remember that patients on chronic replacement therapy for adrenal insufficiency cannot increase endogenous steroid production in times of stress and therefore become relatively adrenally insufficiency unless steroid supplements are administered.

12. MANAGING THE PATIENT ON STEROID THERAPY

Robert C. Fazio, D.M.D., and Leslie S.T. Fang, M.D., Ph.D.

1. Which patients are likely to be on steroids?

The most common indication for steroid use is as an anti-inflammatory drug. Patients with a variety of arthritic conditions, ranging from rheumatoid arthritis to gout, may benefit from short courses of steroids. Patients with collagen vascular diseases such as lupus erythematosus are often on steroids. Patients with severe chronic obstructive pulmonary disease and asthma may also be on intermittent courses of steroids. Other conditions, such as nephrotic syndrome, inflammatory bowel disease, hemolytic anemia, thrombocytopenia, and a variety of dermatologic conditions, may necessitate steroid use. Patients on chemotherapy for some malignancies may also take steroids as part of the chemotherapeutic regimen.

Some patients require long term steroid use. Patients with organ transplants such as kidney, liver, lung and heart transplants require steroids as part of the immunosuppressive regimen. Patients with adrenal insufficiency (Addison's disease) also need long-term steroid therapy.

2. What are the commonly prescribed steroid preparations?

Prednisone is the most commonly prescribed steroid preparation. The usual daily adrenal output of steroids is about the equivalent of 10–20 mg of prednisone, which is reasonable for maintenance therapy but inadequate during periods of stress. In patients with normal adrenal reserves, the maximal output of cortisol in response to severe stress is estimated to be equivalent to about 60 mg of prednisone.

Some of the other steroid preparations available follow.

Steroid Preparations and Potency

DURATION OF ACTION	GLUCOCORTICOID POTENCY
Short-Acting	
Cortisol (hydrocortisone)	1
Cortisone	0.8
Prednisone	4
Prednisolone	4
Methylprednisolone	5
Intermediate-Acting	
Triamcinolone	5
Long-Acting	
Betamethasone	25
Dexamethasone	30

3. How is a steroid generally prescribed?

Because of the side effects of steroids over an extended period of time, the clinician tries to minimize the continuous use of steroids. In patients with adrenal insufficiency, the absence of steroid production mandates continuous administration of steroids. In patients with organ transplants, steroids are necessary to prevent rejection. In most other instances, steroids are generally prescribed for as short a period of time as possible in order to minimize their adverse effects. Whenever feasible, alternate-day steroid therapy is prescribed. In general, steroids should be prescribed at the lowest effective dose for the shortest possible duration.

4. What are the side effects of steroids?

Although steroids are potent anti-inflammatory and immunosuppressive drugs, they have myriad side effects, making their long-term use undesirable.

Change in body habitus with development of moon facies, buffalo hump, and truncal obesity
Increased susceptibility to infections
Adrenal suppression with suppression of the hypothalamic-pituitary-adrenal axis. Patients receiving exogenous steroids stop producing endogenous steroids from the adrenal gland, a process normally controlled by the hypothalamus and the pituitary. This suppression renders the adrenal gland sluggish in the production of steroids under stress and precipitates adrenal insufficiency with resultant cardiovascular instability.

Change in mood: euphoria, psychosis, or depression can develop on steroid therapy
Change in glucose tolerance: this can worsen pre-existing diabetic tendencies
Fluid retention
Hypertension
Gastrointestinal irritation with gastritis, peptic ulceration, and gastrointestinal bleeding
Tendency to bruise easily and poor wound healing
Proximal muscle weakness
Weight gain
Osteoporosis with long-term steroid use
Premature development of cataracts
Development of osteoporosis and pathologic fractures

5. What are the dental concerns about patients on steroid therapy?

It is important to remember that patients on chronic replacement therapy for adrenal insufficiency cannot increase endogenous steroid production in times of stress and therefore become adrenally insufficient unless steroid supplements are administered. For the dentist, it is important to be sure that an adrenally insufficient patient has adequate steroid replacement, since the stress of surgery can precipitate adrenal crisis.

6. What are the general guidelines for the dental management of patients on steroid therapy?

• Steroid supplement in patients who can develop adrenal insufficiency
• Early morning appointments
• Shorter appointments
• Minimize stress
• Use sedation techniques when appropriate
• Modify dental treatment plans when appropriate
• The major goal in these patients is to avoid precipitation of adrenal insufficiency

7. What are the clinical consequences of adrenal insufficiency?

The adrenal glands are responsible for increased production of steroids at times of stress. This ability to produce steroids under physiologic stress is called the stress response. The stress response permits increased cardiovascular tone at times of stress.

Patients with mild adrenal insufficiency experience weakness, weight loss, orthostatic hypotension, nausea, and vomiting.

Patients with severe adrenal insufficiency cannot increase steroid production in response to stress and in extreme situations they may experience cardiovascular collapse.

8. Which patients are likely to become adrenally insufficient?

Although adrenal suppression can result from as little as 20–30 mg of prednisone daily for 7 to 10 days and can persist for 9 to 12 months after the termination of a course of therapy, the stress response from the adrenal glands returns after approximately 11–14 days. For the dentist, the major goal is to avoid causing stress-related adverse events. Therapy should be tailored to supplement patients who cannot adequately mount a steroid response during stress.

Patients who are on alternate day steroid therapy usually do not have significant adrenal insufficiency, since the adrenal glands are still forced to produce some steroids on the "off-steroid day."

Therefore, patients with adrenal insufficiency, patients on daily steroid therapy, and patients who have recently finished a course of steroids should receive steroid supplement for dental procedures.

9. How can adrenal insufficiency be documented?

Adrenal insufficiency can be documented by the use of the cortrisyn stimulation test. The administration of 240 µg of cortrisyn (adrenocorticotropic hormone) is the standard means of testing for suppression. Adrenocorticotropic hormone is the hormone normally produced by the pituitary gland to stimulate steroid production from the adrenal glands. If the serum cortisol level at 60 minutes is above 18 µg/dl or an increase from baseline of at least 10 µg/dl is noted, adrenal responsiveness is sufficient to sustain the patient through a stress equivalent to general anesthesia.

10. How should the dentist address the issue of adrenal insufficiency?

A formal cortrisyn stimulation test is impractical, and the concerns about adrenal insufficiency should be raised on the basis of clinical history. In the majority of cases, the dentist should ask:

• Is it known that the patient's adrenal glands do not function adequately?
• Is the patient on chronic steroid therapy at doses of prednisone higher than 15 mg/day?
• Has the patient been on steroid therapy at doses of prednisone higher than 15 mg/day within the past 2 weeks?

If the answer to any of the above questions is yes, the dentist should assume that the patient will need stress-dose steroids.

11. Which patients should be suspected of having adrenal insufficiency and should be given supplemental steroids for dental interventions?

• Patients with known adrenal insufficiency and inadequate endogenous steroid production: these patients are often maintained on 10 mg of prednisone/day and are incapable of producing more steroid response during stress.
• Patients who are on chronic daily steroid therapy if the daily dose is in excess of 15 mg of prednisone per day
• Patients who have been on daily steroid therapy in excess of 15 mg of prednisone per day within the past 2 weeks

12. What patients are not adrenally suppressed and do not need supplemental steroids for dental interventions?

• Patients on alternate-day steroids
• Patients on low doses of steroid therapy for medical problems other than adrenal insufficiency (less than 15 mg of prednisone per day)
• Patients on inhaled steroids
• Patients with a remote history of steroid use: patients who have been off steroids for longer than 2 weeks. Although adrenal suppression can result from as little as 20–30 mg of prednisone daily for 7–10 days and can persist for 9–12 months after the termination of a course of therapy, the stress response from the adrenal glands returns after approximately 11–14 days.

13. How should supplemental steroids be given?

Supplemental steroids should be given on the morning of the proposed dental intervention. The amount prescribed should be titrated according to the anticipated level of stress of the procedure. In general, the patient should receive 60 mg of prednisone or the equivalent on the morning of the procedure if he or she is anticipated to be under a considerable amount of physiologic stress (e.g., being under general anesthesia). For less stressful procedures, 30–40 mg of prednisone should suffice.

14. Should patients on steroid replacement therapy be given a short course of prophylactic antibiotics?

There are no definitive data regarding prophylactic antibiotics for patients on chronic steroid therapy. However, these patients are at increased risk for developing infection. It is therefore reasonable to prescribe a short course of prophylactic antibiotics if a patient is to undergo interventions that may incur significant soft-tissue or bone trauma. The dentist may consider the use of amoxicillin, 875 mg po bid, for 2–5 days following dental intervention.

15. What are the possible oral manifestations seen in patients on steroid therapy?

Of all the oral manifestations caused by steroids, the most common is oral candidiasis, particularly in patients using inhaled steroids. Oral candidiasis can be treated with antifungal troches, lozenges, or oral solutions (nystatin suspension, 5 ml swish and swallow tid) or oral medication (fluconazole [Diflucan] 200 mg/day for 1 day, then 100 mg daily for 14 days).

16. What are the uses of steroids in the dental setting?

A variety of oral conditions such as erosive lichen planus, aphthous ulcers, benign mucosal pemphigoid, and pemphigus respond to topical or systemic steroids. In some instances, steroids are also used to reduce swelling and inflammation after major oral surgical procedures.

17. How are steroids administered in the dental setting?

Depending on the clinical situation, the dentist may use topical formulations, intralesional and intra-articular injections, or systemic administration.

18. How are topical steroids prescribed in the dental setting?

The topical steroid is the most commonly used formulation by the dentist. Topical steroid preparations are most frequently used to treat erosive lichen planus, aphthous ulcers, and mucous membrane pemphigoid. If used for less than a month, there are usually few associated detrimental effects. However, some of the very high-potency topical steroids can cause suppression of the hypothalamic-pituitary-adrenal axis and should not be prescribed for longer than 2 weeks. Some of the commonly used topical preparations follow. In general, gels adhere better to the oral mucosa and can be applied directly to the lesions. To increase penetration and time in contact with the lesions, gel preparations can be placed inside the affected area. Ointments should be mixed with Orabase in equal amounts in order to better adhere to the oral mucosa. Creams can also be used in the dental setting.

Commonly Prescribed Topical Steroid Preparations in the Dental Practice

GENERIC NAME	BRAND NAME	PREPARATION	DOSAGE
Low Potency			
Aclometasone	Aclovate	Ointment	bid-qid
Hydrocortisone	Ala-Cort	Ointment	bid-qid
	Cort-Dome		
	Delcort		
	Dermacort		
	Hydrocort		
	Hytone		
	Nutracort		
	Penecort		
	Synacort		
Medium Potency			
Fluocinolone	Fluocinolone	Ointment	tid
	Fluosyn		
	Synalar		

(Cont'd. on next page)

Commonly Prescribed Topical Steroid Preparations in the Dental Practice (Continued)

GENERIC NAME	BRAND NAME	PREPARATION	DOSAGE
Medium Potency *(Cont'd.)*			
Hydrocortisone	Hydrocortisone Westcort	Ointment	
Mometasone	Elocon	Ointment	tid
Triamcinolone	Aristocort Delta-Tritex Flutex Kenalog Kenonel Tricet Triderm	Ointment	tid
High Potency			
Amcinonide	Cyclocort	Ointment	tid
Betamethasone	Alphatrex Betamethasone Betatrex Diprosone Maxivate Teladar Valisone	Gel/cream	tid
Desoximetasone	Topicort	Gel	tid
Halcinonide	Halog	Ointment	tid
Triamcinolone	Aristocort Flutex Kenalog Triamcinolone	Ointment	tid
Very High Potency			
Augmented betamethasone	Diprolene	Ointment	qd-bid
Clobetasol	Clobetasol Cormax Embeline Temovate	Ointment	qd-bidf
Diflorasone	Psorcon	Ointment	qd-bid
Halobetasol	Ultravate	Ointment	QD-BID

19. How are intralesional injections used in the dental setting?

Intralesional injections should be used only intermittently. They are usually used for soft-tissue disease. Triamcinolone hexacetonide is the most frequently used preparation for this purpose.

20. How are intra-articular injections used in the dental setting?

Intra-articular injections of triamcinolone are used to decrease bone pathology. These injections should be given no more frequently than every third week in the appropriate circumstances.

21. How are systemic steroids used in the dental setting?

Systemic steroids are infrequently used in the short term before, during and after oral surgery to reduce post-operative edema. Systemic steroids are sometimes necessary in the treatment of severe lichen planus, aphthous ulcers, oral pemphigoid and pemphigus lesions. Treatment beyond

2 weeks should be coordinated with the patient's physician in view of concerns over the suppression of the hypothalamus-pituitary-adrenal axis.

13. THYROID DISORDER

Robert C. Fazio, D.M.D., and Leslie S.T. Fang, M.D., Ph.D.

1. What is the thyroid gland?

The thyroid gland is an endocrine structure located in the neck superior to the suprasternal notch and inferior to the cricoid cartilage. The major function of the gland is the production of the hormone thyroxine, which is important in the regulation of the metabolic rate of the body and affects carbohydrate, protein and lipid metabolism. In addition, thyroxine potentiates the action of other hormones such as catecholamines and growth hormones.

2. How is thyroid function regulated?

Thyroid hormone secretion is regulated in an intricate fashion. The hypothalamus produces a hormone called thyrotropin-releasing hormone (TRH). This stimulates the production of thyroid-stimulating hormone (TSH) from the anterior pituitary gland. TSH, in turn, stimulates the production of thyroxine from the thyroid gland. Circulating thyroxine can negatively feed back to the pituitary and the hypothalamus to halt the secretion of TSH. This feedback mechanism permits fine control of the secretion of the thyroid hormone.

3. How common are thyroid disorders?

Thyroid disorder, after diabetes mellitus, is the second most common class of endocrine disorders and affects approximately 1% of the dental population.

4. What is hyperthyroidism?

Excessive production of thyroxine results in hyperthyroidism. Patients with hyperthyroidism have heat intolerance, nervousness, muscular weakness, excessive sweating, diarrhea, and increased appetite and weight loss. In the elderly patient, excessive thyroxine can present as atrial fibrillation and congestive heart failure.

5. What are the common causes of hyperthryoidism?

In patients under the age of 40, Graves disease accounts for about 90% of all cases of hyperthyroidism. The disease is an autoimmune disorder and is associated with prominent exophthalmos.

Middle-aged and elderly patients are more likely to have hyperthyroidism as a result of toxic multinodular goiter. Less commonly, a single toxic nodule can produce excessive thyroxine.

Transient hyperthyroidism is seen in patients with subacute or chronic thyroiditis. Hyperthyroidism can also result from ingestion of an excessive amount of thyroid hormone.

6. What are the common treatments for hyperthyroidism?

Patients with hyperthyroidism can be treated symptomatically with beta-blockers. Definitive therapy involves the use of antithyroid drugs such as propylthiouracil or methimazole. Side effects of antithyroid drugs include skin rashes, joint pain, and occasionally a decreased white blood cell count (leukopenia).

Patients can receive radioactive iodine or surgery for treatment.

Patients with hyperthyroidism should be monitored closely because hyperthyroidism from inadequate therapy or hypothyroidism from excessive therapy can both occur.

7. What is hypothyroidism?

Hypothyroidism is the result of insufficient production of thyroid hormone. Initially, the patient complains of fatigue, cold intolerance, weakness and excessive weight gain. Subsequently, the patient may become lethargic. In severe cases (myxedema), there is increasing lethargy, culminating in coma.

8. What are the common causes of hypothyroidism?

The majority of patients with hypothyroidism have diseases of the thyroid gland, with chronic thyroiditis (Hashimoto's) being the most common cause. Previous thyroid or neck radiation, thyroid surgery, and idiopathic thyroid atrophy can also result in hypothyroidism.

Rarely, patients with pituitary diseases can have insufficient TSH production, resulting in secondary hypothyroidism.

9. What is the treatment for hypothyroidism?

Patients with hypothyroidism are generally treated with a thyroid preparation such as L-thyroxine (Levoxyl or Synthroid). This treatment is usually begun with 25 to 50 µg of L-thyroxine and slowly increased to a maximal dose of between 150 and 250 µg. Patients are followed clinically, and serial determinations of thyroid function tests and TSH levels are used to monitor adequacy of replacement therapy.

10. What are the common tumors involving the thyroid gland?

Both benign and malignant tumors can occur in the thyroid gland. These are usually detected at the time of a routine examination by the palpation of a nodule in the thyroid. Benign nodules of the thyroid are called adenomas. Malignant tumors of the thyroid include papillary carcinomas, follicular carcinomas, and medullary carcinomas.

Patients with detectable nodules are usually evaluated with a radioactive thyroid scan and thyroid function tests. A nodule that does not take up radioactive iodine is called a cold nodule and is a nonfunctioning nodule. A functioning thyroid nodule would pick up radioactive iodine and would show up in a scan as a hot nodule. Functioning nodules (hot nodules) are much less likely to be malignant. Cold nodules, on the other hand, may be malignant and should be subject to fine-needle biopsy.

11. What is the treatment of tumors of the thyroid?

Benign tumors are followed serially by examination and imaging studies. Large thyroid nodules (larger than 1 cm) should be biopsied using the fine needle aspiration technique. Malignant tumors should be surgically excised. Following thyroid surgery, patients should have serial determinations of thyroid function to monitor for the development of hypothyroidism.

12. What are the dental implications of hyperthyroidism?

Generally, the dentist sees patients who are under long-term control after they have been treated successfully for hyperthyroidism. These patients can be treated with a normal protocol.

The untreated patient or the patient actively being treated for severe hyperthyroidism is particularly susceptible to catecholamines. Catecholamines used as vasoconstrictors in local anesthetic preparations or gingival retraction cords, when coupled with the stress of a dental procedure, can precipitate thyroid storm.

Thyroid storm is characterized by marked exacerbation of the symptoms of hyperthyroidism. Patients can develop high fevers, major central nervous system alterations with confusion, agitation, and delirium, and vomiting and diarrhea. Most important, there is a high risk of life-threatening arrhythmias and congestive heart failure.

The use of catecholamines in patients with hyperthyroidism can aggravate underlying cardiovascular instability and should be done only in consultation with the physician.

13. What are the dental implications of hypothyroidism?

Generally, the dentist sees patients who are under long term control, after they have been treated successfully for hypothyroidism. These patients are typically on longstanding thyroid hormone replacement regimens and can be treated with a normal protocol.

The rare patient with active hypothyroidism who has pre-existing central nervous system depression is acutely sensitive to drugs with central nervous system depressant effects. The use of narcotic analgesics and sedatives is relatively contraindicated.

14. Are there specific concerns that should be raised about patients on chronic thyroid replacement therapy?

The dentist should verify that there has been no recent changes in medication and proceed with dental care using the normal protocol.

14. PREGNANCY

Robert C. Fazio, D.M.D., and Leslie S.T. Fang, M.D., Ph.D.

1. What are the dental considerations for the pregnant patient?

The dentist must be aware of
- Treatment strategies and limitations
- Limitations on radiographic examination
- The safest trimester for dental therapy
- Limitations on drug therapy prescribed by the dentist
- Potential increased risk for periodontal disease during pregnancy
- Potential increased risk to the fetus in the presence of periodontal disease during pregnancy

2. What is the best general treatment strategy for the pregnant patient?

The issue of dental treatment during pregnancy is not clear-cut. Some obstetricians do not restrict dental care for their pregnant patients. Others place significant restrictions on their patients. In general, our approach to therapy is a conservative one. Major elective work should be postponed until after the pregnancy, as the pregnancy has a clear time frame. The sequelae of dental therapy are not always predictable, and the ramifications of problems could be significant. On the other hand, neglecting active periodontal disease, in particular, may have significant negative impact on the fetus (see farther on). The dentist must strike a delicate balance between emergent, near-emergent, and elective therapy during pregnancy.

3. Can radiographs be used?

As a general rule, ordering radiographs should be avoided during pregnancy. The risks are particularly significant during the first trimester. As always, if radiographs must be taken, lead shielding is mandatory for the patient. With proper shielding, the risk to the fetus may be minimal. However, even the slightest risk to the fetus should not be underestimated.

4. What is the safest trimester in which to perform dental therapy?

The short answer is the second trimester. During the first trimester, organ development is most critical. Although most growth occurs during the second and third trimesters, the fetus is especially susceptible to teratogenic influences and abortion during the first trimester. Approximately 15% of pregnancies terminate before the end of the first trimester. The frequency of spontaneous abortion after that period decreases. In the third trimester, risks of syncope and hypertension are greatest. So, too, are cardiovascular demands. Late in pregnancy the fetus may put pressure on the inferior vena cava when the patient is in the supine position. This can result in an impaired venous return, hypotension, and potential syncope in the dental chair. Hypertension as a precursor to eclampsia is most common in the third trimester. Monitoring the blood pressure of the pregnant patient is important. A 2-fold increase in cardiac output in the third trimester is not uncommon. This sometimes creates "flow murmurs" or a heart murmur of pregnancy. Bacterial endocarditis prophylaxis is generally not recommended.

5. Is there an increased risk for periodontal pathology during pregnancy?

Pregnancy alone does not increase the risk of periodontal pathology. However, pregnancy does increase the vascularity of the gingiva and, therefore, exaggerates the response to local factors by the periodontal soft tissues. Therefore, the patient who has pre-existing gingivitis or periodontitis during pregnancy will have an exacerbation of that condition as a result of the increased vascularity of the tissue. Sometimes an area of the gingiva, most frequently a papillary region, responds more emphatically and produces a localized area of intense capillary and inflammatory proliferation. These lesions are identical to pyogenic granuloma and are often referred to as pregnancy tumors.

6. Is periodontal disease a risk to the fetus?

In the setting of significant periodontal disease, there is definitely an increased chronic bacteremia. The relationship between bacteremia and spontaneous abortion is unclear, as is the association of bacteremia with abnormalities in fetal development. However, there is significant evidence that links chronic periodontal infection with preterm, low infant birth weight. These babies are at increased risk.

7. Is it important to treat periodontal disease during pregnancy?

As always, prevention is the most important aspect of periodontal treatment. A pregnant patient with previously healthy gingiva or mild gingivitis should be recommended for a more careful prevention program during pregnancy. Prophylaxis at the beginning of the second and third trimesters is not an unreasonable recommendation.

For patients with significant periodontal disease while they are pregnant, a comprehensive, conservative hygiene phase of treatment should be undertaken. This should include intensive oral hygiene instruction, scaling, root planing, and closed (nonflap) curettage. In view of the association between chronic periodontitis, chronic bacteremia, and preterm low birth weight children, delaying active treatment of periodontitis is ill advised.

On the other hand, the stress of flap surgical therapy, regenerative therapy, or guided tissue regeneration should generally be deferred until after the pregnancy is completed. The key is infection control, the majority of which can be accomplished during conservative therapy. The need for surgical intervention should be driven by the concept of infection control. An acute abscess, therefore, might mandate surgical intervention even during the pregnancy.

8. How are medications prescribed for the pregnant patient?

The dentist must be aware of the pregnancy category risk for each medication he or she considers ordering for the pregnant patient. In general, consultation with the obstetrician/gynecologist is always advisable.

9. What are the pregnancy risk categories?

Generally, a drug is graded category A, category B, category C, category D, or category X, proportional to the potential risk to the fetus. Category D and category X drugs are contraindicated for use by the dentist. Category A drugs are the safest. Unfortunately, no medications commonly used by the dentist fall into category A. Usually, the choice becomes attempting to limit your selection to category B drugs and only judiciously choosing category C drugs in consultation with the physician.

10. How does a drug get into category A, category B, category C, category D, or category X?

Category A medications, the safest drugs, have demonstrated no risk to the fetus in animal model and human studies. Category B drugs had their safety established in animal models without human data, or have shown risk in animal models but safety in human studies. Category C drugs have demonstrated risk in animal models but there are no available human data. A drug is also considered category C if there are no animal or human data to support its safety. Categories D and X drugs have definitive human data demonstrating risk.

11. How should the dentist generally approach prescribing medications for the pregnant patient?

The dentist should theoretically think through the common drugs used in dentistry and his or her preferences and usual alternatives. The dentist should then review those choices based on pregnancy risk categories and be guided by those category designations.

12. Which drugs should the dentist be concerned about?

All medications prescribed by the dentist must be carefully considered. Most commonly, this includes local anesthetics, antibiotics, and analgesics but also includes drugs used topically and systemically for candidiasis, aphthous ulceration, secondary herpes infection, and drugs used to sedate the patient or allay anxiety.

13. What are the pregnancy risk categories for common local anesthetics?

Lidocaine (Octocaine, Xylocaine)	Category B
Prilocaine (Citanest)	Category B
Mepivacaine (Carbocaine, Polocaine)	Category C
Bupivacaine (Marcaine)	Category C
Articaine (Septocaine, Ultracaine)	Category C

The dentist, therefore, should generally limit himself to the use of lidocaine and prilocaine. If mepivacaine, articaine, or bupivacaine is preferred, a consultation with the obstetrician/gynecologist is appropriate. Generally, the dentist should be comfortable prescribing category B drugs but insist on consultation for category C drugs.

14. Can the dentist use vasoconstrictors?

Lidocaine with 1:100,000 epinephrine is a category B local anesthetic. The judicious use of this drug is not contraindicated. Similarly, prilocaine with epinephrine is a category B anesthetic.

Generally, the dentist should limit the use of epinephrine to two Carpules of 1;100,000 solution (four Carpules of 1:200,000 solution).

Solutions of mepivacaine with levonordefrin 1:20,000, and articaine with epinephrine 1:100,000, are category C risk by virtue of the local anesthetic rating and should be avoided when possible or cleared for use by the patient's obstetrician/gynecologist.

15. How should the dentist prescribe antibiotics?

Generally, all penicillins are category B antibiotics, and in the setting of an acute infection are warranted as first-choice drugs. Amoxicillin can be prescribed for the localized infection and augmentin for the spreading infection.

Alternatives for the penicillin-allergic patient with localized infection might include delayed released capsule erythromycin (ERYC) or other simple erythromycins such as enteric-coated erythromycin (E-Mycin) or erythromycin ethylsuccinate (EES). All are category B risk medications. For the spreading infection, for which a broader spectrum antibiotic is desired, azithromycin (Zithromax) can be prescribed as a category B risk drug. It should be noted that clarithromycin (Biaxin) is a category C risk drug, even though its antibiotic spectrum is similar to that of azithromycin. Generally, therefore, clarithromycin is not recommended when a category B alternative drug is available. Other category B drugs include clindamycin (Cleocin) and the commonly prescribed cephalosporins: cephalexin (Keflex) and cefadroxil (Duricef). Also in this category are the extended spectrum cephalosporins—cefuroxime (Ceftin) and loracarbef (Lorabid). Metronidazole (Flagyl) is also a category B risk antibiotic. In addition to clarithromycin, other category C risk drugs mandating a physician consultation include the fluoroquinolones (Cipro or Floxin).

16. Which commonly prescribed antibiotics are contraindicated for the pregnant patient?

All tetracyclines, including tetracycline hydrochloride, doxycyline (Vibramycin) or minocycline (Minocin), are category D risk drugs and are contraindicated for the pregnant patient.

17. Is there a strategy for prescribing analgesics?

For mild pain, acetaminophen (Tylenol) is a category B risk drug and is always approved by the obstetrician/gynecologist. Acetylsalicylic acid (aspirin), on the other hand, is a category D risk drug and is contraindicated for use as an analgesic during pregnancy.

18. How should the pregnant patient with moderate pain be handled?

For nonpregnant patients, the choice of analgesics generally focuses on the selection of a narcotic compounded with aspirin or acetaminophen versus the selection of a nonsteroidal anti-inflammatory drug. Codeine or any of the synthetic codeine preparations, oxycodone and hydrocodone, found in Percocet and Vicodin, respectively, are category C risk drugs when compounded with acetaminophen. This prescription, therefore, would require clearance with the obstetrician/gynecologist. (Percodan is aspirin and oxycodone and, therefore, is rated as a category D risk). Meperidine (Demerol) is a category B risk drug (category D if used for prolonged periods or at high doses at term). The nonsteroidal medications are a wild card. First and foremost, all nonsteroidal anti-inflammatory drugs carry a category D risk in the third trimester. There is significant potential for the occurrence of premature closure of the fetal circulation, and ductus arteriosus and all nonsteroidal drugs are therefore contraindicated in the third trimester. In the first and second trimesters, some nonsteroidal anti-inflammatory drugs carry a category B risk and therefore are preferred over codeine preparations. However, other nonsteroidal drugs carry a category C risk, similar to codeine and acetaminophen and mandate physician consultation. Ibuprofen (Motrin) and naproxen (Naprosyn, Anaprox) are category B drugs. Flurbiprofen (Ansaid), etodolac (Lodine), diflunisal (Dolobid), and rofecoxcib (Vioxx) are category C drugs.

19. Is there any confusion over classification of medications?

Pharmacology references sometimes disagree on risk categories. For example, most pharmacology textbooks rate flurbiprofen (Ansaid) as a category C risk drug in the first two trimesters and as category D in the third trimester. The American Dental Association's therapeutics textbook lists it as a category B risk. Articaine (Septocaine) is a category C anesthetic but is listed as category B in American Dental Association's therapeutics. The clinician is advised to consult the physician whenever there is doubt regarding risk categories and should err on the side of assuming the drug carries a higher risk.

20. Can the dentist use sedative drugs as adjuncts to analgesics, antianxiety medications, and nitrous oxide for inhalation analgesia?

Antianxiety drugs such oral or IV diazepam (Valium), oral alprazolam (Xanax), intravenous midazolam (Versed), and all benzodiazipines are category D drugs and are contraindicated during pregnancy. Nitrous oxide has been shown to be teratogenic among operating room personnel and should not be administered to pregnant patients. It is strictly contraindicated. Hydroxyzine (Vistaril), used as a sedative, is a category C risk. On the other hand, oral promethazine (Phenergan), also a sedative, is a category B risk.

21. What medications can the dentist safely prescribe for intra- and extraoral ulcers?

The extraoral ulcers of secondary herpes virus infection are best treated with penciclovir (Denavir) topical ointment. This is a category B risk drug and can be prescribed routinely. Oral acyclovir (Zovirax) is a category C drug and requires physician clearance. For intraoral aphthous ulcers, amlexanox (Aphthasol) oral paste can be prescribed routinely as a category B drug. Many dentists treat angular cheilitis, prescribing a combination cream of nystatin with triamcinolone (Mycolog cream). This drug, however, is a category C as a combination of antifungal and steroid preparation and requires physician approval. Similarly, all steroid preparations such as 0.1% betamethasone used for desquamative gingivitis are category C risk drugs and require approval. Generally, this is also true for other antifungal drugs such as fluconazole (Diflucan), a category C risk prescription.

22. What should be the dentist's overall strategy for the pregnant patient?

Prevention of periodontal disease and acute odontogenic pathology is paramount. Dental prophylaxis, therefore, is mandated at the beginning of the second and third trimesters minimally. Gross caries must be treated, preferably during the second trimester. All major elective dental care should be deferred. Acute infection should be treated aggressively. Radiographs are contraindicated in all but emergency situations and should be done with mandatory lead shielding. If the patient has significant periodontal disease, an extensive hygiene phase, including conservative scaling and root planing, is indicated. Elective surgical flap therapy and regenerative therapy should generally be deferred unless acute or chronic infection risk is substantial.

23. What should be the dentist's overall drug strategy for the pregnant patient?

My overall drug strategy would include first and foremost a contraindication of all category D or category X drugs. This would include all tetracyclines, all benzodiazipines (e.g., Valium), nitrous oxide, the sedative hydroxyzine (Vistaril), the barbiturate-containing drug Fioricet (acetaminophen, caffeine, butalbital) with codeine, and any aspirin-containing medication. Also any nonsteroidal anti-inflammatory analgesic is strictly contraindicated in the third trimester.

When prescribing medication for the pregnant patient, ideally dentists should limit themselves to category B drugs when possible. Therefore, lidocaine or prilocaine would be my first local anesthetics of choice. With epinephrine, they still remain in category B risk. For analgesics, I would prefer acetaminophen (Tylenol) at any time or category B risk nonsteroidal drugs such as ibuprofen or naproxen during the first two trimesters only. For moderate pain analgesia, a category C drug in the third trimester would include a compound of acetaminophen and codeine with prior clearance from the obstetrician/gynecologist. Meperidine, even when compounded with promethazine, is a category B short-term analgesic option. Because at higher doses meperidine can depress respiratory function, a physician consultation is advisable. For antibiotic choice, my preference is category B penicillins: amoxicillin or augmentin for localized or severe infections, respectively, or simple erythromycins or specifically azithromycin (Zithromax) for the penicillin-allergic patient. Clindamycin (Cleocin) is my first back-up drug, whereas clarithromycin (Biaxin) and ciprofloxacin (Cipro) fall into category C, required physician clearance alternatives. All tetracyclines are strictly contraindicated.

15. ASTHMA

Robert C. Fazio, D.M.D., and Leslie S.T. Fang, M.D., Ph.D.

1. What is asthma?

Asthma is a condition characterized by episodic reversible narrowing of the airways. This results in acute episodes of shortness of breath and wheezing. The disease can begin at any age, but about half of patients develop asthma before the age of 10.

Asthma affects about 2% of the population and is responsible for 50,000 deaths/year in the US.

2. What causes asthma?

The most common cause of asthma is an inherited immunologic disorder that allows inhaled antigens (allergens) to trigger a hypersensitivity response mediated by immunoglobulin E (IgE) and thus produce reversible bronchial narrowing. Asthma can also be precipitated by cold or exercise.

A small subgroup of patients with asthma can experience wheezing and shortness of breath on taking aspirin. These patients often have the clinical triad of asthma, nasal polyps and aspirin sensitivity.

Rarely, asthma may be a manifestation of a systemic vasculitis such as polyarteritis or Churg-Strauss syndrome.

3. What are the crucial issues in the evaluation of the patient with asthma?

A detailed history is crucial in the evaluation of the patient with asthma.

The age at which symptoms of asthma appeared is of some prognostic value because patients who develop asthma in childhood often have amelioration of symptoms as adults. Many patients with severe asthma as children have minimal symptoms in later years. Patients who develop asthma as adults tend to experience less dramatic improvement with time.

The circumstances leading to an asthmatic episode should also be analyzed to identify possible precipitating factors. Some patients develop bronchospasm at times of emotional stress. These patients should be identified and managed with adjunctive sedation techniques for dental procedures. Another common precipitant of asthma is an upper respiratory infection. It is therefore important to avoid elective dental procedures in these patients at the time of an upper respiratory infection. Other precipitants of bronchospasm include exercise, cold air, and air pollutants.

The severity of the patient's asthma should be noted. Patients with a prior history of respiratory insufficiency are obviously problematic and should be managed cautiously.

Knowing the frequency of asthmatic attacks is also important in determining the need for chronic therapy.

4. What are the common inhalational medications used for asthma?

Whenever feasible, asthma is managed with the use of inhalation medications. These are simple to use, have a rapid onset of action, and a short duration of action. Most patients with mild asthma are managed with inhalers alone.

Bronchodilators are often the first-line drugs for patients with mild asthma. These are given in the inhaled form and can have an effect on the airway within minutes. The most commonly prescribed bronchodilators are the beta-2-adrenergic drugs. These drugs selectively relax the smooth muscles lining the airway and have few cardiac side effects. Common selective beta-2-adrenergic bronchodilators include albuterol (Proventil, Ventolin), metaproterenol (Alupent, Metaprel), pirbuterol (Maxair), and salmeterol (Serevent).

Nonselective beta-adrenergic bronchodilators are also commonly prescribed in patients without cardiac contraindications. These include epinephrine preparations (Bronkaid, EpiPen, Primatene Mist, Sus-phrine), isoetharine preparations (Arm-A-Med, Bronkosol), and terbutaline (Brethaire, Brethine). These agents have more cardiovascular side effects and can cause tachycardia, tremulousness, and arrhythmia, but they are very effective agents in patients with no cardiovascular contraindications.

For patients whose asthma is not adequately controlled on bronchodilators alone, low dose inhaled steroids are often helpful. These agents are used because of the increasing understanding that bronchospasm is often mediated via inflammatory responses and can be suppressed by inhaled or systemic steroids. Inhaled steroid preparations include beclomethasone (Beclovent, Vanceril), budesonide (Pulmocort), flunisolide (AeroBid), fluticasone (Flovent), and triamcinolone (Azmacort).

Other inhaled anti-inflammatory drugs inhibit chemical mediators of inflammation and include disodium cromoglycate (Intal) and nedocromil (Tilade). These agents are particularly helpful in patients with cold- or exercise-induced asthma.

Anticholinergic drugs can also be administered in an inhaled form and are effective adjuncts to bronchodilators and steroid inhalers. A common anticholinergic inhaler is ipratropium (Atrovent). These agents act on receptors to prevent smooth muscle contraction.

5. What are the common systemic drugs used in the management of asthma?

Bronchodilators can be administered as oral or parenteral drugs in the treatment of asthma. These include aminophylline (Dilor) and theophylline (Choledyl, Slo-phyllin, Quibron, Slo-bid, Theolair, Uniphyl). The major side effects of these drugs are cardiac, with tachycardia, tremulousness, and arrhythmias as major manifestations.

Some patients with severe asthma may require intermittent courses of steroids. Systemic steroid use has to be minimized because of the significant side effects from these drugs. Nonetheless, steroid therapy may be necessary for management of refractory asthma. The use of steroids and their side effects are discussed in detail in Chapter 12.

Leukotriene antagonists are gaining increasing popularity because of the understanding that these agents can prevent occurrences of asthma. Commonly prescribed leukotriene inhibitors are zafirlukast (Accolate) and montelukast (Singulair).

6. What are the dental implications in the management of the patient with asthma?

The major goal for the dentist in the management of a patient with asthma is to minimize the likelihood of precipitating an asthmatic attack.

A detailed history of the severity of the asthma, the precipitating factors, and the medications used is very helpful in the management of these patients.

7. What are the general guidelines for the management of patients with asthma?

Patients with asthma can occasionally have an exacerbation of symptoms under stress, and efforts should be made to identify patients whose bronchospasms are precipitated by emotional stress.

Minimize stress: Wherever possible, lengthy procedures should be spread over several appointments. Adjunctive sedation techniques should be considered when appropriate for minimization of stress.

Sedation techniques might include the use of N_2O/O_2 inhalation, po diazepam (Valium), or other oral antianxiety medications.

Avoid antihistamines: Antihistamines such as promethazine (Phenergan) or diphenhydramine (Benadryl) should be avoided because they have a drying effect that can exacerbate the formation of tenacious mucus in an acute attack.

Minimize epinephrine use: For patients using methylxanthine preparations (e.g., theophyllin), the dentist should minimize the use of epinephrine in order to avoid additive toxicity and arrhythmia. Local anesthesia up to 2 Carpules of 2% lidocaine with 1:100,000 epinephrine or the equivalent may be used.

Avoid erythromycins and clarithromycin: These drugs should be avoided in patients on methylxanthine preparations (e.g., theophyllin) in order to minimize the likelihood of occurrence of arrhythmias.

Be aware of history of aspirin sensitivity: There is a clinical triad of asthma, nasal polyps, and aspirin sensitivity. It is important to be sure that the patient with asthma does not have this triad when aspirin-containing preparations are prescribed.

8. How should one categorize patients with asthma?

High risk: In patients with symptomatic asthma who manifest audible wheezing and tachypnea and patients with tachycardia, irregular pulse, and other signs of medication side effects, dental intervention is contraindicated.

Significant risk: Despite being on medication, patients with a history of frequent asthma flares have significant risk. The stress of dental procedures may precipitate an asthmatic attack. The dentist may choose to simplify the dental treatment plan in these patients, particularly if a strong component of anxiety is present.

Moderate risk: Patients who have infrequent asthmatic flares on a stable regimen are at lower risk.

9. What are the management issues the dentist should be aware of when treating a patient with asthma?

Patients on bronchodilator therapy deserve special attention. Many bronchodilators have cardiac stimulatory effects and, in patients with underlying cardiac disease, the addition of epinephrine can precipitate arrhythmias. It is therefore prudent to use local anesthetics without epinephrine or to minimize epinephrine use to a maximum of two Carpules of local anesthetic with 1:100,000 epinephrine, or 1:20,000 levonordefrin, or an equivalent.

Because of the risk of increased methylxanthine toxicity with the concurrent use of erythromycin or clindamycin, these antibiotics are relatively contraindicated in patients taking theophylline preparations.

Patients on steroids and patients with a significant history of steroid exposure deserve special attention. Management of patients on chronic steroid therapy is discussed in detail in Chapter 12.

16. CHRONIC OBSTRUCTIVE PULMONARY DISEASE

Robert C. Fazio, D.M.D., and Leslie S.T. Fang, M.D., Ph.D.

1. What is chronic obstructive pulmonary disease (COPD)?

COPD is a disease due to persistent airway obstruction. Two diseases account for the bulk of the patients with COPD: emphysema and chronic bronchitis.

2. What causes COPD?

The major cause of COPD is smoking, which creates irritation and constriction of the smaller airways with resultant damage. On rare occasions, COPD may result from genetic diseases, such as alpha$_1$-antitrypsin deficiency.

3. Discuss the prevalence of COPD.

COPD generally affects men above the age of 40. The prevalence in the general population is almost 30 cases/1000 population. It accounts for over 50,000 deaths per year in the United States.

4. What are the clinical signs of COPD?

Patients may present with coughing, sputum production, wheezing, shortness of breath, or dyspnea on exertion.

5. What is emphysema?

Emphysema is a disease affecting the smaller distal airways, causing destruction of the lung parenchyma with resultant loss of elasticity of the alveolar walls. This process leads to compromise of airflow, particularly during exhalation. Patients experience hyperinflated lungs and formation of emphysematous blebs as tissue destruction progresses. Patients with emphysema complain primarily of shortness of breath, aggravated by exertion. Coughing and sputum production tend to be minor components of the disease.

6. What is chronic bronchitis?

Chronic bronchitis results from oversecretion by the mucous glands of the bronchial tree, resulting in cough and sputum production. The mucus can cause obstruction in the form of plugs, resulting in shortness of breath and dyspnea on exertion.

7. Discuss the sequelae of COPD.

In general, COPD is a progressive disease. Patients have progressive shortness of breath with progressive limitation. The pulmonary disease can lead to right-heart strain and right-heart failure (cor pulmonale). Such patients have limited pulmonary reserve, and even minor infection can cause severe compromises.

8. What are the clinical findings in patients with COPD?

Chest x-ray usually shows hyperinflated lungs and bleb formation. Arterial blood gas shows low oxygen saturation, carbon dioxide retention, and respiratory acidosis. Pulmonary function tests show severe airway obstruction.

9. How is COPD medically managed?

Patients are advised to stop smoking. Patients who are exposed to other pulmonary irritants are told to minimize environmental toxin exposure. Patients with tenacious sputum production are instructed to maintain adequate hydration. Humidifiers are used to maximize the humidity of inhaled air. Various inhalational and systemic drugs are also used to help with airway obstruction.

10. What inhalation medications do patients commonly take?

Bronchodilators are often the first-line drugs for patients with mild asthma. They are given in the inhaled form and may have an effect on the airway within minutes. The most commonly prescribed bronchodilators are the **beta$_2$-adrenergic drugs**. Bronchodilators selectively relax the smooth muscles lining the airway and have few cardiac side effects. Common selective beta$_2$-adrenergic bronchodilators include albuterol (Proventil, Ventolin), metaproterenol (Alupent, Metaprel), pirbuterol (Maxair), and salmeterol (Serevent).

Nonselective beta-adrenergic bronchodilators are also commonly prescribed in patients with no cardiac contraindications. Examples include epinephrine preparations (Bronkaid, Epi Pen, Primatene Mist, Sus-phrine), isoetharine preparations (Arm-a-Med, Bronkosol), and terbutaline (Brethaire, Brethine). These agents have more cardiovascular side effects and can cause tachycardia, tremulousness, and arrhythmia, but they are highly effective in patients with no cardiovascular contraindications.

For patients who are not adequately controlled by bronchodilators alone, low-dose **inhaled steroids** are often helpful. These agents are used because of the increasing understanding that bronchospasm is often mediated via inflammatory responses and can be suppressed by inhaled or systemic steroids. Inhaled steroid preparations include beclomethasone (Beclovent, Vanceril), budesonide (Pulmocort), fluisoide (AeroBid, Flovent), and triamcinolone (Azmacort).

Anticholinergic drugs can also be administered in an inhaled form and are effective adjuncts to bronchodilator and steroid inhalers. Common anticholinergic inhalers include ipratropium (Atrovent). These agents act on receptors to prevent smooth muscle contraction.

11. What systemic drugs are commonly used in the management of COPD?

Bronchodilators can be administered as oral or parenteral drugs in the treatment of asthma. Examples include aminophylline (Dilor) and theophylline (Choledyl, Slo-Phyllin, Quibron, Slo-bid, Theolar, Uniphyl). The major side effects are cardiac manifestations such as tachycardia, tremulousness, and arrhythmia.

Some patients with severe COPD may require intermittent courses of **steroids** during periods of acute exacerbation. Systemic steroid use has to be minimized because of the significant side effects. Nonetheless, steroid therapy may be necessary from management of refractory airway obstruction. The use and side effects of steroids are discussed in detail in Chapter 12.

12. What should the dentist remember when treating a patient with COPD?

Patients should be evaluated to assess the severity of the disease. A review of their medications usually indicates the magnitude of the problem.

It is particularly important to know whether a patient retains carbon dioxide. Such patients have severe disease and are most likely to develop carbon dioxide retention when given oxygen. For patients suspected of having severe disease, the dentist should consult with the physician. For patients with severe disease, the use of nitrous oxide/oxygen in the dental office is contraindicated.

In general, patients who retain carbon dioxide have severe pulmonary compromise and are tachypneic even at rest. They tend to take multiple pulmonary medications. All patients with severe pulmonary disease should consult their physicians and ask specifically about the tendency to carbon dioxide retention.

13. What are the general guidelines for the management of patients with COPD?

Patients with COPD occasionally have an exacerbation of symptoms under stress, and efforts should be made to identify patients in whom bronchospasm is precipitated by emotional stress. Wherever possible, lengthy procedures should be spread over several appointments. Adjunctive sedation techniques should be considered, when appropriate, for minimization of stress.

Sedation techniques might include oral diazepam (Valium). Antihistamines such as promethazine (Phenergan) or diphenhydramine (Benadryl) should be avoided, because they have a drying effect that can exacerbate the formation of tenacious mucus in an acute attack.

14. What are the management issues in treating a patient with COPD?

Patients on bronchodilator therapy deserve special attention. Many bronchodilators have cardiac stimulatory effects, and, in patients with underlying cardiac disease, additional epinephrine can precipitate arrhythmias. It is prudent, therefore, to use local anesthetics without epinephrine. If hemostasis or prolonged anesthesia is required, the dentist should limit the amount of epinephrine to that contained in 2 carpules of local anesthetic preparations with 1:100,000 epinephrine or an equivalent (i.e., 4 carpules of local anesthetic with 1:200,000 epinephrine or 2 carpules of local anesthetic with 1:20,000 levonordefrin).

Because of the risk of increased methylxanthine (theophyline) toxicity (i.e., cardiac arrhythmias) with the concurrent use of erythromycins, these antibiotics are relatively contraindicated in patients taking theophylline preparations.

Patients taking steroids and patients with a significant history of steroid exposure deserve special attention. Management of patients on chronic steroid therapy is discussed in detail in Chapter 12. For the severe stress of general anesthesia, prednisone, 60 mg, should be given orally on the morning of the procedure.

For significant but less stressful procedures in patients for whom adrenal insufficiency is a concern, 30–40 mg of prednisone is often recommended.

17. TUBERCULOSIS

Stephen T. Sonis, D.M.D., D.M.Sc.

1. How common is tuberculosis (TB) in the U.S.?
In 2000, 16,377 cases of TB were reported to the Centers for Disease Control and Prevention. This represents 5.8 cases per 100,000 population. The number of cases reported in 2000 represents a significant decrease (39%) from the number of cases reported in 1992, when the number of TB cases peaked.

2. How does the incidence trend for TB in the U.S. compare with that in other countries?
The case rate among people not born in the U.S. is seven times higher than the case rate for people born in the U.S. Given the mobility of the world's population, this finding has led to public health initiatives to control the disease.

3. How is the tubercle bacillus transmitted?
The tubercle bacillus is transmitted from infected people by small aerosolized droplets that are carried into the respiratory tract of susceptible hosts.

4. Describe the clinical features of primary TB infection.
Mycobacterium tuberculosis generally causes a mild pulmonary disease characterized by fever, chills, cough, and sputum production. Infected foci form granulomas that heal by scarring calcification. The calcification is usually evident on chest x-ray.

5. Where in the lungs are healing granulomata associated with TB most likely to be seen on chest x-ray?
The apices of the lungs.

6. Primary TB infections rarely spread by erosion to contiguous areas. Name the two most common sites of spread and the condition caused by TB.
Pleural space: pleurisy.
Pericardial spaces: pericarditis.

7. Describe the course of TB after primary infection.
After primary infection, TB may remain dormant for years. Reactivation may occur, causing pulmonary or systemic disease. Tubercle bacilli originating in the granulomatous lesions may become disseminated, causing miliary TB and involving the liver, kidneys, vertebral bodies, gastrointestinal tract, or meninges.

8. What is Pott's disease?
TB involving the vertebral bodies of the spine.

9. What are the two most common extrapulmonary forms of TB in HIV-infected patients?
Lymphatic and miliary.

10. What is lymph node involvement called?
Scrofula.

11. What is miliary involvement of the skin called?
Lupus vulgaris.

12. Is TB contagious?
TB is highly contagious.

13. What events generally trigger a medical evaluation for TB?
- History of exposure to the disease
- Positive skin test
- Scar detected on screening chest x-ray
- Symptoms suggestive of the disease (fever, chills, night sweats, weight loss, productive cough)

14. What is the most common presentation of patients for whom a TB work-up is ordered?
Positive skin test but no active infection.

15. About what percentage of people in the U.S. have a positive TB skin test but no sign of active infection?
7%.

16. What skin test is routinely used to test for TB?
The Mantoux or purified protein derivative (PPD) test is typically used to test for TB. The test consists of the intradermal injection of a small volume of liquid PPD that contains 5 tuberculin units and measurement of the patient's delayed hypersensitivity to the antigen. Test material is injected into the forearm, and the diameter of induration is measured 2 or 3 days later.

17. Are the criteria for a positive PPD skin test the same for everyone?
Why would we ask if the answer were yes? The cutoffs in the diameter of induration for a positive PPD test depend on the population tested. For example, for patients at high risk of infection (HIV infection or immunosuppression, recent close contact with TB, prior untreated TB) the bar is lower (> 4 mm) than for patients at no risk (> 14 mm). Health care workers are part of a middle category that includes foreign-born people from high-prevalence countries, low-income populations, intravenous (IV) drug users, and elderly people (positive result = > 9 mm).

18. If a patient has active pulmonary TB and is producing sputum, how can the diagnosis be confirmed?
Examination of the sputum for acid-fast bacilli. Stains that are used to make the diagnosis are the Ziehl-Neelson stain or the Truant fluorescent stain.

19. Can people exposed to TB or people with positive skin tests be effectively treated to prevent the development of active disease?
Yes. Patients with a positive tuberculin skin test can be treated with isoniazid (INH) to prevent active disease. In general, INH prophylaxis is given to all people who have a risk factor for the disease (HIV infection, recent contact with an infected person, abnormal chest x-ray, IV drug abuse, medical conditions that increase risk). For the most part, preventive therapy for other patients with a positive skin test is instituted only in people under the age of 35 years.

20. What is the main toxicity of INH?
INH-induced hepatitis.

21. What is the percent risk that an HIV-positive, PPD-positive person will develop active TB?
Eight percent per year compared with 2.5–4% for someone who has recently converted to a positive PPD test after close contact with a person who has a new case of TB.

22. How should you treat a patient who presents for emergency dental treatment and has a positive skin test but no evidence of active TB?
Such patients patient have had a TB infection, and the disease can be reactivated. Because there is no evidence of active infection, they are thought to be noninfectious. Consequently, dental procedures can be performed using appropriate infection control procedures.

23. Are oral manifestations of TB common?

Even among high-risk populations, the frequency of oral manifestations of TB is low. Fewer than 1% of patients with TB have oral lesions.

24. By what mechanism do oral lesions of TB develop?

It is believed that most oral lesions associated with TB develop when pulmonary organisms are brought to the mouth by coughing.

25. What is the most common presentation of oral TB?

The oral lesions caused by secondary spread of organisms from a primary lung lesion are ulcerative. The ulcers are usually painless and uneven, with jagged, undermined soft borders. The center may be purulent.

26. What are the most common sites for oral TB lesions?

• Base of the tongue (most common)
• Gingiva
• Lip
• Tonsils
• Tooth sockets
• Soft palate

27. What do oral ulcers of TB most closely resemble?

Carcinoma.

28. What is cutix orifacialis?

TB at the corners of the mouth. Lesions present as shallow, granulating ulcerations with pebbly surfaces.

29. What is the best way to make a diagnosis in the patient who presents with an ulcerative lesion of TB?

Biopsy with the demonstration of organisms in the tissue.

18. PEPTIC ULCER DISEASE

Robert C. Fazio, D.M.D., and Leslie S.T. Fang, M.D., Ph.D.

1. What is peptic ulcer disease?

This is a common disorder resulting from damage to the epithelial lining of the stomach or the duodenum.

2. What is the prevalence of peptic ulcer disease?

Prevalence of the disease has been falling because of the widespread use of antacids, histamine (H_2) antagonists (cimetidine [Tagamet], ranitidine [Zantac], famotidine [Pepcid], and nizatidine [Axid]), and proton pump inhibitors (Prilosec, Nexium, and Aciphex). The current estimate is that 1–3% of the population of the US have peptic ulcer disease. The disease usually affects men between the ages of 45 and 65 and women over age 55.

3. What are the symptoms of peptic ulcer disease?

Patients with peptic ulcer disease can present with abdominal pain, gastrointestinal bleeding, bowel obstruction, or bowel perforation.

4. What is the prevalence of gastric versus duodenal ulcer?

- Patients with duodenal ulcers outnumber those with gastric ulcers by 4:1.
- Patients with duodenal ulcers usually have episodic epigastric pain that starts 2–3 hr after a meal. The pain is relieved by food.
- Patients with gastric ulcers often have epigastric pain radiating into the mid-back. The pain is often aggravated by food.
- Patients with either duodenal or gastric cancer may have black tarry stools (melena) secondary to gastrointestinal bleeding.
- Occasionally, patients may have significant scarring from peptic ulcer disease and have symptoms of obstruction, usually at the gastric outlet.
- Patients with severe ulcer disease can have frank perforation of the ulcer and present with bowel perforation and peritonitis.

5. How is peptic ulcer disease diagnosed?

The clinical presentation is usually helpful in the diagnosis of peptic ulcer disease. Confirmation is usually done by endoscopic evaluation of the stomach and the duodenum. This procedure is preferred over performing an upper gastrointestinal series; since cauterization can often be done during endoscopy to stop gastrointestinal bleeding.

6. What would predispose a patient to peptic ulcer disease?

Patients with heavy tobacco or alcohol use are more prone to peptic ulcer disease. A large number of medications such as aspirin, nonsteroidal anti-inflammatory drugs, and corticosteroids can promote ulceration of the gastric and duodenal surfaces.

7. What is *Helicobacter pylori*?

H. pylori is a bacterial infection that results in recurrent symptoms of peptic ulcer disease. These patients have intractable and recurrent symptoms despite being on appropriate therapy. The diagnosis of *H. pylori* infection can be made on the basis of a blood test or by biopsy during endoscopy.

8. How is *H. pylori* infection treated?

H. pylori is responsive to antibiotic therapy. Most frequently, it responds to combinations of proton pump inhibitors and antibiotics, such as Augmentin (amoxicillin/clavulonic acid) and Biaxin (clarithromycin).

Tetracycline and metronidazole are sometimes used as well.

9. **What is the medical management of the patient with peptic ulcer disease?**

Patients with mild symptoms can be managed with over-the-counter antacids.

Patients with more severe disease can be managed with a variety of H_2 antagonists. These are drugs that inhibit the H_2 receptors in the gastrointestinal tract and decrease stomach acid production. Commonly prescribed drugs include cimetadine (Tagamet), ranitidine (Zantac), famotidine (Pepcid) and nizatidine (Axid).

Patients with severe disease can also be managed with proton pump inhibitors. These drugs directly inhibit the acid secreting glands and therefore minimize the amount of acid production. Commonly prescribed drugs include omeprazole (Prilosec), rabeprazole (Aciphex), and esomeprazole (Nexium).

10. **How is peptic ulcer disease addressed surgically?**

With the advent of H_2 antagonists and proton pump inhibitors, surgical intervention for gastric or duodenal ulcer disease has become rare. Some patients who have not been adequately treated may develop severe gastrointestinal bleeding, gastric outlet obstruction, or bowel perforation, necessitating surgical intervention.

11. **How should the dental procedure be altered in patients with peptic ulcer disease?**

- Drugs that cause gastrointestinal irritation should be avoided. This includes aspirin, nonsteroidal anti-inflammatory drugs, corticosteroids, and erythromycin.
- Since stress can accentuate stomach acid production, a stress reduction dental protocol should be employed. Wherever possible, lengthy procedures should be spread over several appointments. Adjunctive sedation techniques should be considered when appropriate for minimization of stress. Sedation techniques might include the use of N_2O/O_2 inhalation, oral antianxiety medications such as diazepam (Valium), or intravenous sedation techniques.
- Antacid therapy is commonly utilized in the medical management of peptic ulcer disease. It should be borne in mind that the efficacy of a number of antibiotics prescribed by the dentist is compromised if given together with antacids. Antibiotics such as tetracycline, ciprofloxacin and other quinolones, and metronidazol (Flagyl) should not be given together with antacids.

12. **Can nonsteroidal anti-inflammatory drugs ever be prescribed for patients with a history of peptic ulcer disease?**

If the patient is currently symptomatic and under active treatment for peptic ulcer disease, nonsteroidal anti-inflammatory drugs are contraindicated.

If the patient gives a history of remote peptic ulcer disease but is no longer symptomatic and is not on active treatment, judicious use of nonsteroidal anti-inflammatory drugs over a short period of time can be considered. The dentist should be aware of any prior problems with these drugs, including some of the over-the-counter preparations such as Motrin and Aleve. In dubious circumstances, it is probably safer to prescribe the selective Cox-2 inhibitors (rofecoxib [Vioxx] and celecoxib [Celebrex]).

19. INFLAMMATORY BOWEL DISEASE

Robert C. Fazio, D.M.D., and Leslie S.T. Fang, M.D., Ph.D.

1. What is inflammatory bowel disease?
Inflammatory bowel disease is the result of autoimmune abnormalities causing inflammation of the bowel. Ulcerative colitis and Crohn's disease account for most of the inflammatory bowel disease. The disease affects patients between the ages of 20 and 45.

2. What is the prevalence of inflammatory bowel disease?
Ulcerative colitis and Crohn's disease have a combined prevalence of 1 in 10,000 population.

3. Why is inflammatory bowel disease important to the dentist?
Inflammatory bowel disease is associated with a number of oral findings. More important, drugs used to manage inflammatory bowel disease can affect dental plans and management.
- Increased risk of aphthous stomatitis
- Increased risk of periodontitis
- Steroid therapy used for inflammatory bowel disease may require dental management
- Patients on therapy may be immunosuppressed
- Some drugs used for inflammatory bowel disease can induce gingival hyperplasia
- Some drugs used for inflammatory bowel disease may have side effects that could alter the selection of dental prescriptions

4. What are the symptoms of inflammatory bowel disease?
Patients with inflammatory bowel disease usually have abdominal pain, fever, and diarrhea. The disease typically begins in young adulthood.

5. What is ulcerative colitis?
Ulcerative colitis is an idiopathic inflammatory disease causing diffuse ulceration of the colon. Ulcerative colitis involves only the colon. Patients may have symptoms ranging from episodic diarrhea to severe abdominal pain, fever, and bloody diarrhea.

6. What is Crohn's disease?
Crohn's disease is a chronic granulomatous inflammation affecting all layers of the bowel wall. The disease can involve any portion of the gastrointestinal tract. About 25% of the patients have involvement of the colon, 25% have involvement of the terminal ileum, and 50% have involvement of both the large and the small bowel. Patients' presenting symptoms are crampy abdominal pain and diarrhea.

7. What are the complications of ulcerative colitis?
Complications of ulcerative colitis include gastrointestinal bleeding and occasionally bowel perforation. More importantly, patients with ulcerative colitis develop carcinoma of the colon about 10 times more frequently than the general population and should be monitored closely.

8. What are the complications of Crohn's disease?
Complications of Crohn's disease include fistulas between loops of the bowel or fistulas extending to the abdominal wall or perineal area. There is also a slightly increased risk of carcinoma over that of the general population.

9. How are patients with ulcerative colitis managed?
Patients with mild disease are often managed with sulfasalazine. The drug appears to be reasonably effective as initial therapy but does have side effects. Side effects include gastrointestinal

upset, hypersensitivity reaction such as rash and fever, and serious idiosyncratic reactions such as agranulocytosis, lupus-like phenomena, and hepatocellular injury.

Patients with more severe disease are managed with sulfapyradine-free-5-aminosalicylate agents. These are administered either orally or by enema, and common preparations include mesalamine and topical 5-aminosalicylic acid enemas. There are few side effects, but interstitial nephritis and idiosyncratic reactions such as pleuropericarditis, pancreatitis, and nephrotic syndrome have been reported.

Patients with severe disease may be placed on steroids, either orally or by enema. The side effects of steroids have been discussed in detail in Chapter 12.

Some patients with severe disease may actually be placed on immunosuppressive agents in order to minimize the use of steroids. Immunosuppressive agents commonly used include azathioprine (Imuran) or cyclosporine (Neoral). These drugs suppress the immune response and make the patients much more susceptible to infections. Suppression of the bone marrow can result in anemia, leukopenia, and thrombocytopenia.

Some patients may be placed on opiates during periods of severe diarrhea. These include codeine, diphenoxylate (Lomotil), tincture of opiate, and loperamide (Imodium A-D).

In patients with very severe disease, total colectomy is a curative procedure. This would be contemplated particularly in instances in which there is a concern about colon cancer.

10. How are patients with Crohn's disease managed?

Patients with Crohn's disease are usually started on sulfasalazine and 5-aminosalicylic acid agents. Metronidazole (Flagyl) can be added to the regimen, particularly in patients with fistulas. Other antibiotics, including ciprofloxacin, have been used. Antibiotics may be effective in decreasing bacterial infection in these fistulas.

In a patient with severe disease, glucocorticoids can be used. The side effects of steroids have been discussed in detail in Chapter 12.

Immunosuppressive drugs such as azathiaprine (Imuran), methotrexate, and cyclosporine have been used in patients with severe disease. Unlike ulcerative colitis, surgery in Crohn's disease does not cure the disease and is usually reserved for bowel obstruction or perforation.

11. What are the oral findings in the patient with ulcerative colitis?

The oral changes that occur in ulcerative colitis are nonspecific and fairly uncommon. Increased risk of aphthous stomatitis has been reported in patients with active disease. Pyoderma gangrenosum and hemorrhagic ulceration have also been reported.

12. What are the oral findings in the patient with Crohn's disease?

Oral manifestations of Crohn's disease include cobblestone architecture of the mucosa, aphthous ulcerations and lymphadenopathy. There is also an increased risk of periodontitis in patients with active disease. The frequency of these lesions has been reported to range from 6–20%. Rapid alveolar bone loss also has been reported in patients with active Crohn's disease.

13. What are the dental management issues for patients with inflammatory bowel disease?

- Patients with inflammatory bowel disease have higher risks of aphthous ulceration and may benefit from amlexanox (Aphthasol), 5% paste in a 5-g tube, applied qid
- Patients with inflammatory bowel disease have increased risk of periodontitis and need a more aggressive recall prophylaxis and examination schedule
- Stress can precipitate flare-ups of disease. It is therefore important to minimize stress in these patients. Wherever possible, lengthy procedures should be spread over several appointments. Adjunctive sedation techniques should be considered when appropriate for minimization of stress. Sedation techniques might include the use of N_2O-O_2 inhalation or oral diazepam (Valium), oral Vistaril, or intravenous sedation.
- Diarrhea is a common symptom of active inflammatory bowel disease. The dentist is therefore advised to avoid prescribing drugs that may cause diarrhea. This would include drugs

such as amoxicillin-clavulonanate potassium (Augmentin) and clindamycin (Cleocin). Whenever feasible, alternate drugs should be prescribed.

- Sulfasalazine can be associated with gastrointestinal upset. The dentist should avoid prescription of drugs that can aggravate this situation, including erythromycin and metronidazole.
- Patients who are on immunosuppressive medications such as azathioprine (Imuran), cyclosporine (Neoral), or methotrexate are much more prone to infections. These patients may need antibiotics postoperatively in order to minimize the likelihood of infection.
- Patients who are on steroid therapy may need stress steroids. The management of patients on steroids is discussed in detail in Chapter 14.
- Some patients may be on cyclosporine. Gingival hyperplasia can occur in these patients, particularly those on high-dose cyclosporine. Strict prevention protocol is therefore recommended.

20. HEPATITIS

Robert C. Fazio, D.M.D., and Leslie S.T. Fang, M.D., Ph.D.

1. What is viral hepatitis?

Viral hepatitis is an infection of the liver by a variety of viruses. It is a contagious disease that affects approximately 500,000 people in the US every year. The majority of patients have symptoms of an acute infection, but a number have disease progression to chronic hepatitis. Equally important, a number of patients become chronic carriers of hepatitis antigen and are potentially infectious. The dentist is particularly at risk because of exposure to the oral secretions and blood of potentially infectious patients.

2. Name the different types of hepatitis.

Many viruses that can potentially infect the liver. The hepatitis A, B, and C viruses cause the most common forms of hepatitis. Hepatitis D and E are less common. Other viruses can cause liver inflammatory response, including cytomegalovirus and Epstein-Barr virus, but the liver disease is usually mild.

3. What is hepatitis A?

Hepatitis A is a relatively common virus that is transmitted by the oral-fecal route. Children and adolescents are more susceptible to infection than adults. The virus has an incubation period of about 30 days. Patients usually have a mild, flulike illness in the prodromal phase, followed by jaundice, nausea, vomiting, and malaise in the clinically icteric phase. Liver function tests show elevation of the transaminases (serum glutamic-oxaloacetic transaminase [SGOT], serum gluta-mase pyruvate transaminase [SGPT]). Infection with hepatitis A can be confirmed by the detection of antibodies to the virus. The disease is self-limited, usually quite mild, and resolves spontaneously over a period of several weeks. Infection produces antibodies that confer lifelong immunity. Hepatitis A infection appears to be a common occurrence, and one survey indicates that more than 80% of patients over the age of 60 have antibodies against hepatitis A virus. There are no chronic carrier states, and fatalities are exceedingly rare. No treatment is necessary.

4. How is a patient with hepatitis A managed?

The patient should be instructed about hepatitis precautions and should continue these precautions until 1 week after the onset of jaundice. The patient should wash hands thoroughly after toilet use and refrain from intimate contact. The patient should not be handling or serving foods to others, but he or she does not need to be confined to home.

5. What is hepatitis B?

Hepatitis B is far more serious than hepatitis A. More important, patients can be chronic carriers and therefore remain infectious for a protracted period of time.

Hepatitis B is predominantly transmitted by a parenteral route. Patients with acute hepatitis B have evidence of the virus in all bodily secretions including blood, sweat, saliva, semen, and vaginal secretions. Hepatitis B is highly infectious and can be passed on from mother to infant and from spouse to spouse.

After exposure to the virus, there is an incubation period of about 12 weeks (range 6 to 24 weeks), during which the infecting virus replicates. The patient then has a prodromal phase when nonspecific symptoms occur. Patients have anorexia, nausea, low-grade fevers, and malaise. Patients then enter into an icteric phase with fevers, chills, malaise, arthralgia, anorexia, nausea, and vomiting, together with clinical icterus. About 10% become chronic carriers and remain infectious after the acute illness. These patients are more prone to development of cirrhosis and hepatoma.

About 2 weeks prior to the onset of symptoms, the surface antigen to hepatitis B (HB_sAg) is detectable in the serum. Shortly thereafter, enzymes associated with hepatocellular damage (SGOT, SGPT) begin to increase, denoting inflammation of the liver. Subsequently, antibodies to hepatitis B develop. Patients with antibodies to hepatitis B (HB_sAb) have protective antibodies and are conferred life-long immunity. Unfortunately, about 10% of patients never develop antibodies. These patients have persistent antigenemia (Hb_sAg-positive) with no antibody formation (Hb_sAb-negative). Infectivity of the virus is usually associated with presence of the e antigen (Hb_eAn-positive). These patients are chronic carriers and remain infectious and continue to have hepatocellular damage.

Active or persistent disease can be detected by the persistence of Hb_eAn, a marker of ongoing viral infection. Viral load can be measured by HB DNA in the blood.

Hepatitis B can be a very serious disease. Some patients with fulminant hepatitis can develop severe hepatocellular damage with resultant hepatic insufficiency and all its complications.

6. How is hepatitis B treated?

The treatment is largely supportive, with the goal of getting the patient through the acute infection. The patient should have a balanced diet with adequate caloric intake and adequate rest, although activity need not be unduly restricted. The patient should omit potentially hepatotoxic agents, especially alcohol. Pruritus should be treated with cholestyramine. Severe nausea and vomiting should be treated with nonphenothiazine antiemetics such as trimethobenzamide (Tigan) suppository. In selected instances, drug treatment with lamivudine (Epivir) should be considered; the usual dose is 100 mg. Liver function tests and HB_sAg levels should be checked at onset and at 12 weeks of the illness.

Patients with severe disease may have to be admitted to the hospital for management. Patients with fulminant hepatitis B should be considered candidates for liver transplant.

Patients with chronic hepatitis B_e antigenemia should also be considered for therapy.

7. What is the treatment for patients with chronic hepatitis B?

For patients with compensated chronic hepatitis B who demonstrate sustained presence of HBV DNA and HB_eAg, alfa-interferon should be considered.

For patients with chronic "replicative" hepatitis B, lamivudine therapy should be considered. This should be continued for 1 year. Patients who lose HBeAg can stop the therapy, while patients who retain HB_eAg should continue lamivudine.

8. What is hepatitis C?

Hepatitis C is a viral hepatitis transmitted largely by blood exposure. Exposure to other body fluids can sometimes cause hepatitis C. Patients with hepatitis C often have mild symptoms of fever, malaise, nausea, vomiting and jaundice. Although the acute disease is usually mild, patients with hepatitis C would often have persistent disease, leading eventually to cirrhosis and liver failure.

Hepatitis C is now one of the leading cause of cirrhosis, following alcoholic liver disease.

Hepatitis C can be detected by determination of hepatitis C antibody in the serum. Extent of infection can be monitored by the determination of the viral load by measuring hepatitis C viral RNA.

9. How is hepatitis C treated?

Those treating patients with hepatitis C should exercise the same precautions as for patients with hepatitis B, with limited exposure to blood and body fluids of infected patients. Alfa-interferon is the mainstay of therapy for hepatitis C and the pegalated interferon (PEG-Intron) also appears to be particularly effective.

Patients with chronic compensated hepatitis C (genotype 1) who have sustained aminotransferase elevations and detectable HCV RNA should be treated with alfa-interferon and oral ribavirin.

In patients with genotypes other than 1 and in patients with low viral titers, consider a 6-month course of therapy, which may suffice.

For patients who do not respond, and for those who relapse whenever therapy is stopped, long-term maintenance therapy should be considered.

Patients on therapy should have close monitoring of their liver function tests, complete blood count, and viral titers.

Patients with worsening liver function tests despite therapy should be considered candidates for liver transplantation.

10. Describe hepatitis D.

Hepatitis D is a viral infection that occurs only in patients with pre-existing hepatitis B. Coinfection with hepatitis D causes marked decline in hepatocellular function in patients with hepatitis B, at times with fulminant hepatic failure. The virus is usually transmitted by needle transmission in drug addicts.

11. What is the treatment for hepatitis D?

The treatment is primarily supportive. Many patients with hepatitis B and D infections have rapid deterioration of the hepatocellular function and may require liver transplantation.

12. What is hepatitis E?

Hepatitis E is a viral hepatitis transmitted by the fecal-oral route. The virus is quite similar to hepatitis A in its infectivity and is usually a mild self-limited illness.

13. What is the treatment of hepatitis E?

The disease is self-limited and is usually managed with supportive care only.

14. What is the implication of viral hepatitis for the dentist?

Because dentists are exposed to the blood and oral secretions of patients, they are particularly at risk for contracting hepatitis. Even with universal precautions, it is important to identify all patients who are potentially infectious.

15. What should the dental evaluation of patients with a history of viral hepatitis entail?

Patients with a history of malaise, low-grade fever, anorexia, nausea and vomiting should be referred for medical evaluation. Patients with scleral icterus or jaundice should have dental procedures deferred and should also be referred for further evaluation.

Patients with a prior history of hepatitis should be carefully evaluated. Liver function tests, complete blood count, prothrombin time, and hepatitis antigen and antibody levels should be carried out.

The dental evaluation should revolve around:
• Does the patient have active hepatocellular disease?
• Does the patient have a chronic infective state?
• Are there compromises in the synthetic function of the liver present with resultant elevation in prothrombin time?
• Are there compromises in the detoxification process?

16. How should the dentist manage the patient with acute viral hepatitis?

All dental procedures should be deferred until the active infection resolves.

17. What is chronic viral hepatitis?

In the circumstances discussed, hepatitis is an acute illness with a symptomatic presentation. However, in a small subset of patients, the patient may not develop protective antibodies and continues to have persistent infectious viral particles circulating in the bloodstream. These patients obviously continue to be infectious and pose a special problem for the dentist. They are by and large completely asymptomatic. Patients often are aware of a previous infection, but only careful blood screening will reveal that they have chronic viral hepatitis.

Chronic hepatitis is most often seen in patients with hepatitis B or hepatitis C infections.

Only a small subset of patients with hepatitis B infection fails to develop protective antibodies and go on to a chronic infectious state. These patients have Hb_sAg and Hb_eAg positivity with no HbsAb detectable; they continue to be infectious.

Patients with hepatitis C, left untreated, remain infectious for life.

18. How should the dentist manage the patient with chronic viral hepatitis?

By and large, the dentist will deal with patients with either chronic hepatitis B or hepatitis C.

For both groups of patients, liver function tests, platelet counts, and prothrombin times should be determined. In the presence of significant liver function abnormalities and/or of a significantly prolonged prothrombin time, planned dental procedures should be deferred.

For patients on interferon-alfa, leukopenia and thrombocytopenia can occur. It is therefore important to have a complete blood count done prior to any intervention. Often, the patient's physician will have recent blood test results

For patients on ribavirin, close monitoring of hemoglobin and hematocrit levels are mandatory. Care should be given to avoid use of any potentially hepatotoxic agent in these patients.

19. What are the dental considerations in the management of patients with hepatitis?

In consultation with the patients' physicians, the dentist should:

a. Determine the type of hepatitis the patient has had
b. Determine whether the patient is still potentially infectious
c. Evaluate the patient for the risk of bleeding
d. Evaluate the severity of the liver insufficiency in order to assess the ability of the patient to metabolize medications and to synthesize clotting factors
e. Be familiar with the management of a potential bleeding diathesis
f. Consider the various choices for antibiotics, analgesics, and sedatives, depending on the degree of liver dysfunction.

20. How should the dentist approach the bleeding diathesis in patients with hepatitis?

Most patients with hepatitis have normal coagulation capabilities. Some patients with hepatitis (active or chronic) may have enough hepatic compromise to affect hemostasis.

- A detailed history of previous bleeding difficulties is very helpful.
- A complete blood count with platelet count and prothrombin time should be known prior to any dental procedures.
- The dentist should assess the status of the soft tissue and gauge the degree of soft tissue and bone trauma anticipated.
- The patient should be instructed to completely abstain from alcohol both before and after the procedure.
- Patients with normal platelet counts and normal prothrombin/partial thromboplastin times can undergo dental intervention with careful attention to hemostasis.
- Patients may have coagulopathy related to decreased synthesis of factors produced by the liver (factors I, II, V, VII, IX, and X). Only some of these factors are vitamin K–dependent. Patients with significant coagulopathy need replacement of factors in the form of fresh frozen plasma. This should be coordinated with their physicians, and infusion should be given shortly before the intended dental procedure.
- Acute alcohol consumption can suppress the bone marrow and can result in thrombocytopenia. It is therefore important to reinforce the "no alcohol" rule.

21. What if the dentist finds a low platelet count?

Most patients with hepatitis have normal platelet counts. A small percentage of patients may develop enough hepatic disease to have portal hypertension, hypersplenism, or thrombocytopenia.

If the platelet count is between 50,000 and 100,000, the patient should be able to form a hemostatic plug, but this ability is usually mildly compromised. The dentist should expect some clinical bleeding. Minor surgical interventions, such as the atraumatic removal of one or two teeth, can proceed using careful technique with attention to hemostasis. Local anesthesia, including regional block injections, can be done safely. Major surgical interventions should probably be done under platelet coverage. Platelets should be transfused in a medical center. Each unit of platelets is expected to raise the platelet count by 10,000. Inadequate response to platelet transfusion should raise a concern about increased destruction of platelets, either by an immunologic mechanism or by hypersplenism. Postoperatively, a 4.8% tranexamic acid mouthwash, 10 ml three to four times a day for 3 to 7 days, may be helpful.

If the platelet count is less than 50,000, platelet transfusion is necessary for dental procedures. Platelet count should be optimized prior to local analgesia and surgery. Block analgesia is contraindicated if the platelet count is less than 50,000.

If the platelet count is less than 20,000, the patient should be referred for medical evaluation and management. All dental procedures should be deferred.

Aspirin and most nonsteroidal anti-inflammatory drugs should be avoided.

Rofecoxib (Vioxx) and celecoxib (Celebrex) appear to be safer choices for analgesia in these patients. These Cox-2 inhibitors do not interact with platelet function and in this regard are unique among NSAIDs.

22. What should a dentist do if he or she finds an abnormal prothrombin time in the patient with hepatitis?

Most patients with hepatitis have a normal prothrombin time. A small percentage of patients may have enough hepatic compromise to have difficulties synthesizing an adequate amount of coagulation factors, These patients may need replacement therapy.

Briefly, the guidelines should be

• The dentist must consult the patient's physician.
• Patients with heavy alcohol consumption may have a dietary deficiency of vitamin K and may be coagulopathic with deficiency of vitamin K–dependent factors (factors II, VII, IX, and X). These patients respond to vitamin K therapy, and this should be coordinated with their physicians. Normally, vitamin K repletion is done by either IV or IM injections of vitamin K, 10 mg each day for 3 days.
• Patients may have coagulopathy related to decreased synthesis of factors produced by the liver (factors I, II, V, VII, IX, and X). Only some of these factors are vitamin K–dependent. Patients with significant coagulopathy need replacement of factors in the form of fresh frozen plasma. This should be coordinated with their physicians, and infusion should be given shortly before the intended dental procedure.
• Generally, dental surgical procedures can be carried out safely if the INR is less than 2.2.
• Most dental procedures can be safely carried out at even higher INRs, up to 3.0 or more.
• Acute alcohol consumption can suppress the bone marrow and result in thrombocytopenia. It is therefore important to reinforce the "no alcohol" rule.

23. How should the dentist modify the use of antibiotics in the patient with hepatitis?

The dentist should be careful in prescribing antibiotics because of the possibility of compromised hepatic clearance of the drugs. Some patients with hepatitis may have completely normal hepatic function, and no substantive changes are necessary for these patients. Others, however, may have significant problems with drug metabolism. In patients with significant hepatic compromise:

• Penicillins and cephalosporins are generally safe to use.
• Clarithromycin (Biaxin) is primarily excreted by the kidneys and only partially metabolized by the liver. It is safe to use in patients with hepatic compromise.
• Erythromycin preparations and azithromax (Zithromax) are metabolized by the liver and should be avoided in patients with hepatic compromise.

- Tetracycline and minocycline are excreted by the kidneys and are safe to use in patients with hepatic compromise.
- Doxycycline is primarily metabolized by the liver and should be avoided.
- Clindamycin (Cleocin) is relatively contraindicated and should be avoided. In instances of severe infection in which clindamycin is the drug of choice, the dose should be reduced in patients with significant hepatic compromise
- Metronidazole (Flagyl), if indicated, should be dose-adjusted in patients with hepatic compromise.

24. How should the dentist modify the use of analgesics in the patient with hepatitis?

The dentist should be careful in prescribing analgesics because of the possibility of compromised hepatic clearance of the drugs. Some patients with hepatitis may have completely normal hepatic function, and no substantive changes are necessary for these patients. Others, however, may have significant problems with drug metabolism. In these patients with significant hepatic compromise:

- If the patient has thrombocytopenia, all aspirin-containing compounds and nonsteroidal anti-inflammatory drugs are contraindicated because of their adverse effect on platelet function.
- COX 2 inhibitors such as rofecoxib (Vioxx) and celecoxib (Celebrex) are safe since they do not affect platelet function
- Acetaminophen (Tylenol) and all compounds containing acetaminophen are contraindicated because of toxicity to the liver. The maximal recommended dose of acetaminophen in a patient with normal liver function is 4000 mg/day. Patients who consume alcohol tolerate a much lower dose before liver toxicity is encountered. Patients with pre-existing liver function compromise should avoid taking any acetaminophen-containing compounds.
- Narcotics should be prescribed in reduced doses because of the concern over decreased drug metabolism. Demerol, codeine, and tramadol (Ultram) should be prescribed in reduced doses.
- All sedatives and tranquilizers should be avoided if possible because of compromised hepatic clearance.

25. How should the dentist protect himself against hepatitis B?

Ideally, all dentists should receive hepatitis B vaccine since they are among some of the highest risk groups for contracting hepatitis B in the work environment. Prior to vaccination, the dentist should have hepatitis B Ag and Ab determinations. Dentists who have positive Ag or antibody responses do not need vaccination. Those with negative hepatitis B Ag and Ab test results are candidates for the vaccine.

Hepatitis B vaccine utilizes a recombinant DNA vaccine and is free of infectious complications. Usually a series of three injections is administered. The dentist should have a follow-up serologic determination to ensure conversion to hepatitis B antibody positivity.

On rare occasion, a second series may be necessary if the dentist remains antibody-negative after the first series.

Hepatitis B vaccine does not confer protection against hepatitis C. There is currently no vaccine for hepatitis C.

26. Does one series of injections of hepatitis B vaccine confer lifelong immunity?

No, it is advisable to receive a booster shot every 5–10 years.

27. If the dentist inadvertently received a needle stick from a patient with acute or chronic hepatitis B, what are the appropriate procedures?

If the dentist has had hepatitis B vaccine and has hepatitis B antibody, he or she should be protected and no further measures are necessary.

If the dentist is hepatitis Ag- and Ab-negative, there is concern about possible infection. The next step is to find out if the patient is indeed infectious. If the patient has infectious hepatitis B and is Hb_sAg- and Hb_eAg-positive, the needle stick carries a 5–8% chance of transmitting hepatitis B.

The dentist should receive hepatitis B immunoglobulin (HBIG) as soon as possible after the needle exposure. Although globulin injections are recommended up to 7 days after inoculation, their efficacy is poor beyond the first 2 days. The dentist should then complete a 3-injection series of hepatitis B vaccine starting immediately after the needle stick in order to confer active immunity.

28. If the dentist inadvertently received a needle stick from a patient with hepatitis C, what are the appropriate procedures?
- There is no vaccine for hepatitis C.
- All patients with hepatitis C remain infectious.
- Unfortunately, immunoglobulin injection after needle exposure has not been proved efficacious in the prevention of hepatitis C transmission.
- Fortunately, hepatitis C transmissibility via needle stick appears to be quite low (less than 1%).
- Other than thorough cleansing of the wound, no other interventions are efficacious.

29. Should the dentist provide hepatitis B vaccine to the employees?
All employees who are likely to come into contact with blood and salivary secretions should be given the option of receiving hepatitis B vaccine. Since the recombinant DNA vaccine carries no infectious complications, there should be little reluctance about receiving the vaccine. It is important to check Hb_sAb a month after the last of the three injections to ensure seroconversion.

21. CIRRHOSIS

Robert C. Fazio, D.M.D., and Leslie S.T. Fang, M.D., Ph.D.

1. What is cirrhosis?

Cirrhosis is the result of severe or protracted injury to the liver causing loss of liver cells and progressive scarring. It is the fourth leading cause of death in young men between the ages of 35 and 54. The major cause of cirrhosis is alcoholic liver disease.

2. Discuss the consequences of cirrhosis.

The liver is a vital organ responsible for synthesis and detoxification. With destruction of hepatic cells, the liver has a diminished capacity to synthesize plasma proteins such as albumin, clotting factors, and lipoproteins. With hepatic insufficiency, the ability to detoxify substances also becomes compromised, and drugs and toxins normally metabolized by the liver may accumulate.

With hepatic insufficiency, the patient may become encephalopathic because of the inability to detoxify even normal products of metabolism.

Furthermore, with scarring of the liver, the portal circulation is blocked, resulting in portal hypertension. This, in turn, leads to the development of ascites and portosystemic collaterals including esophageal varices, a source of frequent massive hemorrhage.

3 Explain the significance of cirrhosis to the dentist.

The patient with cirrhosis presents a special problem for the dentist, Inadequate synthesis of clotting factors may result in prolongation of prothrombin time and clinical bleeding. The inability to detoxify drugs may result in drug accumulation, and the use of even minor sedatives must be carefully weighed.

4. What are the causes of cirrhosis?

The most common cause of cirrhosis is alcoholic liver disease with resultant Laennec's cirrhosis. Cirrhosis can also occur as a result of hepatitis, particularly chronic hepatitis B or hepatitis C. Toxic hepatitis as a result of drug or toxin exposure can also result in cirrhosis. In patients with severe congestive heart failure, passive congestion of the liver can result in cirrhosis. Less commonly, cirrhosis may be a result of inborn error of metabolism. Patients with abnormal iron deposition (hemachromocytosis) or copper deposition (Wilson's disease) may develop cirrhosis. Rarely, patients with autoimmune disease of the liver such as primary biliary cirrhosis can develop cirrhosis.

5. What are the clinical manifestations of cirrhosis?

Cirrhosis may be totally asymptomatic and be found as an incidental finding at autopsy, or it may be clinically compromising. Cirrhosis often becomes clinically apparent late in life, manifesting itself as portal hypertension, fluid retention, and encephalopathy.

Portal hypertension is the result of compromised flow of the portal circulation through a scarred liver. The increase in portal pressure leads to splenomegaly and the formation of a system of collateral veins, which are fragile and can cause severe bleeding (e.g. variceal bleeding). Portal hypertension can also result in ascites.

Fluid retention is the result of hypoalbuminemia. Compromised hepatic synthesis of albumin leads to decreased intravascular oncotic pressure and resultant third-spacing of fluid with ascites and peripheral edema.

Failure to detoxify even normal products of metabolism results in hepatic encephalopathy. Severe encephalopathy can produce coma and seizures.

6. What are the laboratory findings of cirrhosis?

Because of splenomegaly, there is increased sequestration and destruction of platelets in the spleen, and patients often have thrombocytopenia with significant clinical bleeding.

Compromises in hepatic synthesis can result in abnormalities in the levels of clotting factors. Patients often have elevated prothrombin times, accentuating the bleeding diathesis. The poor synthetic capability also results in decreased serum albumin levels. The degree of hypoalbuminemia and of prolongation of prothrombin time gives the clinician an idea of the degree of compromise of synthetic activity.

Patients with cirrhosis may have abnormal liver function test results with elevated transaminases (serum glutamic-oxaloacetate transaminase [SGOT], serum glutamate pyruvate transaminase [SGPT]), alkaline phosphatase, and bilirubin levels. These abnormalities can reflect the degree of ongoing inflammation and portal disruption.

In patients with alcoholic liver disease, dietary deficiency may result in decreased folate and vitamin B_{12} levels, causing macrocytic anemia. Vitamin B_{12} and folate deficiency may also compromise platelet production.

In patients with cirrhosis whose cause is unclear, a liver biopsy is helpful in delineating the degree of scarring and the possible cause.

7. How are patients with cirrhosis managed?

Patients are advised to maintain caloric intake of >2000 to 3000 kcal/day. The use of alcohol and other hepatotoxic agents is prohibited. Tranquilizers and sedatives should be avoided.

Specific therapy is designed to manage ascites, encephalopathy, and variceal bleeding.

8. How is ascites managed in patients with cirrhosis?

Patients with ascites are instructed to restrict daily sodium intake to less than 2 g/day. They should consume >50 g of protein each day. Fluids should be restricted to less than 1.5 L per day.

In patients with symptomatic ascites, spironolactone (Aldactone) is begun to initiate diuresis. If spironolactone is inadequate for fluid mobilization, a diuretic such as furosemide (Lasix) may be added.

Diuretics should be held at the first sign of intravascular volume depletion. Potassium supplement may be necessary in patients on diuretics.

In some instances, large-volume paracentesis may be necessary for patient comfort.

9. How is encephalopathy managed in patients with cirrhosis?

At the first sign of encephalopathy, protein intake should be reduced to 20–30 g/day. Dietary supplement with ornithine, aspartate, benzoate or phenylacetate can be considered. When protein restriction is inadequate, lactulose is often used to control encephalopathy. Lactulose dose is titrated to allow 2–3 loose stools/day. In severe cases, neomycin or metronidazole may be added.

10. How is variceal bleeding managed in patients with cirrhosis?

Patients with variceal bleeding have a precarious and life-threatening condition. They are often managed on low doses of beta-blocker such as propranolol for primary prevention. Beta-blockers appear to be effective in lowering portal pressures. In patients with significant bleeding, endoscopic sclerotherapy and banding may be considered. In patients with severe bleeding, shunting procedures that would decrease portal pressure may be necessary. Currently, transhepatic intravascular placement of a portosystemic shunt (TIPS) is probably the least invasive way of establishing a portosystemic shunt.

In patients with significant clinical bleeding, platelet and fresh frozen plasma replacements may be necessary

11. What are the dental concerns in patients with cirrhosis?

Patients with cirrhosis pose a special problem for the dentist. Inadequate synthesis of clotting factors may result in prolongation of prothrombin time and clinical bleeding. Splenic sequestration and destruction of platelets lead to thrombocytopenia with resultant bleeding. Inability of the liver to detoxify drugs may result in drug accumulation and the use of even minor sedatives must be carefully weighed.

12. **How should a dentist evaluate a patient with cirrhosis?**
    • Potential bleeding problems: The patient should be asked about any history of abnormal bleeding. Clotting factor abnormalities and thrombocytopenia may be present in the patient with severe liver disease. Clotting factor deficiency is the result of inability of the cirrhotic liver to synthesize factors. Platelet deficiency is the result of platelet production difficulties and problems with sequestration in the patient with hypersplenism.
    • The patient should be asked specifically about a history of encephalopathy or variceal bleeding, since these patients are at much higher risk for any intervention.
    • Knowledge of their dietary restrictions and the medications patients are on also provides important clues about the severity of the liver disease. Patients with ascites are likely to have salt and fluid restrictions and to be on spironolactone and furosemide. Patients with a history of encephalopathy are likely to have protein restrictions and are likely to be on lactulose, neomycin, or metronidazole.
    • Labwork for a complete blood count with platelet count, prothrombin time and liver function tests should be available prior to dental intervention.

13. **How should the dentist manage a patient with cirrhosis?**
    The patient with cirrhosis presents a special problem for the dentist:
    • Potential bleeding diathesis: thrombocytopenia and factor deficiencies can result in significant bleeding diathesis
    • Restrictions on the choice of analgesics
    • Restrictions on the choice of antibiotics
    • Restrictions on the use of a number of sedatives

14. **How should a dentist approach a patient with cirrhosis and a bleeding diathesis?**
    Patients with cirrhosis can have significant bleeding diathesis because of abnormal synthesis of clotting factors and thrombocytopenia.
    • A complete blood count with platelet count and prothrombin time should be done prior to any dental procedures.
    • The patient should be instructed to completely abstain from alcohol both before and after the procedure.
    • Patients with normal platelet counts and normal prothrombin times can have dental intervention with careful attention paid to hemostasis.
    • Patients may have decreased platelet count because of hypersplenism, and this should be corrected prior to any dental intervention.
    • Patients with heavy alcohol consumption may have dietary deficiency of vitamin K and may be coagulopathic, with deficiencies of vitamin K–dependent factors (factors II, VII, IX, and X). These patients respond to vitamin K therapy, and this should be coordinated with their physicians. Normally, vitamin K repletion is done by either IV or IM injections of vitamin K, 10 mg each day for 3 days.
    • Dietary deficiency of vitamin B_{12} and folate can also result in macrocytic anemia and thrombocytopenia related to bone marrow suppression.
    • Patients may have coagulopathy related to decreased synthesis of factors produced by the liver (factors I, II, V, VII, IX and X). Only some of these factors will be vitamin K–dependent. Patients with significant coagulopathy require replacement of factors in the form of fresh frozen plasma. This should be coordinated with their physicians and infusions should be given shortly before the intended dental procedure.
    • Acute alcohol consumption can suppress the bone marrow and can result in thrombocytopenia. It is therefore important to reinforce the "no alcohol" rule.

15. **What if the dentist finds a low platelet count?**
    Most patients with cirrhosis have a normal platelet count. Some patients with severe cirrhosis may develop portal hypertension, hypersplenism, and thrombocytopenia.

- If the platelet count is between 50,000–100,000, the patient should be able to form a hemostatic plug but this ability is usually mildly compromised. The dentist should expect some clinical bleeding. Minor surgical interventions, such as the atraumatic removal of one or two teeth, can proceed using careful technique with attention to hemostasis. Local analgesia, including regional block injections, can be done safely. Major surgical interventions should probably be performed under platelet coverage. Platelets should be transfused in a medical center. Each unit of platelet is expected to raise the platelet count by 10,000. Inadequate response to platelet transfusion should raise the concern about increased destruction of platelets, either by an immunologic mechanism or by hypersplenism. Postoperatively, a 4.8% tranexamic acid mouthwash, 10 ml three to four times a day for 3 to 7 days, may be helpful.
- If the platelet count is less than 50,000, platelet transfusion is necessary for dental procedures. Platelet count should be optimized prior to local analgesia and surgery. Block analgesia is contraindicated if the platelet count is less than 50,000.
- If the platelet count is less than 20,000, the patient should be referred for medical evaluation and management. All dental procedures should be deferred.
- Aspirin and nonsteroidal anti-inflammatory drugs should be avoided.
- Rofecoxib (Vioxx) and celecoxib (Celebrex) appear to be safer choices for analgesia in these patients.

16. What should the dentist do if the patient with cirrhosis has an abnormal prothrombin time?

Most patients with cirrhosis should have a normal prothrombin time. Some patients, however, have enough hepatic compromise to have difficulties synthesizing adequate amount of coagulation factors, These patients may need replacement therapy.

Briefly, the guidelines are
- The dentist must consult the patient's physician.
- Patients with heavy alcohol consumption may have dietary deficiency of vitamin K and may be coagulopathic, with deficiency of vitamin K–dependent factors (factors II, VII, IX, and X). These patients will respond to vitamin K therapy and this should be coordinated with their physicians. Normally, vitamin K repletion is done by either IV or IM injections of vitamin K, 10 mg each day for 3 days.
- Patients may have coagulopathy related to decreased synthesis of factors produced by the liver (factors I, II, V, VII, IX, and X). Only some of these factors are vitamin K–dependent. Patients with significant coagulopathy need replacement of factors in the form of fresh frozen plasma. This should be coordinated with their physicians, and infusions should be given shortly before the intended dental procedure.
- Generally, dental surgical procedures can be carried out safely if the INR is less than 2.2.
- Most dental procedures can be safely carried out at even higher INRs, up to 3.0 or more.
- Acute alcohol consumption can suppress the bone marrow and can result in thrombocytopenia. It is therefore important to reinforce the "no alcohol" rule.

17. How should the dentist modify the use of antibiotics in the patient with cirrhosis?

The dentist should be careful in prescribing antibiotics because of the possibility of compromised hepatic clearance of the drugs. Some patients with cirrhosis may have completely normal hepatic function, and no substantive changes are necessary for these patients. Others, however, may have significant problems with drug metabolism. In these patients with significant hepatic compromise:
- Penicillins and cephalosporins are generally safe to use.
- Clarithromycin (Biaxin) is primarily excreted by the kidney and only partially metabolized by the liver. It is safe to use in patients with hepatic compromise.
- Erythromycin preparations and azithromycin (Zithromax) are metabolized by the liver and should be avoided in patients with hepatic compromise.

- Tetracycline and minocycline are excreted by the kidneys and are safe to use in patients with hepatic compromise.
- Doxycycline is primarily metabolized by the liver and should be avoided.
- Clindamycin (Cleocin) is relatively contraindicated and should be avoided. In instances of severe infection in which clindamycin is the drug of choice, the dose should be reduced in patients with significant hepatic compromise.
- Metronidazole (Flagyl), if indicated, should be dose-adjusted in patients with hepatic compromise.

18. How should the dentist modify the use of analgesics in the patient with cirrhosis?

The dentist should be careful in prescribing analgesics because of the possibility of compromised hepatic clearance of the drugs. Some patients with cirrhosis may have completely normal hepatic function, and no substantive changes are necessary for these patients. Others, however, may have significant problems with drug metabolism. In these patients with significant hepatic compromise:

- If the patient has thrombocytopenia, all aspirin-containing compounds and nonsteroidal anti-inflammatory drugs are contraindicated because of their adverse effect on platelet function.
- COX 2 inhibitors such as rofecoxib (Vioxx) and celecoxib (Celebrex) are safe because they do not affect platelet function.
- Acetaminophen (Tylenol) and all compounds containing acetaminophen are contraindicated because of toxicity to the liver. The maximal recommended dose of acetaminophen in a patient with normal liver function is 4000 mg/day. Patients who consume alcohol tolerate a much lower dose before liver toxicity is encountered. Patients with pre-existing liver function compromise should avoid taking any acetaminophen-containing compounds.
- Narcotics should be prescribed in reduced doses because of the concern over decreased drug metabolism. Demerol, codeine, and tramadol (Ultram) should be prescribed in reduced doses.
- All sedatives and tranquilizers should be avoided if possible because of compromised hepatic clearances.

19. How should a dentist manage a patient with a history of hepatic encephalopathy?

Although the dentist should be exceedingly judicious in the use of any drug metabolized by the liver in a patient with cirrhosis, this should be of particular concern in the patient who has already had a history of hepatic encephalopathy. Sedatives, tranquilizers, and analgesics commonly used in the dental practice cannot be prescribed because of possible aggravation of encephalopathy. The patient's physician should be consulted before medication is prescribed.

22. ANEMIA

Robert C. Fazio, D.M.D., and Leslie S.T. Fang, M.D., Ph.D.

1. What is anemia?

Anemia is defined as a decrease in the number of circulating red blood cells, a decrease in hemoglobin concentration, and/or a decrease in hematocrit. Anemia is a relatively common condition with a reported incidence of 17–18 cases per 1000 population annually.

2. What are the common causes of anemia?

Anemia can result from excessive blood loss, decreased red cell production, or increased destruction of red blood cells. Blood loss is the most common cause of anemia. In young women, excessive blood loss during menstruation is a frequent cause. Blood loss can also result from structural lesions in the gastrointestinal tract, such as polyps, ulcers, or cancers.

Decreased production of red cells can occur as dietary deficiency of iron, folate, or vitamin B_{12}. Other causes include decreased erythropoietin production as a result of renal disease or other chronic diseases, or defects in stem cell proliferation, hemoglobin synthesis, or DNA synthesis. A number of drugs can compromise the ability of the bone marrow to produce adequate red cells.

Increased destruction of red cells can result from disorders of red cell membrane (hereditary spherocytosis), disorder of hemoglobin synthesis (thalassemia, sickle cell anemia), deficiency of enzymes such as glucose-6-phosphate dehydrogenase (G-6-PD), or antibody mediated hemolysis. Hypersplenism, with a resultant increase in reticuloendothelial system activity, can result in increased sequestration and destruction of red cells.

3. What are the clinical manifestations of anemia?

Patients with anemia may be asymptomatic and have the disease discovered during a routine evaluation. Patients are generally asymptomatic until the hematocrit falls below 30 ml/dl. At lower levels of hematocrit, patients may develop fatigue, weakness, dizziness, and dyspnea on exertion. With severe anemia, significant orthostatic symptoms may appear, and patients may have dyspnea even at rest.

4. What are the oral findings in patients with anemia?

The patient may have atrophic glossitis and angular cheilitis on oral examination.

5. What laboratory tests are useful in the evaluation of anemia?

The medical evaluation of anemia requires a systematic approach because there are a great many possible causes and a vast array of diagnostic tests are available. In most instances, the initial laboratory tests include a complete blood count and determination of mean corpuscular volume (MCV) and mean corpuscular hemoglobin concentration (MCHC). A blood smear is done to examine the morphologic appearance of the blood cells under the microscope. Based on all the morphology, the causes of the anemia can be categorized. Under the microscope, the red cells may be small (microcytic), normal (normocytic), or large (macrocytic), and they may contain low (hypochromic) or normal (normochromic) amounts of hemoglobin.

6. What are the causes of microcytic hypochromic anemia?

By far the most common cause of microcytic hypochromic anemia is iron deficiency resulting from excess blood loss. Inadequate intake or poor absorption of iron can also result in microcytic hypochromic anemia. In menstruating women, excessive blood loss and inadequate dietary iron replacement can result in anemia. In one study, iron deficiency anemia was found in 10 to 20% of women studied. In men and nonmenstruating females, blood loss is usually from an occult source in the gastrointestinal tract, such as gastritis, ulcer, polyps, or cancer. It is important to assess the cause of the iron deficiency anemia in these patients because many can result in other serious complications.

Patients with poor dietary habits may become iron-deficient. In some instances, iron deficiency is the result of poor gastrointestinal absorption. This can happen in patients with tropical sprue and in those who have had a partial gastrectomy. Microcytic hypochromic anemia can also occur in patients with chronic disease. Patients with thalassemia can also have microcytic hypochromic anemia. This is a genetic disorder that results in abnormal hemoglobin production and occurs more frequently in patients of Mediterranean descent. Some patients with sideroblastic anemia may also have macrocytic hypochromic anemia.

7. How is a patient with microcytic hypochromic anemia evaluated?

Since the majority of patients with microcytic hypochromic anemia have iron deficiency, a thorough history should be obtained to examine the possible sources of blood loss. The evaluation should include a ferritin test, which is an accurate way of determining iron stores. Patients with iron deficiency have low serum ferritin levels. However, since ferritin is an acute phase reactant, it may be elevated in patients with an underlying inflammatory condition. In these instances, an iron and iron binding capacity should be obtained. Patients with iron deficiency should have a low serum iron (Fe) level and a high total iron binding capacity (TIBC), with a resultant iron saturation (Fe/TIBC) that is less than 15%.

Patients with normal iron studies should be evaluated for anemia of chronic disease, sideroblastic anemia, and thalassemia.

The diagnosis of thalassemia can be made on the basis of a family history of anemia and Mediterranean extraction. Determination of the hemoglobin A_2 level will lead to the diagnosis of thalassemia. In instances in which the diagnosis is unclear even after the above evaluation, a bone marrow biopsy may be necessary.

8. How is microcytic hypochromic anemia treated?

In patients with iron deficiency, the patient is advised to eat a diet high in dietary iron (e.g., liver, lean red meat, veal, oysters, iron-enriched cereals, and beans). In patients with severe anemia or in patients who have responded poorly to dietary repletion, an oral iron supplement can be prescribed. It is important not to prescribe excessive amount of iron for prolonged periods of time because it is associated with increased risk of malignancy and atherosclerotic disease.

Parenteral iron is usually not recommended unless there is a demonstrated problem with gastrointestinal absorption of iron.

Patients with anemia of chronic disease should have the underlying disease addressed. In some instances, erythropoietin injections may be helpful in patients with symptomatic anemia.

Patients with Mediterranean anemia usually have very mild anemia and do not require therapy.

9. How is a patient with macrocytic anemia evaluated?

Macrocytic anemia is often the result of dietary folate or vitamin B_{12} deficiency. Less commonly, it may be associated with aplastic anemia, acute hemolysis, or hemorrhage with brisk reticulocytosis, chronic liver disease, myelodysplastic syndrome, and severe hypothyroidism.

On blood smear, vitamin B_{12} and folate deficiencies are associated with hypersegmented polymorphonuclear white cells and macrocytes.

A blood smear will also allow the clinician to make the diagnosis of brisk reticulocytosis and chronic liver disease. Vitamin B_{12} and folate levels should be obtained. In instances where the diagnosis is elusive, a bone marrow biopsy may be necessary.

10. How is macrocytic anemia treated?

Once the diagnosis is made, dietary deficiency can be aggressively replaced. Folate can be given orally. Vitamin B_{12} deficiency is usually secondary to an inherent lack of an intrinsic factor necessary for vitamin B_{12} absorption. For these patients, vitamin B_{12} has to be administered monthly by injection for the remainder of their lives. This is important because vitamin B_{12}

deficiency is associated not only with anemia but also with severe and sometimes permanent neurologic damage.

11. How is a patient with normocytic anemia evaluated?
Normocytic anemia can be associated with chronic diseases, chronic renal insufficiency, and hemolysis. Rare causes of normocytic anemia include hypothyroidism, myelofibrosis, and sideroblastic anemia.
Evaluation should begin with a blood smear. Diagnosis of hemolysis can be readily made on the basis of increased reticulocytes. Anemia associated with chronic disease and renal insufficiency is associated with low reticulocyte counts.

12. How is anemia of chronic disease treated?
Anemia of chronic disease is treated by management of the underlying disease. In some instances, such as renal insufficiency, erythropoietin therapy may be necessary.

13. How is a patient with hemolysis evaluated?
Hemolysis can be the result of drugs, an autoimmune mechanism, a hereditary mechanism (sickle cell anemia and hereditary spherocytosis), a cold-agglutinin–induced mechanism (viral infection, lymphoma), or microangiopathy (heart valve, vasculitis, disseminated intravascular coagulopathy). These various causes can be differentiated on the basis of a battery of tests, including Coomb's test, cold agglutinin, hemoglobin electrophoresis, or determination of G-6-PD activity.

14. How is hemolytic anemia treated?
Drugs that can potentially cause hemolysis should be stopped. In instances of autoimmune hemolysis, a brief course of steroids is often very helpful. In patients with hemoglobinopathy, specific therapy can be directed to the disease. Patients with severe hemolysis may benefit from splenectomy.

15. What is the significance of the various kinds of anemia to the dentist?
Anemia can complicate dental management since most patients with significant anemia are in a hypermetabolic state. Additional stresses can tip the patient over, particularly patients with coronary disease.

16. What is the correct dental evaluation of patients with anemia?
The dentist may suspect anemia in a patient presenting with pallor who complains of fatigue, weakness and dizziness. These patients should have a complete blood count prior to dental intervention.
More commonly, the dentist has a patient with a known history of anemia. The patient should be asked about the exact cause of the anemia, the therapeutic interventions undertaken, and the medications used. Assessment should also include a determination of whether symptoms are present in the patient. A recent complete blood count is important in the overall evaluation.

17. How should the dentist manage the patient with anemia?
The dental management of individuals with anemia should be tailored to the patient's clinical status. The dentist should be aware of the cause and the extent of the patient's anemia and determine the proper course of dental intervention. Patients who are symptomatic from their anemia should have their clinical status stabilized prior to elective dental intervention.
Patients with significant anemia are not candidates for outpatient general anesthesia or intravenous sedation. For these patients, a medical consultation is necessary.
It is important to understand the cause of the anemia, since the management of the patient with iron deficiency is very different from the management of this patient with bone marrow suppression secondary to malignancy.

18. Which patients with anemia are at the highest risk?
• Patients with a low hemoglobin or abnormal MCV and MCHC and an undiagnosed anemia
• All patients with a hematocrit of less than 30mg/dl (hemoglobin of less than 10 g/dl) with no clear cause
• Patients with anemia and a coagulopathy
• Patients who require repeated blood transfusions

19. Which patients with anemia are at low risk?
• Patients with a history of anemia that has been treated and corrected
• Patients with mild anemia (hematocrit higher than 30 mg/dl and hemoglobin higher than 10 g/dl) who require no intervention
• Patients with identified causes of anemia who are asymptomatic and under treatment
• Asymptomatic patients with anemia of chronic disease and a hematocrit of higher than 30 ml/dl

20. How should a dentist manage an anemic patient at low risk?
In general, normal dental protocols can be employed.

21. Is angular cheilitis always associated with vitamin B_{12} deficiency?
No; other common causes include fungal infection. Lost vertical dimension can also lead to angular cheilitis. Treatment of angular cheilitis can therefore range from vitamin B_{12} replacement to use of Mycolog cream to denture replacement.

22. What is Mycolog cream?
A combination of the steroid, triamcinolone acetate, and the antifungal, nystatin. It should be applied to the affected area bid, not to exceed 25 days. If the dentist has ruled out lost vertical dimension as the etiology, this drug is a reasonable first-line treatment. Patients are often advised to add a multivitamin. If there is no response, the patient should be referred for an anemia workup.

23. BLEEDING DISORDERS

Robert C. Fazio, D.M.D., and Leslie S.T. Fang, M.D., Ph.D.

1. Why do patients have bleeding disorders?

Hemostasis is a complicated process involving a number of physiologic events. When a blood vessel is damaged, marked vasoconstriction results. Platelets adhere to the damaged surface and aggregate to form a temporary hemostatic plug. Through two separate pathways, the intrinsic and the extrinsic pathways, involving a cascade of 12 circulating plasma proteins called clotting factors, the conversion of fibrinogen to fibrin is completed. Fibrin binds to the aggregated platelets to form a definitive hemostatic clot. Finally, anticlotting mechanisms in the fibrinolytic pathway are activated to prevent propagation of the clot and to allow for clot dissolution and repair of the damaged vessel. The fibrinolytic pathway is designed to limit the amount of clot that can form during the healing process. Successful hemostasis is therefore dependent on adequate numbers of platelets, proper functioning of the platelets, adequate levels of clotting factors, and proper functioning of the fibrinolytic pathway.

In brief, platelets are responsible for the formation of a temporary plug, and clotting factors are responsible for the formation of a permanent clot.

2. What are the major causes of bleeding?

Bleeding can be the result of inability to form a temporary clot or the inability to form a definitive clot. Inability to form a temporary clot results from inadequate platelet count (thrombocytopenia) or abnormal platelet function (thrombocytopathy). Inability to form a definitive clot results from abnormalities in the clotting factors.

3. What are the dental concerns with respect to bleeding diathesis?

Although there are myriad problems that can cause bleeding, the most common reasons for abnormal clotting in the dental setting revolve around patient ingestion of aspirin and nonsteroidal anti-inflammatory drugs, which interferes with platelet function, and the ingestion of coumadin, which interferes with clotting factor synthesis.

It is important to stress to the patient that alcohol can further accentuate bleeding diathesis.

It is also important for the dentist to know how to manage patients with hemophilia.

4. What are the tests available to evaluate hemostasis?

The most common defects in hemostasis involve abnormalities of platelets or coagulation factors. These defects can be diagnosed with a few simple laboratory tests: platelet count, bleeding time, which measures the function of the platelets and prothrombin time (PT) and partial thromboplastin time (PTT), which measure the integrity of the clotting factors.

5. What is an abnormal platelet count (thrombocytopenia)?

The platelet count provides a quantitative evaluation of platelet function. The normal platelet count should be 100,000 to 400,000 cells/mm^3. A platelet count of less than 100,000 cells/mm^3 is called thrombocytopenia. Mild thrombocytopenia (platelet count of 50,000 to 100,000 cells/mm^3) can result in abnormal bleeding postoperatively. Severe thrombocytopenia (less than 50,000 cells/mm^3) can be associated with major postoperative bleeding, and for these patients platelet transfusion is often necessary prior to any dental intervention.

6. How is platelet function assessed?

The bleeding time provides an assessment of the adequacy of platelet count and function. The test measures how long it takes for a standardized skin incision to stop bleeding by the formation of a temporary plug. Using the standard Ivy method, the normal bleeding time is 5–9 minutes. The bleeding time is prolonged in patients with either thrombocytopenia or abnormal platelet function.

A patient taking aspirin may have a bleeding time of 9–12 minutes. This can lead to mild intra-operative and postoperative bleeding. A patient on clopidogrel (Plavix) may have a bleeding time longer than 12 minutes and can have significant bleeding intraoperatively and postoperatively.

7. How is the integrity of the clotting factors assessed?
Two tests, the PT and the PTT, provide a reasonable measure of the integrity of the clotting factors.

8. What does the PT measure?
The PT measures the effectiveness of the extrinsic pathway to mediate fibrin clot formation. A normal PT indicates normal levels of factor VII and those factors common both to the intrinsic and the extrinsic pathways (factors V, X, prothrombin, and fibrinogen). PT can be expressed in a number of ways: as PT in seconds with a value for control; as PTR, which is the ratio of the patient's PT in comparison to the control PT; or as INR, which is the most accurate way of following PT. INR takes into account reagent variability and allows for the most accurate monitoring of PT. A normal INR is 1, and an INR above 2 usually denotes coagulopathy.

Patients taking coumadin have a prolonged PT/INR because of the interference of coumadin with the synthesis of vitamin K clotting factors. PT/INR are monitored frequently in these patients (weekly to monthly). A normal therapeutic range of INR would usually be in the 2 to 3 range. Patients requiring high-intensity anticoagulation may have an INR in the 2.5 to 3.5 range.

9. What does the PTT measure?
PTT measures the effectiveness of the intrinsic pathway in mediating fibrin clot formation. This tests for all factors except factor VII. PTT is usually expressed in seconds. A normal PTT is usually 25 to 40 seconds. Prolongation of the PTT by 5 to 10 seconds above the upper limit of normal may be associated with mild bleeding abnormalities. Further prolongation may be associated with significant clinical bleeding.

PTT is commonly used to monitor heparin therapy. It is sometimes used to screen for hemophilia A and B.

10. What are the bleeding disorders associated with platelet problems?
In general, the disorders are either attributable to a decrease in platelet count (thrombocytopenia) or to a disorder in platelet function (thrombocytopathy).

11. What are the common causes of thrombocytopenia?
• Drug-induced thrombocytopenia: A number of drugs can cause thrombocytopenia. This can be mediated by some marrow suppression or by increased destruction of platelets. Cytotoxic drugs (such as chemotherapeutic agents or immunosuppressive drugs), alcohol, and thiazide diuretics are the most common drugs implicated in the suppression of platelet production from the bone marrow. Drugs that are associated with increased peripheral destruction of platelets include quinine, quinidine, sulfonamides, and methyldopa. Gold, penicillamine, and p-aminosalicylic acid can also cause enhanced platelet destruction. The peripheral destruction of platelets is usually mediated via immunologic mechanisms.
• Immune thrombocytopenic purpura (ITP): ITP is a rare autoimmune disease causing rapid destruction of platelets, usually an acute illness that resolves either spontaneously or with treatment. In rare instances, ITP may recur. Severe ITP can be associated with profound thrombocytopenia (platelet counts < 5000 cells/mm^3) and can be associated with significant clinical bleeding.
  The dentist is more likely to encounter a patient giving a history of prior ITP that has completely resolved. The dentist should defer all elective procedures in a patient with active ITP.

- Thrombotic thrombocytopenic purpura (TTP): This is also a rare autoimmune disease but is much more serious than ITP because of related other systemic complications. Patients with TTP not only have thrombocytopenia but also have fevers, hemolytic anemia, and renal and neurologic complications. Severe TTP can be associated with profound thrombocytopenia (platelet counts < 5,000 cells/mm^3) and can be associated with significant clinical bleeding.

  The dentist is more likely to encounter a patient giving a history of prior TTP that has completely resolved. The dentist should defer all elective procedures in a patient with active TTP.

- Bone marrow failure: thrombocytopenia can occur because of failure of the bone marrow. Bone marrow failure can be secondary to drugs, a deficiency of vitamin B$_{12}$ or folate, or involvement of the bone marrow by infiltrative diseases. Widely metastatic cancer, leukemia, and myeloma can cause bone marrow suppression. In other patients, bone marrow failure may be the result of myelofibrosis. In most instances, bone marrow failure can be recognized because the other cell lines are also affected, causing pancytopenia.

- Hypersplenism: thrombocytopenia can be the result of hypersplenism. The most common cause of hypersplenism is portal hypertension secondary to cirrhosis. Other causes, such as chronic infection, inflammatory diseases, neoplasm, and storage disease, are considerably less common.

- Human immunodeficiency virus (HIV) infection: Patients with HIV infection can develop thrombocytopenia. The thrombocytopenia may precede other symptoms. Thrombocytopenia in these patients is believed to be related to the bone marrow suppressive effect of the virus.

  Furthermore, drugs used to treat HIV infection can often have suppressive effects on the bone marrow, further accentuating thrombocytopenia.

12. What are the common causes of thrombocytopathy?

In thrombocytopathy, despite the normal number of platelets, the platelets do not function normally and form a temporary ineffective hemostatic plug, with resultant clinical bleeding. Thrombocytopathy can be the result of either inherited or acquired disorders.

13. What are the inherited disorders of platelet function?

Several inherited disorders affect platelet function. The most common is von Willebrand's disease. In this disease, there is both an abnormality in the function of platelets and a deficiency in the production of factor VII. Patients with this disease can therefore bleed both from a platelet abnormality and from factor VII deficiency. Other inherited disorders of platelet function include Bernard-Soulier syndrome and storage pool diseases.

14. What are the acquired disorders of platelet function?

Acquired disorders of platelet function are far more common than inherited disorders.

- Drug-induced defects: by far the most common reason for thrombocytopathy is drug-induced. Aspirin and aspirin-containing compounds are the most common drugs to cause platelet function abnormalities. Aspirin inhibits cyclo-oxygenase in the platelets in an irreversible fashion. Once a platelet is exposed to aspirin, its function is irreversibly compromised. The effect of aspirin in susceptible patients therefore lasts the lifetime of the platelet population exposed. Patients exposed to even low doses of aspirin can have platelet function abnormalities for 7–10 days. This is not a dose-dependent phenomenon, and patients on 81 mg of aspirin can have as much platelet function abnormality as patients taking a much higher dose.

  Clopidogrel (Plavix) is another agent that inhibits cyclo-oxygenase irreversibly and causes platelet function abnormalities for 7–10 days after last exposure.

  Nonsteroidal anti-inflammatory drugs, on the other hand, cause reversible inhibition of cyclo-oxygenase. The effect of the nonsteroidal anti-inflammatory drugs on platelet function therefore lasts only the lifetime of the drug, and thrombocytopathy is usually reversed 24 to 48 hours after the last exposure to the drugs.

The newer COX-2-specific inhibitors (rofecoxib [Vioxx] and celecoxib [Celebrex]) do not affect platelet function.

Concurrent ingestion of alcohol with aspirin or nonsteroidal anti-inflammatory drugs can markedly enhance thrombocytopathy.

Other drugs that have been rarely reported to cause thrombocytopathy include the tricyclic antidepressants, phenothiazines, carbenicillin, nitrofurantoin, dipyridamole, and some cephalosporins.

- Uremia: chronic renal insufficiency is a common reason for platelet function abnormalities. Platelet function is impaired by a circulating toxin, which can be cleared by dialysis. Uremic platelet dysfunction usually occurs at blood urea nitrogen above 50 (normal levels 10–20 mg/dl).
- Myeloproliferative disorders: less commonly, patients with myeloproliferative disorders such as essential thrombocythemia, polycythemia vera, chronic lymphocytic lymphoma and myeloid dyplasia can have impaired platelet function.

15. What are the common disorders of blood coagulation?

Coagulation factor deficiency is caused either by a congenital disorder or by acquired disorder.

16. What are the common congenital disorders of factor deficiency?

A number of congenital clotting factor deficiencies have been described, but three diseases account for more than 90% of all inherited coagulation factor deficiencies.

- [a] Hemophilia A: hemophilia A, or classic hemophilia, is caused by a deficiency of factor VIII. The disorder is inherited in a sex-linked recessive fashion and is therefore more common in males. The severity of the disease closely parallels the level of circulating factor VIII. Patients with severe disease have less than 1% factor VIII. Patients with moderate disease have 1–5% factor VIII, and patients with mild disease have levels of factor VIII ranging from 5–30%.
- Hemophilia B: hemophilia B, or Christmas disease, is secondary to factor IX deficiency. The disorder is also transmitted in a sex-linked recessive fashion.
- von Willebrand's disease: there are many modes of inheritance of this disease. Patients with this disease have evidence of both abnormal platelet function and deficiency of factor VIII.

17. What are the acquired disorders of blood coagulation?

Deficiency of vitamin K–dependent coagulation factors is the most common acquired disorder of coagulation. Factors II (prothrombin), VII, IX, and X are made in the liver and require vitamin K for synthesis of their active forms. Among these factors, factor VII has the shortest half-life (3–5 hours). Therefore, prolongation of PT (which measures factor VII activity) is the first indicator of deficiency of vitamin K-dependent factors. Common causes of acquired disorders of coagulation include:

- Oral anticoagulants: Coumarin anticoagulants competitively inhibit vitamin K action. Patients on anticoagulants therefore have a prolonged PT.
- Liver disease: With significant liver disease, synthesis of a number of coagulation factors is impaired. Vitamin K–dependent factors (II, VII, IX, and X) as well as factors I and V are all synthesized by the liver. Patients with severe liver disease can therefore have significant compromise in their blood's ability to clot.
- Heparin therapy: Heparin acts by accelerating the inactivation of thrombin. It is usually administered intravenously for the treatment of thromboembolic diseases.

  Low-molecular-weight heparin (delteparin or Fragmin) is now used as a subcutaneous preparation and has the same effect as intravenous heparin. Low-molecular-weight heparin has a half-life of about 12 hours and can be administered subcutaneously. Because it is administered subcutaneously, the medication can be given on an outpatient basis, usually on a twice a day regimen. The use of low-molecular-weight heparin now allows for discontinuation of coumadin and for heparinization to be carried out in the outpatient setting.

- Malabsorption: Vitamin K is a fat-soluble vitamin and requires bile acids for absorption. Patients with intestinal diseases that would interfere with fat absorption have problems with vitamin K absorption. Vitamin K deficiency can result in insufficient synthesis of vitamin K–dependent factors.
- Long-term use of broad-spectrum antibiotics: on rare occasion, patients on long-term broad-spectrum antibiotics can alter the colonic flora sufficiently to cause decreased vitamin K synthesis.

18. How should the dentist approach the patient with regard to bleeding diathesis?

By far the most important process in the dental evaluation is a detailed history from the patient. Identification of the susceptible patient greatly decreases the likelihood of severe bleeding. The dental history should include:

- Known bleeding disorders: Patients with hemophilia, liver disease, bone marrow disease, and uremia should be carefully assessed for hemostatic abnormalities prior to any dental intervention.
- History of abnormal bleeding: patients should be asked specifically about prior history of abnormal bleeding. Gingival bleeding is not an infrequent indicator of a bleeding diathesis. Abnormal bleeding associated with prior surgeries, history of easy bruising, history of frequent nosebleeds, and history of excessive menstrual bleeding should all be red flags for further evaluation.
- Family history of abnormal bleeding: careful history of family history of bleeding can lead to identification of patients with inherited disorder of hemostasis
- Medication history: all drugs that can cause thrombocytopenia, thrombocytopathy, bone marrow suppression, and interference with the coagulation pathways should be identified and stopped at appropriate times prior to dental intervention. The key medications to specifically identify include aspirin, aspirin-containing compounds, nonsteroidal anti-inflammatory drugs, coumadin, and clopidogrel.

19. What are the basic tests the dentist should order to assess hemostasis?

In general, complete blood count with platelet count, bleeding time, PT, and PTT should address most of the concerns with hemostasis. In rare instances, specific tests such as platelet aggregation tests or factor levels may be appropriate. The latter tests have to be coordinated with the patient's physician.

20. When should the dentist order these tests?

- A patient who has a strong personal or family history of bleeding should be screened.
- A patient known to be on medications that can cause thrombocytopenia should be screened.
- Patients with prior history of illnesses that can interfere with hemostasis should be screened (e.g., ITP, TTP).
- Patients on coumadin must be screened.

21. What should the dentist do in a patient identified to have thrombocytopenia (platelet count < 100,000)?

By far the most important issue is the identification of the cause of the thrombocytopenia. If the cause is not obvious, the patient should be referred to his or her physician for further evaluation prior to any dental intervention.

- Is the patient on drugs that can interfere with platelet production?
- Is the patient on drugs that can accelerate platelet destruction?
- Does the patient have liver disease and portal hypertension?
- Does the patient have other diseases that can cause hypersplenism?
- Does the patient have diseases that can cause bone marrow failure?

22. What should the dentist do if a patient is found to have a prolonged bleeding time (BT > 9 minutes)?

Again, it is important to identify the cause of the thrombocytopathy.

- All medications taken within the preceding 2 weeks should be reviewed. Specifically, patients should be asked about use of any product that may contain aspirin, non-steroidal anti-inflammatory drugs, and clopidogrel (Plavix).
- Patients with renal disease should be identified.
- Patients with inherited disorders of platelet function should be identified. Patients should be screened for von Willebrand's disease.

23. What should the dentist do if a patient is found to have a prolonged PT (INR > 1.5)?

It is important to identify the cause of the prolongation of PT

- Is the patient on medications that can cause abnormalities in the synthesis of coagulation factors? Is the patient on an anticoagulant?
- Does the patient have liver disease?
- Does the patient have intestinal diseases that can interfere with bile salt production?
- Does the patient have malabsorption?
- Is the patient on long-term broad-spectrum antibiotics?

24. What should the dentist do if a patient is found to have a prolonged PTT (> 40 sec)?

It is important to identify the cause of the prolongation of PTT.

- Does the patient have liver disease?
- Is the patient on heparin?
- Is the patient on low-molecular-weight heparin?
- Does the patient have hemophilia (classic or Christmas disease)?
- Does the patient have von Willebrand's disease?

25. How should the dentist manage a patient with thrombocytopenia?

Management is in part dictated by the underlying cause of thrombocytopenia and in part by the degree of thrombocytopenia. In all instances, if the thrombocytopenia is caused by a reversible process, dental procedures should be deferred until the platelet counts return to normal. In instances where the thrombocytopenia is deemed irreversible, management should be dictated by the degree of thrombocytopenia.

- If the platelet count is between 50,000 and 100,000 cells/mm^3, the patient should be able to form a hemostatic plug but this ability is usually mildly compromised. The dentist should expect some clinical bleeding. Minor surgical interventions, such as the atraumatic removal of one or two teeth, can proceed using careful technique with attention to hemostasis. Local anesthesia, including regional block injections can be done safely. Major surgical interventions should probably be done under platelet coverage. Platelet should be transfused in a medical center. Each unit of platelet is expected to raise the platelet count by 10,000 cells/mm^3. Inadequate response to platelet transfusion should raise the concern about increased destruction of platelets, either by an immunologic mechanism or by hypersplenism. Postoperatively a 4.8% tranexamic acid mouthwash, 10 ml three to four times a day for 3 to 7 days, may be helpful.
- If the platelet count is less than 50,000 cells/mm^3, platelet transfusion is necessary for dental procedures. Platelet count should be optimized prior to local anesthesia and surgery. Block anesthesia is contraindicated if the platelet count is less than 50,000 cells/mm^3.
- If the platelet count is less than 20,000 cells/mm^3, all dental procedures should be deferred.

26. In the thrombocytopenic patient, how should platelet transfusion be carried out?

Platelets can be replaced or supplemented by platelet transfusion, but the sequestration of platelets is very rapid. When given prophylactically, half the platelets should be given before surgery to control capillary bleeding and the other half after operation to facilitate the placement of adequate sutures.

27. What should the dentist do to control bleeding in the thrombocytopenic patient?
If bleeding occurs post-operatively, additional platelet transfusions should be carried out to minimize bleeding. Local hemostatic measures with the use of tranexamic acid topically or platelet concentrates locally may be helpful. A 4.8% tranexamic acid mouthwash, 10 ml three to four times a day for three to seven days, may be helpful.

28. How should the dentist manage a patient with thrombocytopathy?
• Most of the problem with thrombocytopathy that the dentist would encounter comes from exposure to drugs that can impair platelet function. The most common drugs include aspirin, clopidogrel (Plavix), and nonsteroidal anti-inflammatory drugs. Stopping these drugs at appropriate intervals prior to dental intervention should reverse the thrombocytopathy.
• In instances where the patient has a known underlying disease causing thrombocytopathy, careful attention to hemostasis should be employed. Specific recommendations depend on the underlying disease and the degree of the platelet function abnormalities.
• In patients likely to have thrombocytopathy (e.g., a patient with renal insufficiency), determining a bleeding time is helpful in management.
• A normal bleeding time using the Ivy method is between 5 and 9 minutes. A bleeding time of 9–12 minutes denotes a mild thrombocytopathy. Minor dental procedures can proceed with attention to hemostasis. Bleeding time longer than 12 minutes denotes a significant degree of platelet dysfunction. Dental procedures should be delayed until the bleeding time is corrected.
• Local measures that will help hemostasis should be employed.

29. What are local measures that can help hemostasis?
• Compressive packing and dressing
• Extra sutures
• Microfibrillar collagen hemostat
• Oxidized cellulose
• 4.8% tranexamic acid mouthwash

30. How should the dentist manage a patient taking aspirin or aspirin-containing medications?
Aspirin binds the cyclo-oxygenase system in the platelet irreversibly and impairs platelet function for the duration of the lifetime of the exposed platelets. Aspirin and aspirin-containing medications should therefore be stopped 7–10 days prior to planned elective dental procedures. In urgent situation, surgery can proceed with careful hemostatic protocol. Most patients would have only mild prolongation of bleeding time (9–12 minutes) on aspirin. However, a rare patient may have an idiosyncratic response and have a bleeding time of longer than 12 minutes.

Local hemostatic measures using compressive packing and dressing, extra sutures, microfibrillar collagen hemostat, oxidized cellulose, tranexamic acid topically, or platelet concentrates locally may be helpful. A 4.8% tranexamic acid mouthwash, 10 ml three to four times a day for 3 to 7 days, may be helpful.

31. How should the dentist manage a patient taking nonsteroidal anti-inflammatory drugs?
Because the inhibition of cyclo-oxygenase by nonsteroidal anti-inflammatory drugs is reversible, most dentists may elect to proceed with dental interventions using careful hemostatic protocol. Based on intraoperative assessment of bleeding, local hemostatic measures using compressive packing and dressing, extra sutures, microfibrillar collagen hemostat, oxidized cellulose, tranexamic acid topically, or platelet concentrates locally may be helpful. A 4.8% tranexamic acid mouthwash, 10 ml three to four times a day for 3 to 7 days, may be helpful. When maximum hemostasis is required, all NSAIDs should be stopped 72 hours prior to the planned dental surgery. The selective Cox-2 inhibitors (Vioxx, Celebrex) can be continued in all circumstances.

32. How should the dentist manage a patient taking clopidogrel (Plavix)?
Clopidogrel (Plavix) should be stopped 7–10 days prior to planned dental procedures. Since clopidogrel can sometimes cause anemia and leukopenia in addition to the thrombocytopathy, a complete laboratory blood count should be obtained. Unlike aspirin, patients on clopidogrel may have a significantly prolonged bleeding time (>12 minutes) and significant bleeding can occur if the drug is continued through dental surgery.

Local hemostatic measures using compressive packing and dressing, extra sutures, microfibrillar collagen hemostat, oxidized cellulose, or tranexamic acid topically may be helpful. A 4.8% tranexamic acid mouthwash, 10 ml three to four times a day for 3 to 7 days, may be helpful.

33. What should the dentist do if a patient with thrombocytopathy has postoperative bleeding?
Desmopressin (DDAVP), a synthetic analogue of vasopressin that induces the release of factor VIIIC, von Willebrand's factor, and tissue plasminogen activator from storage sites in the endothelium can be given as a slow intravenous infusion (0.4 µg/kg) and repeated every 12 hours for up to 4 days. Local hemostatic measures using compressive packing and dressing, extra sutures, microfibrillar collagen hemostat, oxidized cellulose, or tranexamic acid topically may be helpful. A 4.8% tranexamic acid mouthwash, 10 ml three to four times a day for 3 to 7 days, may be helpful.

34. How should the dentist manage a patient with chronic renal disease?
Renal insufficiency can be gauged by knowing the patient's blood urea nitrogen (BUN) or creatinine level. Normal patients have a BUN level in the 10–20 range. Patients with moderate compromise in renal function often would have a BUN level greater than 50. Patients with BUN levels higher than 50 can have abnormalities in platelet function with resultant bleeding diathesis. The dentist should therefore be concerned about the possibility of bleeding complications in these patients.

To assess the degree of thrombocytopathy, the dentist should coordinate with the patient's physician and obtain an Ivy bleeding time.

The interference with platelet function is usually mild and no specific interventions are necessary for patients with bleeding time less than 12 minutes.

In a small subset of patients with renal disease, the bleeding time may be markedly prolonged. Although there are a number of approaches to these patients, the most practical is the use of desmopressin (DDAVP) (0.4 µg/kg) intravenously prior to the planned dental procedures. This obviously must be coordinated with the patient's physician utilizing a medical center for infusion. DDAVP can be repeated every 12 hours as necessary for up to 4 days.

Patients on hemodialysis or chronic peritoneal dialysis have adequate removal of the uremic toxin that causes thrombocytopathy and DO NOT need determination of bleeding times prior to dental interventions.

If clinical bleeding occurs postoperatively, DDAVP infusion is helpful. Local hemostatic measures with the use of tranexamic acid topically or platelet concentrates locally may improve the bleeding. A 4.8% tranexamic acid mouthwash, 10 ml three to four times a day for 3 to 7 days, may be helpful.

35. How should the dentist approach a patient with a history of ITP?
In the majority of instances, the dentist would be seeing a patient with a prior history of ITP. After the acute illness, patients have normal platelet count and can be managed using the normal protocol. However, a small percentage can have recurrent disease. It is therefore important to order a platelet count prior to planned dental intervention.

Very rarely, a patient with active disease may require emergency dental intervention. These patients are often on prednisone. It is important to have an up-to-date platelet count prior to dental intervention. Management of patients on steroid therapy is covered in Chapter 12.

36. How should the dentist approach a patient with a history of TTP?

More commonly, the dentist would be seeing a patient with a past history of TTP as opposed to a patient with active disease. Since TTP can recur, it is important to check a platelet count prior to dental intervention. Patients with active TTP are critically ill and should not have any dental interventions.

37. How should the dentist approach a patient with von Willebrand's disease?

There are two defects in patients with von Willebrand's disease. One is a qualitative defect in platelet function, and the other is factor VIII deficiency. Most of the time, the factor VIII deficiency is mild, and patients with von Willebrand's disease can be managed with DDAVP. DDAVP has to be administered at 4 µg/kg intravenously shortly before the dental procedure. This has to be coordinated with the patient's physician. In patients with severe von Willebrand's disease, infusion of factor VIII may be necessary prior to dental intervention. Concentrated factor VIII with fibrinogen is available as a cryoprecipitate. The available units of factor VIII in cryoprecipitate are 10 times those found in fresh-frozen plasma. Currently, lyophilized or other purified preparations of factor VIII are available. Recombinant synthetic factor VIII, although more expensive, has no infectious risks and is therefore the preferred product.

If clinical bleeding occurs postoperatively, DDAVP infusion can be administered. Local hemostatic measures using compressive packing and dressing, extra sutures, microfibrillar collagen hemostat, oxidized cellulose, or tranexamic acid topically may be helpful. A 4.8% tranexamic acid mouthwash, 10 ml three to four times a day for 3 to 7 days, may be helpful.

38. How should the dentist approach a patient on oral anticoagulant therapy?

Because of the complexity of anticoagulation therapy, a separate chapter addresses the patient taking oral anticoagulant (Chapter 24).

39. How should the dentist approach a patient with hemophilia A (classic hemophilia)?

Patients with hemophilia A have varying degrees of hemostatic dysfunction, depending upon the degree of factor VIII deficiency. The patient's physician should be consulted and actively involved in treatment.

Although patients with hemophilia were previously managed as in-patients, most dental procedures are now carried out in the outpatient setting. In general, all dental procedures should be carried out under adequate coverage with factor VIII concentrate. This has to be coordinated with the patient's physician. Factor VIII should last about 12 hours, and it is important to give the patient factor VIII replacement on the morning of and in the evening of the procedure. A small percentage of patients may need additional factor replacements during days 2 and 3 following the dental intervention. This depends on the dental procedure performed, the amount of soft tissue and bone trauma, and the amount of pre-existing soft-tissue inflammation or infection. The patient's physician should be carefully informed of any concern over protracted bleeding in order to coordinate aggressive factor replacement.

Fresh frozen plasma contains all the procoagulants and can be used in the therapy of patients with clotting factor deficiencies. However, concentrated factor VIII preparations are usually given for management of bleeding disorder in patients with hemophilia A. Concentrated factor VIII with fibrinogen is available as a cryoprecipitate. The available units of factor VIII in cryoprecipitate are 10 times that found in fresh-frozen plasma. Currently, lyophilized or other purified preparations of factor VIII are available in the management of patients with hemophilia A. Most of the factor VIII currently used is a recombinant product synthesized in vitro, since this minimizes the possibility of transmission of infection.

E-aminocaproic acid (Amicar) can be used orally to help with hemostasis. Amicar works on the fibrinolytic pathway and blocks lysis of formed clots by blocking activation of the fibrinolytic system. The fibrinolytic pathway is a system designed to stop the clotting process. It prevents inappropriate propagation of clots. Medications such as Amicar interfere with this process and therefore promote clot formation. However, Amicar should be used as adjunctive therapy and not as replacement for factor deficiency. Amicar should be started an hour after the dental procedure. The loading dose is 5 g orally and 1 g orally every hour thereafter for six doses, or until bleeding has stopped.

Tranexamic acid (Cyklokapron) is another agent that acts on the fibrinolytic pathways. The medication is prescribed at 25 mg/kg every 6 hours, starting on the day prior to dental procedures and continued after surgery until bleeding has ceased.

Bleeding postoperatively in patients with hemophilia has to be assessed to make sure that there is no anatomic reason for the bleeding. However, in the majority of the cases of delayed bleeding, the cause is inadequate factor VIII level and aggressive replacement therapy is necessary. E-aminocaproic acid and tranexamic acid can be used adjunctively.

Local hemostatic measures using compressive packing and dressing, extra sutures, microfibrillar collagen hemostat, oxidized cellulose, or tranexamic acid topically may be helpful. A 4.8% tranexamic acid mouthwash, 10 ml three to four times a day for 3 to 7 days, may be helpful.

40. How should the dentist manage the patient with hemophilia B?

Patients with hemophilia B have varying degrees of deficiency of factor IX. They need infusion of concentrated factor IX prior to dental procedures.

Prothrombin complex concentrates (Proplex T) are lyophilized concentrates of factors II, VII, IX, and X and were used as factor replacements in patients with Christmas disease. Proplex is problematic because of risks of infection transmission as it is a plasma concentrate. Synthetic factor IX, although more expensive, is now available for factor replacement and is the preferred product because it carries no infectious complications.

Although patients with hemophilia were previously managed as in-patients, most dental procedures are now carried out in the outpatient setting. In general, all dental procedures should be carried out under adequate coverage with factor IX concentrate. This has to be coordinated with the patient's physician. Factor IX should last about 24 hours, and it is important to give the patient factor IX replacement on the morning of the procedure. A small percentage of patients may need further factor replacement during days 2 and 3 following the dental intervention. This depends on the dental procedure performed, the amount of soft tissue and bone trauma, and the amount of pre-existing soft-tissue inflammation or infection. The patient's physician should be informed of any concerns over protracted bleeding in order to coordinate aggressive factor replacement.

Post-operative bleeding must be assessed to ensure that there is no anatomic reason for the bleeding. However, in the majority of cases of delayed bleeding, the cause is inadequate factor IX levels, and aggressive replacement therapy is necessary. In some instance, ε-aminocaproic acid (Amicar) can be used intravenously to help with hemostasis. Amicar works on the fibrinolytic pathway and blocks lysis of formed clots by blocking activation of the fibrinolytic system. However, Amicar should be used as adjunctive therapy and not as replacement for factor deficiency. Local hemostatic measures with the use of tranexamic acid topically may be helpful. A 4.8% tranexamic acid mouthwash, 10 ml three to four times a day for 3 to 7 days, may be helpful.

41. How should the dentist manage the bleeding disorders of patients with liver disease?

• Tests of CBC with platelet count and PT should be done prior to any dental procedures.
• The patient should be instructed to completely abstain from alcohol both before and after the procedure.
• Patients with normal platelet counts and normal PTs can undergo dental intervention with careful attention to hemostasis.
• Patients may have decreased platelet counts because of hypersplenism, and this should be corrected prior to any dental intervention.
• Patients with heavy alcohol consumption may have dietary deficiency of vitamin K and may be coagulopathic, with deficiency of vitamin K–dependent factors (factors II, VII, IX,

and X). These patients respond to vitamin K therapy, and this should be coordinated with their physicians. Normally, vitamin K repletion is done by either intravenous or intramuscular injections of vitamin K, 10 mg each day for 3 days.

- Dietary deficiency of vitamin B_{12} and folate can also result in macrocytic anemia and thrombocytopenia related to bone marrow suppression.
- Patients may have coagulopathy related to decreased synthesis of factors produced by the liver (factors I, II, V, VII, IX, and X). Only some of these factors are vitamin K–dependent. Patients with significant coagulopathy need replacement of factors in the form of fresh-frozen plasma. This should be coordinated with their physicians, and infusion should be given shortly before the intended dental procedure.
- Acute alcohol consumption can suppress the bone marrow and can result in thrombocytopenia. It is therefore important to reinforce the "no alcohol" rule.

24. ANTICOAGULATION THERAPY

Robert C. Fazio, D.M.D., and Leslie S.T. Fang, M.D., Ph.D.

1. Why are patients on anticoagulation therapy?
Primarily for prevention and management of thromboembolic diseases.

2. What is the impact of anticoagulation therapy on the dental practice?
It is estimated that about 2% of the dental population is on anticoagulation therapy. Since anticoagulation implies some degree of interference with the clotting mechanism, there is always the concern of trying to balance the risk of bleeding against the risk of anticoagulation.

3. What is the controversy in managing patients on anticoagulation therapy?
Although the traditional view has been to err on the side of minimizing bleeding, the more recent practices in anticoagulation therapy allow for continuation of some degree of anticoagulation through all except for the most complicated dental surgery. The physician is more worried about precipitating a thromboembolic event, whereas the dentist is more concerned about significant intraoperative and postoperative bleeding. The overall trend in anticoagulation therapy has been toward less anticoagulation and more resistance to interrupting the anticoagulation.

4. What are thromboembolic diseases that necessitate anticoagulation therapy?
Thromboembolic diseases are diseases that involve clot formation. Clots can form in a variety of vessels and can have a wide variety of manifestations and complications.

Clots form either because there is a hypercoagulable state or because there is an anatomic problem with the vessel. Clots can form either in the venous or in the arterial circulation.
- In the venous circulation, clots can form in the deep venous system with resultant deep venous thrombophlebitis. This occurs most commonly in the deep venous system of the pelvis and the lower extremities.
- Clots can form in the chambers of the heart if there is enlargement or stasis of the chambers. Therefore, patients with atrial fibrillation are at risk for clot formation in the left atrium because of a dilated and static atrium. Similarly, clots can form in the ventricles in a patient with a low cardiac output and dilated ventricles. This is usually the result of ischemic heart disease and multiple myocardial infarctions. Dilated cardiomyopathy can also occur in patients with severe myocarditis.
- Clots can form on abnormal heart valves. Patients with mitral stenosis, particularly if they are in atrial fibrillation, have a high propensity for clot formation.
- Clots can form on mechanical heart valves. Clots are infrequent in biocompatible valves such as porcine valves but occur frequently in mechanical valves. Anticoagulation should not be interrupted in patients with mechanical heart valves because of the very serious sequelae of thrombotic and embolic complications. These patients tend to need more intense anticoagulation (i.e., higher International Normalized Ratios [INRs]) because they have a higher risk of clot formation.
- Clots can also form in other portions of the arterial circulation. Patients with carotid artery disease or peripheral vascular disease are sometimes placed on anticoagulation to prevent occlusion of vessels.
- There is also an increasing trend to anticoagulating patients with ischemic heart disease to prevent myocardial infarctions. These patients usually have multiple risk factors, such as diabetes mellitus, obesity, hyperlipidemia, hypertension, a history of smoking, or a strong family history of myocardial infarction. They are usually maintained on low intensity anticoagulation (INR 1.5–2.0).
- Not only can the clots create problems locally by occlusing vessels, but they can also be launched and cause an embolic event.

- Patients with deep venous thrombophlebitis can have an embolic event with a clot traveling from the lower extremity or the pelvis into the lung, a phenomenon called pulmonary embolism.
- Patients with clots in the heart or who have mechanical heart valves can have embolic cerebrovascular accidents and emboli traveling to other organs, including kidneys, spleen, and bowel, with profound sequelae.

5. What are hypercoagulable states?

Some patients have abnormal clotting mechanisms and are therefore more prone to recurrent episodes of thrombosis and emboli. These patients often have either a clotting factor abnormality or an immunologic abnormality. They have abnormal clots in the arterial and venous circulation, pulmonary emboli, cerebrovascular accidents, and spontaneous abortions.

Patients with inherited protein S deficiency, protein C resistance, factor V Leiden defect, antithrombin III antibodies, and anticardiolipin antibodies can all have serious thromboembolic complications.

These disorders were once thought to be rare, but with increased testing for hypercoagulable states, more and more patients have been found to have these defects.

Because of the significant propensity for clot formation in these patients, high intensity anticoagulation (INR 2.5–3.5) is usually prescribed, and anticoagulation should rarely be interrupted.

6. What are the durations of anticoagulation?

Duration of anticoagulation varies according to the indication for anticoagulation therapy. Patients with minor or transient problems are anticoagulated for short periods of time. Patients with serious thromboembolic disease need lifelong anticoagulation.

- Patients with deep venous thrombophlebitis are usually anticoagulated for 3–6 months.
- Patients with pulmonary embolism are usually anticoagulated for 6–12 months.
- Patients with porcine replacement valves are usually anticoagulated for 3 months following cardiac surgery. Because of the biocompatibility of the valves, anticoagulation is not necessary thereafter.
- Patients with atrial fibrillation are on anticoagulation therapy for life.
- Patients with dilated cardiomyopathy are anticoagulated for life
- Patients with embolic cerebrovascular accidents are often on anticoagulation therapy for the remainder of their lives.
- Patients with mechanical heart valves are on anticoagulation therapy for life.
- Patients with hypercoagulable states are on anticoagulation therapy for life.

7. How is anticoagulation therapy monitored?

Coumadin therapy is monitored by blood testing of PT (prothrombin time) and the determination of INR. Instead of using either the PT or the PT ratio, anticoagulation is now monitored using the INR, which takes into account reagent differences and is a more standard approach to monitoring.

At the beginning of anticoagulation therapy, patients may have to have frequent determinations of INR in order to determine the appropriate range of anticoagulation. Once a patient has settled into the desirable range, INR may be monitored as infrequently as once a month. With intercurrent illness or antibiotic therapy, INR may change, and the frequency of blood monitoring may have to be increased.

The dentist should be aware of a recent INR reading in patients on anticoagulation and should also be aware of the likelihood of increasing INR with the use of broad-spectrum antibiotics.

8. What governs the intensity of anticoagulation?

In the majority of instances, PT/INR is maintained in the 2.0–3.0 range. In instances where intense anticoagulation is necessary, INR ranges of 2.5 to 3.5 may be necessary.

The intensity of anticoagulation is dictated by the propensity towards clotting. Patients at high risk of clot formation, in general, will need a higher intensity of anticoagulation.

A. Patients at moderate risk of clot formation (INR 2–3):
- Those with deep venous thrombophlebitis
- Those with atrial fibrillation
- Patients with low ejection fraction and dilated cardiomyopathy
- Patients with cerebrovascular accidents and transient ischemic attacks
- Those with vascular disease such as carotid artery disease and peripheral vascular disease

B. Patients at high risk for clot formation (INR 2.5–3.5)
- Those with mechanical heart valves
- Those with hypercoagulable states

9. What should a dentist do when managing a patient on Coumadin?

There should be three sets of considerations:
- What is the risk of stopping anticoagulation therapy for a short period of time? Why is the patient on anticoagulation?
- What is the proposed dental procedure?
- What is the state of the soft tissue with respect to inflammation?

These three sets of considerations will govern the recommendation for the management of patients on Coumadin.

10. What is the risk of stopping anticoagulation for a short period of time?

Stopping anticoagulation therapy puts the patient at risk for whatever underlying thromboembolic condition exists. Therefore:
- Patients at moderate risk have minimal risk with a brief interruption of anticoagulation therapy.
- Patients at high risk should not have interruption of anticoagulation therapy if at all possible.

11. What is the dental procedure planned?

Procedures that incur significant soft tissue trauma obviously result in more bleeding, and thought should be given to transiently interrupting anticoagulation therapy.

12. What is the state of the soft tissue with respect to inflammation?

The more soft-tissue inflammation the patient has, the more likely it is that the dental procedure will incur bleeding. Consideration should be given to transiently interrupting anticoagulation therapy in patients who may have significant soft-tissue and bone trauma.

The patient with mild to moderate inflammation can generally undergo a scaling procedure at therapeutic levels of INR. However, a patient with severe inflammation who requires deep scaling probably should have his or her anticoagulation interrupted so that the procedure can proceed at a lower INR (INR < 2.2).

13. How should the dentist approach the patient on routine anticoagulation (INR 2.0–3.0)?

- The dental office should contact the physician's office and request recent INR results.
- If the INRs have been stable and in the therapeutic range (INR 2.0–3.0), the dentist can proceed with nonsurgical and minor surgical procedures as planned.
- For surgical dental therapy, especially involving significant soft-tissue and bone trauma, anticoagulation should be stopped for 2–3 days prior to the procedure so that the INR will drop below 2.2. In general, the surgical procedures can be safely carried out at that level.

   The risk of thrombosis is low with this brief an interruption, and most physicians have no difficulty with this regimen.

   The dentist should emphasize to the physician that he or she does not desire complete normalization of INR. The proposed protocol will have the INR to the low end of the therapeutic range. Some patients taking Coumadin have INRs of 2.0–2.2 and require no interruption when undergoing dental surgery.

- For very extensive dental surgery, the dentist should maneuver the INR into the subthera-peutic range (INR <1.5 in some instances). In these patients, another INR reading on the morning of surgery is needed to ensure safety.
- The decision to interrupt anticoagulation should also be modified according to the degree of inflammation of the soft tissue.

    In general, the higher the degree of inflammation of the soft tissue the patient has, the lower the dentist would want the INR to be at the time of intervention.

    Also important is the amount of bone trauma anticipated. Extensive bone trauma would call for a lower INR and transient interruption of anticoagulation.
- Local hemostatic measures, including compression packing, application of oxidized cellu-lose, and microfibrillar collagen hemostat, should be used. Tranexamic acid used topically may be also be helpful. A 4.8% tranexamic acid mouthwash, 10 ml used three to four times a day for 3 to 7 days, may be helpful.

14. How should the dentist approach the patient at high risk for clotting and on high-inten-sity anticoagulation therapy?

Patients with mechanical valves and patients in a hypercoagulable state generally should not have their anticoagulation therapy interrupted.

- It is important to verify that the INR is in the 2.5–3.5 range.
- All nonsurgical dental therapy should be completed with no interruption in coumadin ther-apy. If the INR is in the 3.0–3.5 range, block anesthesia should be approached cautiously. Infiltrative local anesthesia is preferred in this setting.
- The dentist should be able to do **minor** dental surgical procedures in patients with an INR of up to 3.0, with careful attention to hemostasis. A brief interruption of Coumadin therapy may be required.

    For extensive surgery, patients' INRs should be in ranges less than 2.2. Because of the high risk of leaving the patient without anticoagulation, therapy should involve the physi-cian in designing a short-term heparin regimen.
- The decision to interrupt anticoagulation should also be modified according to the degree of inflammation of the soft tissue.

    In general, the higher the degree of inflammation of the soft tissue of the patient, the lower the dentist would want the INR to be at the time of intervention.
- Local hemostatic measures, including compression packing, application of oxidized cellu-lose, and microfibrillar collagen hemostat, should be used. Tranexamic acid given topically is also recommended. A 4.8% tranexamic acid mouthwash, 10 ml given three to four times a day for 3 to 7 days, may be helpful.

15. What is short-term heparinization?

Heparin has a very short half-life, whereas coumadin has a long half-life. The goal is to be able to keep the patient anticoagulated on heparin until several hours before the dental procedure. Heparin is then stopped, and the patient undergoes surgery with reversed anticoagulation. Heparin is resumed shortly after the surgical procedure, and Coumadin is restarted. Heparin is continued until the PT/INR is back in the therapeutic range.

In the past, the patient had to be admitted to the hospital for heparin infusion, and heparin was stopped 2 hours prior to surgery. Heparin was then resumed about 4 hours thereafter and then Coumadin therapy was resumed. This required an in-patient hospital stay of 5–7 days.

Currently, a low-molecular-weight heparin preparation allows for the administration of heparin subcutaneously on an outpatient basis. The preparation, dalteparin (Fragmin), is given on an every 12-hour regimen. Coumadin is stopped 4 days prior to the intended surgical procedure, and Fragmin is started. Fragmin is held back on the morning of surgery, and the dental procedure is car-ried out about 12 hours after the last dose of Fragmin. Both Fragmin and Coumadin are resumed the evening of the procedure. Fragmin therapy is continued until the INR is back in the 2.5–3.5 range.

All of this requires extensive involvement of the patient's physician.

16. What drugs interact with Coumadin?
Unfortunately, many drugs interact with coumadin. For the dentist, the choice of antibiotics and analgesics would be complicated if coumadin were continued.

17. What commonly prescribed antibiotics are "safe" with Coumadin?
• Prolonged courses of any antibiotic can affect the intestinal flora, alter vitamin K synthesis, and prolong the INR in patients on Coumadin. It is therefore important to make the course of antibiotic administration as short as possible.
• Among the antibiotics commonly prescribed for treatment of dental infection:
  • Tetracycline is contraindicated.
  • Erythromycin, clarithromycin, metronidazole, ciprofloxacin, ofloxacin, and levofloxacin interact with Coumadin and should be avoided.
  • "Safer" antibiotics include penicillins, commonly used cephalosporins, clindamycin, and azithromycin. Azithromycin is an interesting macrolide that does not interfere with cytochrome p450 and has less effect on anticoagulation therapy. Although there is one negative case report, azithromycin is generally not known to interact with Coumadin.

18. Among the commonly prescribed analgesics, what are the "safer" drugs for the patient on oral anticoagulation therapy?
• Aspirin should be avoided.
• All nonsteroidal anti-inflammatory drugs should be avoided.
• Among the COX-2 inhibitors, rofecoxib (Vioxx) interacts with coumadin but does not interfere with platelet function. Data on celecoxib (Celebrex) are unclear.
• Propoxyphene plus acetaminophen (Darvocet) interacts with coumadin and is therefore contraindicated.
• Tramadol (Ultram) interacts with coumadin in an idiosyncratic fashion. Although most patients on Ultram show no change in INR, a few patients have been found to have markedly elevated INRs on the drug.
• There are data that suggest that even acetaminophen can interact with Coumadin to a finite extent. Hylek (JAMA 1998) and Bell (JAMA 1998), in two independent studies, suggested that several doses of acetaminophen can increase the INR of patients on stable doses of Coumadin.
• Dentists are therefore advised to prescribe the "safer" analgesics in patients on Coumadin. This includes codeine and codeine derivatives, probably with lower doses of the acetaminophen component (i.e., Percocet 5/325 or 10/325 with 325 mg of acetaminophen per dose). Other analgesics that are deemed safe include meperidine (Demerol) or meperidine (Demerol) plus promethazine (Phenergan)

25. HEMATOLOGIC MALIGNANCIES

Stephen T. Sonis, D.M.D., D.M.Sc.

1. What is leukemia?

Leukemia refers to a number of neoplastic diseases of the blood-forming elements of the body.

2. How are leukemias classified?

Leukemias are classified by clinical course (acute or chronic) and histologic origin in bone marrow (lymphoblastic or nonlymphoblastic).

3. What is the prognosis for survival in patients with untreated leukemia?

Less than 1 year.

4. What is the most common form on nonlymphoblastic leukemia? What cell line does it affect?

The most common form of nonlymphoblastic leukemia is myelogenous leukemia, which affects cells of the granulocyte line.

5. Are leukemias essentially a single disease?

No. In many ways they behave like individual diseases, striking different patient populations and varying in their clinical course.

6. What are some of the possible causes of leukemia?

- Chemicals and drugs
- Ionizing radiation
- Genetic predisposition
- RNA viruses

7. Describe the specific presenting signs and symptoms for leukemia.

There are none. The onset is often insidious and nonspecific. Patients often complain of symptoms suggesting a low-grade viral infection, including fatigue, malaise, and fever. However, unlike a viral infection, the condition persists and usually worsens.

8. What precipitates the majority of symptoms in patients with leukemia?

For the most part, presenting signs and symptoms are related to the replacement of normal bone marrow elements with neoplastic leukemia cells. As a consequence, patients are anemic with neutropenia and thrombocytopenia, which create an increased risk for infection and bleeding. In cases in which large numbers of leukemic cells spill into the peripheral blood, infiltrates may occur in the lymph nodes, spleen, and gingiva.

9. What is the easiest laboratory test to evaluate a patient suspected of having leukemia?

A complete blood count (CBC) that includes a white blood cell (WBC) count, a differential white blood cell count, hemoglobin, and hematocrit is easy and usually diagnostic. Marked increases in the WBC count are typical, although the extent of leukocytosis can vary. Platelets are often reduced, and the presence of immature blast forms is noted. Because patients with leukemia are often anemic, red blood cell production is reduced, resulting in lowered hemoglobin and hematocrit. Platelet production is also adversely affected, resulting in thrombocytopenia.

10. Give the average WBC count (cells/mm^3) for the following: normal patient, patient with acute myelogenous leukemia (AML), patient with chronic lymphocytic leukemia (CLL), and patient with chronic myelogenous leukemia (CML).

Normal:	4,000–10,000	CLL:	50,000–100,000
AML:	10,000–100,000	CML:	100,000–500,000

11. What is the normal percent of blast forms in the peripheral blood of a healthy patient? Of a patient with AML?

Normal: 0%

AML: 50–80%

12. Contrast the percent of lymphocytes in a patient with CLL and a healthy person.

Patients with CLL have a higher percentage of lymphocytes in peripheral blood (80%) compared with normal individuals (30–40%).

13. What technique is used to make a definitive diagnosis of leukemia?

Bone marrow biopsy.

14. What modality of treatment is typically used to treat leukemia?

Although chemotherapy is used to treat all forms of leukemia, the specific agent varies with the type of leukemia. For patients with acute leukemia, therapy is divided into an induction phase, in which the goal is to eliminate or reduce the leukemic cell population. Often induction chemotherapy is initiated emergently. When no leukemia cells are detectable in the marrow, the patient is said to be in remission. To prevent recurrence, the patient is given a long course (up to 2 years) of maintenance therapy. Acute leukemia usually requires more aggressive treatment than chronic forms of the disease.

15. Bone marrow transplant offers the opportunity to treat patients with lethal doses of antineoplastic drugs. Because the source of the transplant must be another person (allogeneic transplant), patients are at risk for what condition?

Graft vs. host disease (GVHD), which occurs when immunocompetent cells in the grafted bone marrow attack the immunologically inert recipient (host). Among the tissues most commonly targeted by GVHD are the mouth, skin, lungs, gastrointestinal tract, and liver.

16. What is the most common cause of death in patients with AML?

Most deaths result from infection (70%). Uncontrollable bleeding results in 10% of AML-related deaths.

17. What form of leukemia is associated with the Philadelphia chromosome?

Chronic myelogenous leukemia.

18. What is the most common leukemia in adults? At what age is it typically noted?

Chronic lymphocytic leukemia is the most common form and is seen most often in elderly patients.

19. True or false: Oral pathoses are frequent signs or symptoms in patients with undiagnosed leukemia. Provide statistics to support your answer.

Oral pathoses are frequent presenting signs or symptoms associated with acute leukemias. Of patients with ALL, almost all (90%) have oral problems. Of importance, almost one-fourth seek primary medical evaluation because of mouth problems.

Among patients with other forms of acute leukemia, about two-thirds have oral changes during the early stages of the disease; of these, one-third seek medical attention because of oral problems.

20. List the typical oral and head and neck manifestations of AML.

• Spontaneous gingival bleeding or oozing

• Petechiae formation

• Oral soft tissue or gingival infection

• Pharyngitis

• Lymphadenopathy

21. Gingival bleeding is common among healthy patients with periodontal disease. When should you suspect that gingival bleeding is of systemic origin and possibly represents the presenting signs of leukemia?

Most gingival bleeding associated with periodontal disease is a consequence of some type of provocation, such as tooth-brushing or flossing. Patients who are profoundly thrombocytopenic (platelet count < 20,000 cells/mm^3) may demonstrate almost constant spontaneous gingival oozing. Consequently, when the signs and symptoms outweigh the local factors or do not follow the normal clinical course, you should consider a possible systemic etiology.

22. What are the major considerations in providing dental treatment to patients with leukemia?

Prevention of infection and bleeding is the major consideration. It is imperative to communicate with the patient's physician before contemplating any treatment.

23. What is the major concern in performing an extraction in a patient who has successfully completed induction therapy for AML and is currently undergoing maintenance therapy?

You need to be concerned about the patient's level of chemotherapy-induced myelosuppression, which is likely to produce both neutropenia and thromocytopenia.

24. Fortunately the treatment of leukemia often results in cure. How should you treat an 18-year-old woman who had leukemia when she was 4 years old?

A patient in this category can be treated normally.

25. What are lymphomas?

Lymphomas are malignancies of lymphoreticular origin that most often involve the lymph nodes. Lymphomas are not a single type of neoplasm but rather represent a variety of clinical and histologic entities.

26. What is the major significance of lymphomas for dentists?

1. Because a significant number of lymphomas initially involve the head and neck nodes, dentists can play an important role in diagnosis.

2. The chemotherapy and radiation therapy used to treat lymphomas often affect the mouth.

3. Children who are treated for lymphoma may have altered growth and development of structures in the head and neck.

27. What is Hodgkin's disease?

Hodgkin's disease is a fairly common form of lymphoma with variety of subtypes based on histologic evaluation. It affects about 7/100,000 of the U.S. population.

28. What is the age predilection for Hodgkin's disease?

It is most common between the ages of 15 and 34 years and after the age of 50 years.

29. How does Hodgkin's disease present clinically?

Lymphadenopathy is the most common presenting sign of Hodgkin's disease. The lymph nodes are usually well defined, rubbery, and painless. The nodes of the neck and axilla are most commonly involved. Progressive disease involving the mediastinal nodes may result in shortness of breath. Progressive itching may be noted, a symptom most ofter reported in younger women. Constitutional symptoms of night sweats, fatigue, fever, and weight loss may be present.

30. How is a patient suspected of Hodgkin's disease evaluated?

Medical evaluation of the patient suspected of having Hodgkin's disease consists of history, physical examination, and biopsy of the involved lymph node. Once a histologic diagnosis is made, the next step in the work-up is to determine the extent of the disease. This step is accomplished by imaging studies, using x-rays, computed tomography (CT), and magnetic resonance imaging (MRI) to evaluate the extent of the disease so that it can be staged.

31. How is Hodgkin's disease staged? Why is staging important?
Staging provides information about the clinical behavior of the disease and is important in helping to decide therapy. With Hodgkin's disease, staging defines whether the disease involves a unifocal site or has spread to more distant sites (spleen, extralymphatic sites). There are four stages of Hodgkin's disease:
　　Stage I: involvement of a single lymph node region or a single extralymphatic organ or site.
　　Stage II: involvement of two or more lymph node regions on the same side of the diaphragm or localized involvement of an extralymphatic organ or site and one or more lymph node regions on the same side of the diaphragm.
　　Stage III: involvement of lymph node regions on both sides of the diaphragm.
　　Stage IV: disseminated or diffuse involvement of one or more extralymphatic organs or tissues, with or without associated lymph node involvement.

32. What is the significance of substages 1A and 1B?
Substaging refers to symptoms that accompany anatomic findings. Patients who are asymptomatic are substage A, and patients who have fever, night sweats, or unexplained weight loss > 10% are classified as substage B.

33. What cells do pathologists look for in making a diagnosis of Hodgkin's disease?
Reed-Sternberg cells.

34. How does survival correlate with stage?
The higher the stage the lower the survival rate. Whereas the 5-year disease-free survival for patients with stage I disease is about 90%, it is only about 65% for patients with stage IV disease.

35. How is Hodgkin's disease treated?
Multiagent chemotherapy and radiation are the primary treatments. Surgery is usually limited to diagnosis and, in some cases, splenectomy.

36. Lymphadenopathy of the head and neck is common and may be due to many causes— most often an inflammatory process. List 10 questions that help to differentiate lymphadenopathy due to an inflammatory process from lymphadenopathy due to a noninflammatory process such as malignancy.
　　1. Are the nodes tender?
　　2. How long has the patient been aware of the lymphadenopathy?
　　3. Have the nodes changed in size?
　　4. Does the patient have a sore throat or upper respiratory infection?
　　5. Are the nodes movable?
　　6. Are the involved nodes unilateral or bilateral?
　　7. What is the texture and density of the nodes?
　　8. Is there evidence of intraoral or facial infection?
　　9. Is there evidence of oral lesions?
　　10. Has the patient had recent contact with cats?

37. Why the interest in feline contact?
Benign lymphoreticulosis or cat-scratch fever may result in unilateral lymph node enlargement in the head and neck.

38. Does bilateral lymphadenopathy always indicate a benign process?
Absolutely not. But bilateral, tender nodes are more likely to be associated with an inflammatory process.

39. What should you do if a patient presents with a firm, nonmovable, enlarging cervical node?

Because this presentation may be associated with a neoplastic process, the patient should be referred for biopsy.

40. Besides lymphomas, what other head and neck malignancies may result in lymphadenopathy?

Any squamous cell cancer of the head and neck may spread to the lymph nodes. Besides oral cancers, cancers of the nasopharynx or larynx may result in lymphadenopathy.

41. What are the dental management considerations in patients with Hodgkin's disease?
- Immunosuppression may result in an increased risk of infection.
- Radiation therapy to the neck may involve the salivary glands and produce xerostomia.
- Chemotherapy may result in myelosuppression or mucositis.

42. What disease should you be wary of 5–10 years after a patient has been successfully treated for Hodgkin's disease?

Leukemia.

43. Are non-Hodgkin's lymphomas important to the dentist?

Non-Hodgkin's malignancies occur twice as often as Hodgkin's disease and may present as nonhealing ulcers or masses in the mouth either as a primary lesion or as a secondary manifestation. Diagnosis is made by biopsy.

26. ARTHRITIS

Robert C. Fazio, D.M.D., and Leslie S.T. Fang, M.D., Ph.D.

1. What is arthritis?

Arthritis is the result of inflammatory or degenerative processes involving the joints. Patients with arthritis can have pain, swelling, limitation of motion or frank deformity of the joints.

2. What causes inflammatory arthritis?

Inflammatory arthritis can result from infection (septic arthritis and gonococcal arthritis), crystal deposits (gout, pseudogout), and a number of immunologically mediated diseases, such as rheumatoid arthritis, systemic lupus erythematosus, scleroderma, and spondyloarthropathies.

3. What causes noninflammatory arthritis?

Noninflammatory arthritis results from degenerative changes in the joints. Osteoarthritis is by far the most common form of noninflammatory arthritis.

4. What forms of arthritis is the dentist most likely to see?

Osteoarthritis or degenerative joint disease—by far. The dentist also may see patients with gout or rheumatoid arthritis.

5. Define osteoarthritis.

Osteoarthritis is the most common form of arthritis. It results from wear and tear on the joint cartilage and secondary mechanical disruption of the joint. The disease process usually results from aging, but occasionally trauma is the underlying cause. Osteoarthritis most commonly affects the weight-bearing joints such as the hips, knees, and spine. Joints of the hands also may be involved. Typically, the disease has an insidious but progressive course. Early symptoms include stiffness, which can progress to pain and swelling with resultant limitation of range of motion.

The involved joints are often enlarged and deformed. Deformities in the joints of the hands include enlargement of the terminal interphalangeal joints (Heberden's nodes) and, less commonly, the proximal interphalangeal joints (Bouchard's nodes). The diagnosis can usually be made on clinical grounds. Radiologic evaluation may reveal deformities, including formation of osteophytes, reduced joint space, and cysts.

6. How is osteoarthritis treated?

1. Exercise, weight loss, and physical therapy are important interventions for patients with osteoarthritis.

2. Acetaminophen, in doses up to 4 gm/day, is often prescribed for pain control.

3. For patients not responding to acetaminophen, aspirin or nonsteroidal anti-inflammatory drugs (NSAIDs) are prescribed.

4. If gastritis or peptic ulcer disease prohibits use of standard NSAIDs, COX-2 specific inhibitors, such as celecoxib (Celebrex) and rofecoxib (Vioxx), may be prescribed.

5. During periods of acute and debilitating joint flares, narcotics may have to be used for a defined period.

6. For patients with severe degenerative joint disease, orthopedic intervention with joint replacement may be necessary.

7. What is gout?

Gout is an acute inflammatory arthritis usually involving a single joint (monoarticular arthritis). The disease results from deposition of uric acid crystals into the joint fluid, which induces an inflammatory response. The disease primarily affects men over the age of 40. The onset of the attack is abrupt, and symptoms peak within 24 hours. The proximal interphalangeal joint of the great toe is the classic site of involvement, but ankles, wrists, olecranon bursae, and knees also may be involved. The involved joint is usually red, warm, and acutely inflamed. Considerable pain and tenderness result in limited range of motion. The diagnosis usually can be made on clinical grounds. Aspiration of the inflamed joint can yield uric acid crystals.

8. How is gout treated?
For an acute flare of gout
1. Begin with either colchicine or an NSAID.
2. Continue full-dose therapy until symptoms resolve, then taper to cessation.
3. For refractory cases of acute gout, a short course of steroids (7–10 days) may be necessary.

For patients with recurrent episodes of gout
1. Advise weight reduction and exercise.
2. Instruct patients how to follow a diet low in purine; this diet usually involves avoidance of red meat and red wine.
3. Avoid drugs that can raise uric acid levels, such as thiazide diuretics and loop diuretics.
4. Use allopurinol to prevent recurrent attacks.
5. In some patients, the use of an agent such as probenecid to promote uric acid excretion may be beneficial.

9. What is rheumatoid arthritis?
Rheumatoid arthritis is an autoimmune disease affecting primarily women. The disease typically has its onset in the third or fourth decade of life. Rheumatoid arthritis usually has a subacute presentation with symmetric involvement of multiple joints (polyarticular arthritis). Joints of the hands and wrists are most commonly affected. Patients initially notice stiffness in these joints in the morning. Stiffness progresss to pain and swelling with limited range of motion. Joint deformity is seen in the later stages of the disease. Of interest to the dentist is the occasional involvement of the temporomandibular joint.

Examination during an acute episode reveals involvement of multiple, symmetric joints, particularly the small joints of the hands. Patients with long-standing rheumatoid arthritis may have deviation of the fingers, swan-neck deformity of the wrist, and deposits of subcutaneous nodules (rheumatoid nodules). Laboratory evaluation reveals a positive rheumatoid factor in about 75% of patients. The erythrocyte sedimentation rate (ESR) is often elevated. Radiographic evaluation may reveal changes such as osteoporosis, reduction in joint space, and bone erosions. The American College of Rheumatology has established specific criteria for the diagnosis of rheumatoid arthritis. They are classified as major criteria or minor criteria and involve a combination of clinical findings and serologic abnormalities.

Characteristically, rheumatoid arthritis is a smoldering disease with intermittent flares. Asymptomatic periods may be followed by severe flares.

10. Describe the treatment of rheumatoid arthritis.
1. Patients should be given an exercise and physical therapy regimen.
2. At the time of initial diagnosis, disease-modifying treatment (e.g., methotrexate, hydroxychloroquine, sulfasalazine) should be promptly implemented. The goal is to minimize the likelihood of disease progression.
3. A rheumatologist should be involved to provide prompt intervention.
4. While waiting for disease-modifying treatment to take effect (often as long as 6 months), NSAIDs are often used.
5. Selective COX-2 inhibitors are used only in instances when nonselective agents are not well tolerated or the patient is at high risk for peptic ulceration or gastrointestinal bleeding.
6. For patients with highly active disease whose symptoms are inadequately controlled by NSAIDs or COX-2 inhibitors, a short course of steroids may be used.
7. For patients with severe and refractory disease, Embrel or Remicade injections are often quite beneficial.
8. For patients with joint deformities and limitation, surgery may be necessary.

11. How should the dentist evaluate patients with a history of arthritis?
1. Find out what kind of arthritis the patient has.
2. Be sure that the disease is not active.
3. Ask about the kind of medications the patient is taking.
4. Ask whether the patient has a history of steroid use.

12. How should the dentist approach the patient taking aspirin?
Aspirin binds the cyclo-oxygenase system in the platelet irreversibly and impairs function for the lifetime of exposed platelets. Aspirin and aspirin-containing medications, therefore, should be stopped 7–10 days before elective dental procedures. In urgent situation, surgery can proceed with a careful hemostatic protocol. Most patients have either no significant changes or only mild prolongation of bleeding time (9–12 minutes). However, a rare patient may have an idiosyncratic response with a bleeding time of more than 12 minutes. It is important, therefore, to determine whether another drug can be substituted for 7–10 days before elective dental procedures. Generally, a patient can substitute an NSAID. Although NSAIDs can affect platelet function, the effect is generally less than that of aspirin because NSAIDs bind to cyclo-oxygenase in a reversible fashion and have an antiplatelet effect only when they are still in the circulation.

Recently, anti-inflammatory drugs with predominantly COX-2 inhibitory effects have been introduced, including celecoxib (Celebrex), rofecoxib (Vioxx), and valdecoxib (Bextra). Because these drugs do not significantly inhibit the COX-1 enzyme, they have little effect on platelet function. Their efficacy is similar to that of the traditional NSAIDs, and they may be an ideal substitute for aspirin before elective dental procedures. If the patient cannot discontinue aspirin without clinical compromise, the dentist should order an Ivy template bleeding time. If the bleeding time is less than 10 minutes, the dentist can proceed using a normal protocol. If the bleeding time is in the range of 10–12 minutes, the dentist should anticipate increased but manageable bleeding.

Local hemostatic measures using compressive packing and dressing, extra sutures, microfibrillar collagen hemostat, oxidized cellulose, and topical tranexamic acid may be helpful. A 4.8% tranexamic acid mouthwash, 10 ml 3–4 times/day for 3–7 days, may be helpful. If the bleeding time is longer than 12 minutes, the dentist should anticipate the potential of excessive bleeding. If the bleeding time is significantly longer than 12 minutes, platelet transfusion may have to be used for emergency procedures. All elective procedures should be deferred.

13. How should the dentist approach the patient taking NSAIDs?
Because the inhibition of cyclo-oxygenase by NSAIDs is reversible, most dentists elect to proceed with dental interventions using careful hemostatic protocol. If the patient experiences significant intraoperative bleeding, local hemostatic measures using compressive packing and dressing, extra sutures, microfibrillar collagen hemostat, oxidized cellulose, and/or topical tranexamic acid may be helpful. Most often, however, the dentist simply recommends short-term discontuance of the NSAID or substitutes a selective COX-2 NSAID that does not interact with platelet function.

14. How should the dentist approach the patient taking methotrexate?
The methotrexate dose used in managing arthritis is quite low, and patients usually have a normal complete blood count (CBC) and normal liver function tests. They can be managed without modification of normal dental protocols. However, because methotrexate therapy can be complicated by drug-induced hepatitis and pancytopenia, a recent CBC and recent liver function tests should be reviewed. Generally, the dentist can get such information from the patient's physician. For patients with anemia, leukopenia, thrombocytopenia, or liver function abnormalities, dental procedures should be postponed. The dentist should consult with the patient's physician and discuss the treatment plan.

15. How should the dentist approach the patient with a history of corticosteroid use?
Practical issues to consider for patients on steroid therapy include:
• Early morning appointments
• Shorter appointments

• Minimized stress
• Use of sedation techniques when appropriate
• Modification of dental treatment plans when appropriate
The major goal is to avoid precipitation of adrenal insufficiency. Details pertaining to management of patients with a history of corticosteroid use are discussed in Chapter 12. Generally, in patients receiving prednisone in daily doses of 15 mg or more, the dose should be increased to 30–40 mg on the day of moderately stressful dental procedures. For more stressful procedures, including general anesthesia, the dose should be increased to 60 mg on the day of the procedure. For patients receiving less than 15 mg/day of prednisone, supplemental steroids are usually not necessary.

16. Should patients on chronic steroid maintenance therapy receive antibiotics after the dental procedure?

Although no sound data address the need for postoperative antibiotics in patients on maintenance steroid therapy, most patients who have undergone a dental procedure with significant soft tissue trauma may benefit from a short course of antibiotics. Choice of antibiotics should be individualized, but first-line antibiotics, such as amoxicillin (875 mg 2 times/day) can be prescribed for 3 days.

17. How should the dentist approach the patient with gout?

Special considerations should be taken into account when prescribing medications for patients with gout. Some drugs, such as aspirin and aspirin-containing compounds, have a uricosuric effect and should be avoided because they can raise the serum uric acid level and precipitate an acute flare.

18. How should the dentist approach patients with prosthetic joints?

The use of prophylactic antibiotics for patients with prosthetic joints undergoing dental procedures has been controversial for many years. Unlike the high risk of infection for an intravascular prosthetic heart valve, the prosthetic joint is an extravascular prosthesis that is usually not exposed to bacteremia. For many years, studies showed that most orthopedic surgeons recommend prophylactic antibiotics, but few believed that convincing data supported such a recommendation. Before 1997, the American Association of Orthopedic Surgeons (AAOP) made no formal recommendations.

19. What are the current recommendations of the AAOP?

In 1997 the AAOP and American Dental Association (ADA) made the following recommendations:
1. Prophylactic antibiotics are not recommended for patients with prosthetic joints undergoing routine dental procedures.
2. Prophylactic antibiotics are recommended if the patient is undergoing a procedure likely to induce significant bacteremia *and* the patient has a joint at high risk for infection. Both criteria must be fulfilled for prophylaxis to be required.
3. High-risk dental procedures are those that are likely to incur "significant bleeding." Procedures listed by the AAOS are identical to those identified as "at-risk procedures" for subacute bacterial endocarditis in the American Heart Associations Guidelines.
4. A joint at high risk for infection is defined as
   • A joint that has been placed within the past 2 years
   • Any joint with a history of prior joint infection
   • Any prosthetic joint in a patient with hemophilia
   • Any prosthetic joint in a patient with type 1 diabetes mellitus
   • Any prosthetic joint placed in a patient with rheumatoid arthritis
   • Any prosthetic joint placed in a patient on immunosuppressive therapy.

20. What antibiotics are generally recommended for patients with prosthetic joints?

Antibiotics for prophylaxis in a patient with a high-risk prosthetic joint undergoing a high-risk dental procedure include the following:

1. Cephalexin (Keflex), 2 gm (500 mg × 4)
2. Clindamycin (Cleocin,) 600 mg (150 mg × 4)
3. Azithromycin (Zithromax), 500 mg (250 mg × 2)
4. Clarithromycin (Biaxin), 500 mg
5. Amoxicillin, 2 gm (500 mg × 4)

21. Which of the above regimens is most suspect?

Although all of the listed regimens are recommended, the dentist should be mindful that two-thirds of all prosthetic joint infections are caused by staphylococcal species. Amoxicillin does not cover staphylococcal species well and perhaps should not be the first-line drug of choice.

22. Many orthopedic surgeons still recommend across-the-board coverage for all dental procedures. What should the dentist do?

Unless the patient has been specifically instructed by the orthopedic surgeon to receive prophylactic antibiotics, the dentist should proceed using the AAOS/ADA guidelines. If the patient has been specifically instructed by the orthopedic surgeon to receive antibiotic prophylactically, the dentist should discuss the specific indications for prophylaxis with the surgeon and review the guidelines of the physician's national organization.

23. What should be included in the dental records of a patient with a prosthetic joint?

It is important to record the date of placement of the prosthetic joint. For most patients in whom a prosthetic joint has been placed for osteoarthritis, antibiotic prophylaxis is no longer necessary 2 years after the joint replacement.

24. What are the oral findings in patients with arthritis?

The temporomandibular joint (TMJ) may be affected by arthritis. Patients complain of joint tenderness and trismus and may have swelling and erythema over the affected joint. Not infrequently, patients with TMJ syndrome may present to the dentist thinking that the pain is related to a dental problem. Such patients should be referred to their physicians for evaluation and management.

25. What is Sjögren's syndrome?

Sjögren's syndrome is a chronic autoimmune disorder consisting of xerostomia, dry eyes, and connective tissue disease. Rheumatoid arthritis occurs in 50% of patients with Sjögren's syndrome. The most striking oral findings are xerostomia, bilateral parotid gland enlargement, and atrophy of filiform and fungiform lingual papillae. Angular cheilitis also has been noted.

The treatment of Sjögren's syndrome is palliative. When necessary, saliva substitute may be used. In addition, because of the high frequency of caries in patients with impaired parotid gland function, the use of topical fluorides and frequent dental prophylaxis should be considered. Neutral sodium fluoride in a 1.1% gel can be applied as a re-brush after normal oral hygiene protocols. The patient should spit out but not rinse out the gel and avoid eating or drinking for 30 minutes. If the patient previously had a high caries index, the dentist may consider fabricating custom fluoride trays for a more sustained application 7 minutes). Acid pH fluoride gels are to be avoided because of their potential to etch porcelain restorations and compromise esthetics.

27. CHRONIC RENAL FAILURE AND DIALYSIS

Robert C. Fazio, D.M.D., and Leslie S.T. Fang, M.D., Ph.D.

1. Describe the role of the normal kidney.

The normal kidney is involved in a number of specialized functions, including maintenance of fluid and electrolyte balance, acid-base balance, excretion of nitrogenous waste, and clearance of drugs. In addition, the kidney is also responsible for production or metabolism of a number of hormones, including renin, vitamin D, prostaglandins, and erythropoeitin.

2. What are the consequences of renal dysfunction?

- Patients can have problems with uremic symptoms related to accumulation of nitrogenous waste. Accumulation of nitrogenous waste can impair platelet function and result in uremic bleeding.
- Patients have problems with excretion of many drugs and drug metabolites, and toxicity may develop.
- Patients can retain fluid and develop hypertension and congestive heart failure.
- Patients can have problems with metabolic acidosis due to accumulation of sulfates and phosphates.
- Endocrine abnormalities can result in hypertension from excessive production of renin.
- Patients can be quite anemic because of insufficient erythropoeitin.
- Inability to metabolize vitamin D to the active metabolite results in hypocalcemia. This, together with hyperphosphatemia from phosphate retention, can result in hyperparathyroidism with demineralization of bone and renal dystrophy.

3. What causes renal insufficiency?

The most common cause of chronic renal failure is nephrosclerosis due to long-standing hypertension. Diabetes mellitus is the second most common cause of renal dysfunction. A large number of other diseases also can result in chronic renal insufficiency, including chronic inflammatory diseases of the kidneys, pyelonephritis, and nephrotoxicity due to various drugs, including analgesic excess (e.g., nonsteroidal anti-inflammatory drugs).

4. What are the symptoms of renal insufficiency?

Normally, the blood urea nitrogen (BUN) level is less than 20 mg/dl, and creatinine level is less than 1.5 mg/dl. Higher values denote some degree of renal dysfunction. However, patients usually do not have symptoms until the BUN is above 50 mg/dl or the creatinine level is above 5 mg/dl. Severe renal insufficiency is usually associated with BUN level greater than 100 mg/dl or creatinine level greater than 10 mg/dl.

Early symptoms of renal insufficiency include fatigue, lassitude, and weakness. Later patients may develop itching, easy bruisability, and anorexia. Fluid retention usually occurs later in the disease: patients may develop hypertension and congestive heart failure. Patients with severe azotemia develop lethargy, encephalopathy, and vomiting. Dialysis is usually necessary at this stage. Untreated patients can develop seizures, coma, and death.

5. What are the signs of renal insufficiency?

Patients with chronic renal insufficiency are often hypertensive. The skin is sallow and pale. Patients may have evidence of fluid retention and congestive heart failure. They have peripheral edema, elevated jugular venous pressure, rales in the lung bases, and a third heart sound. Patients with severe renal insufficiency may be lethargic with encephalopathy and asterixis.

6. What laboratory abnormalities are commonly seen in patients with chronic renal insufficiency?

Patients with renal insufficiency are usually anemic. BUN and creatinine are elevated. The electrolyte profile often reveals metabolic acidosis and hyperkalemia. Patients often have hyperphosphatemia secondary to phosphate retention, which results in hypocalcemia. Compromise in vitamin D synthesis further accentuates hypocalcemia. Hyperphosphatemia and hypocalcemia result in an elevated level of parathyroid hormone (PTH) with renal osteodystrophy. Uremic toxins can result in compromises of platelet function with prolongation of bleeding time.

7. Describe the clinical course of chronic renal insufficiency.

The clinical course depends on the underlying cause of the renal disease. Some diseases, such as diabetic nephropathy, are associated with rapid deterioration. Others, such as polycystic kidney disease, involve a much slower rate of decline.

8. Describe the medical management of anemia due to chronic renal insufficiency.

Anemia of chronic renal insufficiency is due to deficiency of erythropoietin, which is normally synthesized by the kidneys. Symptomatic patients with anemia (hematocrit less than 30% or hemoglobin level less than 10 gm/dl) are usually managed with the administration of either erythropoietin (Epogen or Procrit) or darebopoietin (Aranesp). Erythropoietin is administered subcutaneously, usually 3 times/week. Aranesp has a much longer half-life and can be administered every other week. Aranesp is also administered subcutaneously.

Do not assume that anemia is caused only by erythropoietin deficiency. Uremic patients have prolonged bleeding time and may have gastrointestinal oozing and blood loss. It is therefore important to ensure that patients do not have iron deficiency.

9. How is hypertension due to chronic renal insufficiency managed?

Blood pressure has to be aggressively managed in patients with any renal disease. Inadequate blood pressure control (to levels of 130/70 mmHg) can result in more rapid progression of renal disease. Among the many agents used to manage blood pressure, angiotensin-converting enzyme (ACE) inhibitors such as enalopril (Vasotec), captopril (Capoten), and lisinopril (Zestril, Prinivil) have been shown to slow progression of renal disease. Similar data are emerging for the angiotensin receptor blockers (ARBs), such as losartan (Cozaar), irbesartan (Avapro), and valsartan (Diovan). These agents are preferred for patients with chronic renal insufficiency.

10. How is azotemia managed in patients with chronic renal insufficiency?

The kidney is responsible for the removal of nitrogenous waste. Accumulation of these wastes in renal failure causes some of the uremic symptoms. Usually, reduction of protein intake to 0.75 gm/day/kg body weight is sufficient. For patients with creatinine greater than 7 mg/dl, reduction of protein intake to 0.5 gm/day/kg body weight allows sufficient amounts for daily requirements while slowing progression of renal failure.

11. Describe the management of sodium and fluid balance in patients with chronic renal insufficiency.

In patients with **moderate renal insufficiency**, salt and water intake must be adequate to match the excessive loss that results from deterioration of tubular function. Patients cannot concentrate their urine, and rigid restriction may actually accelerate renal damage by causing dehydration.

In patients with **severe renal insufficiency**, salt and water retention results from limited excretion. Sodium and water restriction and use of diuretics may become necessary.

12. How is acidosis managed in patients with chronic renal insufficiency?

Acidosis is in part related to phosphate retention; thus, aggressive binding of phosphate is important. After phosphate binding, sodium bicarbonate is used to treat acidosis. Caution is necessary to avoid sodium overload and congestive heart failure.

13. How is hyperkalemia managed in patients with chronic renal insufficiency?

Hyperkalemia is a serious complication that can precipitate cardiac arrhythmia. Dietary potassium intake should be carefully restricted in patients with hyperkalemia. Acidosis should be reversed. In some instances, hyperkalemia may necessitate use of sodium polystyrene sulfonate (Kayexelate). In patients with severe hyperkalemia (potassium greater than 6.5 mg/dl), dialysis may be necessary.

14. Describe the management of hyperphosphatemia in patients with chronic renal insufficiency.

Hyperphosphatemia is managed by stringent restriction of dietary phosphate. Aggressive phosphate binding is usually done by the use of calcium carbonate, calcium citrate, calcium acetate (PhosLo), or Renagel.

15. How is hypocalcemia managed in patients with chronic renal insufficiency?

Hyperphosphatemia must be addressed first because a high level of phosphate precludes successful treatment of hypocalcemia. After phosphate is normalized, hypocalcemia is managed with calcium supplement and the use of vitamin D or vitamin D analogs.

16. Among the many medical problems of patients with chronic renal insufficiency, what are the most important issues for the dentist?

1. By far the most common concern for the dentist is the management of bleeding diathesis in uremic patients with thrombocytopathy.

2. The kidneys excrete many drug and drug metabolites. It is important to adjust dosages of renally excreted drugs in patients with chronic renal insufficiency.

3. Hyperkalemia is a life-threatening complication. It is important for the dentist to be sure that hyperkalemia is corrected before to any dental procedures.

17. How should the dentist evaluate patients with chronic renal insufficiency?

1. The dentist should be concerned about risks associated with hypertension.

2. The dentist should be aware of the possibility of platelet function abnormalities.

3. The dentist should be aware of drugs that require dose adjustment because they are excreted by the kidneys.

4. The dentist should be aware of drugs that are contraindicated in patients with chronic renal insufficiency.

5. The patient should have close, ongoing medical follow-up.

6. Recent complete blood count and electrolyte, BUN, and creatinine levels should be available to assess the degree of renal insufficiency.

7. Medications should be carefully reviewed.

8. The patient's blood pressure should be measured before any dental intervention.

18. How should the dentist approach a patient with chronic renal insufficiency?

1. In patients with significant hypertension, blood pressure should be under better control before any dental intervention is performed.

2. The dentist should be aware of the thrombocytopathy associated with renal insufficiency.

3. Care should be exercised when drugs are prescribed because the kidneys excrete many drugs and drug metabolites.

19. How should a dentist approach the possible bleeding diathesis of patients with chronic renal insufficiency?

1. Renal insufficiency can be gauged by knowing the patient's BUN or creatinine level. The normal range of BUN is 10–20. Patients with moderate compromise in renal function often have BUN greater than 50. Patients with BUN greater than 50 may have abnormalities in platelet function with resultant bleeding diathesis. The dentist should be concerned about the possibility of bleeding complications in patients who have BUN greater than 50.

2. To assess the degree of thrombocytopathy, the dentist should coordinate with the patient's physician and obtain an Ivy bleeding time using a standard template.

3. The interference with platelet function is usually mild, and the typical patient has slightly elevated bleeding times (< 12 minutes vs. normal time <10 minutes). For such patients, no specific intervention is necessary unless the surgical procedure involves significant soft tissue and bone trauma. Local hemostatic measures, including extra suturing, compression packing, application of oxidized cellulose, and microfibrillar collagen Hemostat, can be used. In rare cases, a 4.8% tranexamic acid mouthwash, 10 ml 3 or 4 times/day for 3–7 days, may be helpful.

4. For advanced surgical procedures, the dentist may elect to consult the physician and use 1-desamino-8-D-arginine vasopressin (DDAVP) to correct the thrombocytopathy.

5. In a small subset of patients with renal disease, the bleeding time may be markedly prolonged (> 12 minutes). The most practical approach is the use of DDAVP (0.4 μg/kg) intravenously before the planned dental procedures. (A 70-kg patient would receive 70 × 0.4 = 28 μg DDAVP intravenously). This approach obviously must be coordinated with the patient's physician, using a medical center for infusion. DDAVP can be repeated every 12 hours as necessary for up to 4 days.

20. What is dialysis?

Dialysis is the procedure used to remove nitrogenous waste and excessive fluid from patients with severe renal insufficiency. Dialysis also helps with management of hypocalcemia and acidosis. Two major kinds of dialysis are available: hemodialysis and peritoneal dialysis. Most patients on peritoneal dialysis undergo ambulatory peritoneal dialysis, but some patients are on chronic cycling peritoneal dialysis.

21. What is hemodialysis?

Hemodialysis is the procedure by which a machine is used to clear waste and excessive fluid from patients with chronic renal insufficiency. Vascular access is necessary. Patients are generally dialysed 3 times/week for 3 hours at each session. Most patients go to a dialysis center for treatments. A small minority of patients undergo the procedures at home.

During dialysis, blood is accessed from the patient's circulation and passed into the dialysis machine. Drugs such as erythropoeitin and vitamin D can be administered during the treatment. To avoid clotting of blood in the machine, heparin is usually administered. Heparin is a short-acting anticoagulant that can cause bleeding complications only on the day of dialysis. Usually the heparin effect is eliminated from the system in 2–3 hours.

22. What methods of vascular access are commonly used for patients on hemodialysis?

The most commonly used method is a **fistula**. A vein, usually in the forearm, is connected end-to-side to an artery. The resultant vessel gradually matures over about 3 months to provide access for hemodialysis.

In some patients, **grafts** are placed for dialysis. The grafts are made of synthetic material such as Gortex and PTFE. These foreign grafts in the circulation have to be accessed repeatedly for dialysis. Grafts are more susceptible to infection and clotting.

In some patients who have difficulty with establishment of vascular access, **in-dwelling catheters** are used. They are usually tunneled subcutaneously into the internal jugular vein. They are highly susceptible to infection and clotting.

23. What should the dentist be concerned about when treating a patient on hemodialysis?

1. The dentist should be aware of the type of access used for hemodialysis.
2. The dentist should be aware of the dialysis schedule.
3. The dentist should decide whether dental prophylaxis is necessary.

24. Which hemodialysis patients require dental prophylaxis?

1. In general, patients with an arteriovenous fistula have a native vessel for access and do not require antibiotic prophylaxis.

2. Patients with grafts and indwelling catheters have a high risk of infection of the access devices from bacteremia and should receive antibiotic prophylaxis.

25. What antibiotics should be used for prophylaxis in patients on hemodialysis?
1. Standard antibiotic prophylaxis can be used. These regimens are identical to those recommended by the American Heart Association for prophylaxis of subacute bacterial endocarditis.
2. The major concern is staphylococcal infection of the access. It is therefore reasonable to consider use of antistaphylococcal antibiotics for dental prophylaxis. Cephalexin (Kelfex, 2000 mg), clindamycin (Cleocin, 600 mg), azithromycin (Zithromax, 500 mg), or clarithromycin (Biaxin, 500 mg) may be used for better staphylococcal coverage. The standard amoxicillin regimen is less effective against staphylococcal species and therefore less desirable.
3. Another convenient way of giving antistaphylococcal antibiotic prophylaxis involves the use of vancomycin.
4. The dentist should inform the patient's nephrologist that dental prophylaxis is desired.
5. Vancomycin may be given intravenously during the patient's dialysis.
6. Vancomycin stays in the bloodstream of a patient on dialysis for 5–7 days and should be considered only when multiple dental appointments are needed within a short period.

26. How should the dentist modify the scheduling of patients on dialysis?
1. The dentist should plan the dental procedure on a nondialysis day to avoid the heparin used during dialysis, which can significantly aggravate bleeding tendencies. Heparin is a short-acting anticoagulant that causes bleeding complications only on the day of dialysis. Usually the heparin effect is eliminated from the system in 2–3 hours.
2. If vancomycin is the preferred antibiotic, arrangements should be made with the patient's nephrologist for administration during dialysis on the day before the planned procedure.

27. What modifications should be made to medications commonly prescribed in dentistry for patients on hemodialysis?
1. Among the analgesics, acetaminophen is safe to prescribe. Aspirin should be avoided because patients already have thrombocytopathy. Nonsteroidal anti-inflammatory drugs and COX-2 inhibitors should be used judiciously. Selective COX-2 inhibitors (Vioxx, Celebrex) are the preferred NSAID choice for analgesia of very short duration. Unlike conventional NSAIDS, the COX-2 inhibitors do not compromise platelet function and therefore do not exacerbate uremia-induced thrombocytopathy.
2. Among the narcotics, codeine, oxycodone, and hydroxycodone can be prescribed, but care should be taken to minimize oversedation in patients with preexisting encephalopathy.
3. Among the antibiotics, penicillin, cephalosporins, clindamycin, erythromycin, macrolides, and metronidazole are safe to use.
4. Tetracyclines, with the exception of doxycycline, are contraindicated because of potential renal toxicity.
5. Doxycycline is metabolized in the liver and can be safely prescribed for patients on peritoneal dialysis.
6. The quinolones (ciprofloxacin, ofloxacin, levofloxacin, and etafloxacin) are renally excreted and have to be dose-adjusted.

28. What is peritoneal dialysis?
Although 90% of the patients with end-stage renal disease are treated with hemodialysis, 10% are on peritoneal dialysis. A catheter is placed surgically into the peritoneal cavity. Specially mixed fluid is infused into the peritoneal cavity and allowed to dwell for a number of hours. Through the peritoneal membrane, waste and excessive fluid are removed. The fluid is drained from the peritoneal cavity, and the process is repeated. On average, the patient has to do 4 or 5 exchanges each day to ensure adequate clearances of waste.

29. Define CAPD and CCPD.

Patients on CAPD (continuous ambulatory peritoneal dialysis) undergo 4 or 5 manual exchanges per day, whereas patients on CCPD (continuous cycling peritoneal dialysis) are attached to a machine (cycler) that makes the exchanges at night while the patient sleeps.

30. What are the complications of peritoneal dialysis?

The major risk for patients on either CAPD or CCPD is peritonitis.

31. What are the dental concerns for patients on peritoneal dialysis?

Bacteremia can seed the peritoneal fluid. Patients on peritoneal dialysis, therefore, should have dental prophylaxis. In general, standard dental prophylaxis is appropriate.

32. What modifications should be made to medications commonly prescribed in dentistry for patients on peritoneal dialysis?

The six guidelines in question 27 also apply to patients on peritoneal dialysis. Although most sedatives are metabolized by the liver, they must be used judiciously to avoid aggravation of encephalopathy.

28. TRANSPLANTATION

Robert C. Fazio, D.M.D., and Leslie S.T. Fang, M.D., Ph.D.

1. Who receives an organ transplant?
Appropriate patients with end-stage renal, liver, cardiac, and pulmonary diseases are candidates for transplantation.

2. What is the most common organ transplant?
Renal transplantation is the most common organ transplant, followed by liver, heart, and lung transplants.

3. Where are donor organs obtained?
About 30% of renal transplants are from living related or living unrelated donors. A very small percentage of patients with liver or lung transplants get the organs from a living source. All other transplants are done with organs from a cadaveric source.

4. What should the dentist be concerned about in patients who have received an organ transplant?
Regardless of the organ transplanted, the dentist should be aware of the issues surrounding immunosuppressive drugs. Patients are much more prone to infection and should have antibiotic prophylaxis. They also should be carefully monitored and aggressively treated for infections. Most of the patients take steroids, and the dentist should follow the protocol for patients on steroid therapy (see Chapter 12).

5. What are the common immunosuppressive drugs used in organ transplantation?
1. Most patients take steroids.
2. Patients often take azathiaprine (Imuran) or mycophenolate mofetil (Cellcept).
3. Patients often take various preparations of cyclosporine (Sandimmune, Neoral).
4. Some patients take tacrolimus (Prograf) instead of cyclosporine.

6. Should transplant patients receive antibiotic prophylaxis?
Although transplant patients do not have underlying cardiac defects, antibiotic prophylaxis is appropriate because of the increased risk of infection. In most cases, standard antibiotic prophylactic therapy is appropriate.

7. How should the dentist manage patients on steroid therapy?
Transplant patients are continuously on steroid therapy and are adrenally suppressed. The following strategies are recommended:
1. Steroid supplement is necessary for more complex dental procedures.
2. Early morning appointments are best.
3. Shorter appointments are preferred.
4. Minimize stress.
5. Use sedation techniques when appropriate.
6. Dental treatment plans may require notification as appropriate.
7. The major goal is to avoid precipitation of adrenal insufficiency.

8. What is the clinical consequence of adrenal insufficiency?
The adrenal glands are responsible for increased production of steroids at times of stress. The ability to produce steroids under physiologic stress is called the stress response. The stress response permits increased cardiovascular tone at times of stress.

Patients with mild adrenal insufficiency experience weakness, weight loss, orthostatic hypotension, nausea, and vomiting. Patients with severe adrenal insufficiency cannot increase steroid production in response to stress and in extreme situations may have cardiovascular collapse.

9. How should supplemental steroids be given?

Supplemental steroids should be given on the morning of the proposed dental intervention. The dosage should be titrated according to the anticipated level of stress from the procedure. In general, patients should receive 60 mg of prednisone on the morning of the procedure if they are expected to be under considerable physiologic stress (e.g., general anesthesia). For less stressful procedures, 30–40 mg of prednisone will suffice.

10. How should the dentist approach patients taking Imuran or Cellcept?

Both agents can suppress the bone marrow and alter the patient's immune response. It is important, therefore, to consider antibiotic prophylaxis. It is also important to treat infections aggressively.

11. How should the dentist approach patients taking cyclosporine therapy?

1. Patients taking cyclosporine are much more prone to gingival hyperplasia.

2. Cyclosporine can cause hypertension. It is important to measure blood pressure before any dental intervention.

3. Cyclosporine can cause hyperkalemia. It is important to have a recent serum potassium before complex dental procedures.

4. Cyclosporine can cause nephrotoxicity. It is important to have a recent assessment of blood urea nitrogen and creatinine.

12. What should the dentist know about gingival hyperplasia in patients taking cyclosporine?

As many as 40% of patients taking cyclosporine develop gingival hyperplasia. Younger patients taking the drug are more likely to be affected than older patients. The severity of gingival hyperplasia appears to be dose-related. With progressive decreases in doses of cyclosporine, the incidence of hyperplasia also decreases. However, the addition of a second at-risk drug, such as a calcium channel blocker, markedly accentuates the predisposition to gingival hyperplasia.

Because the phenomenon is dose-related, patients who take higher doses of cyclosporine are more likely to develop gingival hyperplasia. In general, patients with cardiac, liver, and lung transplant tend to be at higher risk than patients with renal transplant because of the doses of cyclosporine prescribed.

It appears that the development of hyperplasia is most active for the first 3 months after initiation of therapy. The hyperplasia usually plateaus by 9 months to 1 year.

Because poor oral hygiene and the presence of plaque increases the severity of cyclosporine-induced hyperplasia, patients who receive the drug should have intensive oral hygiene instructions and more frequent recall prophylaxes and examinations. The use of an antimicrobial mouth rinse such as chlorhexidine may be helpful.

13. How should the dentist approach the patient taking Prograf?

Prograf is similar to cyclosporine in its physiologic function. However, gingival hyperplasia is uncommon in patients taking Prograf. Prograf is also less likely to cause renal dysfunction and hyperkalemia.

14. How should the dentist approach the patient with a renal transplant?

It is important to have a reasonable assessment of the status of the patient with a renal transplant. The following guidelines are recommended:

1. Dental procedures should not be done at a time when renal function is in flux: Patients who have active renal rejection should have dental treatment deferred until renal function has stabilized.

2. It is important to know what medications the patient takes. Not infrequently they take antihypertensives and diuretics (see Chapters 3 and 6) in addition to immunosuppressive agents.

3. It is important to know whether the patient is taking antibiotics prophylactically. Not infrequently, patients take trimethoprim/sulfamethoxazole (Bactrim) for prophylaxis against *Pneumocystis carinii*. This may influence antibiotic choices. Oral flora often are altered by chronic low-dose Bactrim.

4. It is important to avoid nephrotoxic drugs. Among drugs commonly prescribed by dentists, the following should be avoided:
- Nonsteroidal anti-inflammatory drugs
- COX-2 inhibitors (i.e., Vioxx, Celebrex)
- Tetracycline and derivatives (except for doxycycline)
- Erythromycins
- Macrolides

5. It is important to adjust doses of medications that are renally excreted in patients with any degree of renal dysfunction.

15. What adjustments should the dentist make in choices of antibiotics in patients with renal transplants?

1. Penicillin, cephalosporins, and clindamycin are safe to use.

2. Erythromycin and all of the macrolides are contraindicated because they raise cyclosporine and Prograf levels by interfereing with their metabolism via the cytochrome p450 system, even with a short course. Although azithromycin (Zithromax) does not affect the cytochrome p450 system, it carries a labeling warning because it is classified as a macrolide.

3. Tetracyclines, with the exception of doxycycline, are contraindicated because of potential renal toxicity. Doxycycline is metabolized in the liver.

4. The quinolones (ciprofloxacin, ofloxacin, levofloxacin, and etafloxacin) are renally excreted and have to be dose-adjusted.

16. How should the dentist adjust analgesic usage in patients with renal transplant?

1. Acetaminophen is safe to prescribe.

2. Aspirin should be avoided because many patients with renal dysfunction already have thrombocytopathy. Furthermore, aspirin further aggravates the gastropathy induced by steroids.

3. Nonsteroidal anti-inflammatory drugs are contraindicated because they can worsen renal insufficiency. For similar reasons, even the COX-2 inhibitors have to be avoided.

17. How should the dentist adjust the use of narcotics and sedatives in patients with renal transplant?

1. Codeine, oxycodone, and hydrocodone can be prescribed, but care should be taken to minimize oversedation.

2. Although most sedatives are metabolized by the liver, it is important to use these drugs judiciously.

18. How should the dentist approach patients with liver transplant?

1. The stability of liver function should be established. No dental procedures should be done in patients with evidence of organ rejection.

2. A recent set of liver function tests, including prothrombin time, should be reviewed with the physician.

3. A recent complete blood count and platelet count should be available.

4. The complete list of medications should be reviewed.

19. How should the dentist modify antibiotic dosing in patients with liver transplant?

1. Penicillins and cephalosporins are generally safe to use.

2. Erythromycin preparations and macrolides should be avoided. These drugs interfere with metabolism of cyclosporine and Prograf by the cytochrome p450 system, and even a short course can markedly elevate drug levels and result in toxicity. Azithromax (Zithromax) is metabolized by the liver and should be avoided in patients with hepatic compromise.

3. Tetracycline and minocycline are excreted by the kidneys and are safe to use in patients with hepatic compromise.

4. Doxycycline is metabolized primarily by the liver and should be avoided.

5. Clindamycin (Cleocin) is relatively contraindicated and should be avoided. In instances of severe infection when clindamycin is the drug of choice, the dose should be reduced in patients with significant hepatic compromise.

6. Metronidazole (Flagyl), if indicated, should be dose-adjusted in patients with hepatic compromise.

20. How should the dentist modify the use of analgesics and sedatives in patients with liver transplant?

The dentist should be careful in prescribing analgesics because of the possibility of compromised hepatic clearance of the drugs. Some patients with liver transplant may have completely normal hepatic function; no substantive changes are necessary. Others, however, may have varying degree of problems with drug metabolism. In patients with any extent of hepatic compromise, the following guidelines are recommended:

1. Acetaminophen (Tylenol) and all compounds containing acetaminophen are contraindicated because of toxicity to the liver. The maximal recommended dose of acetaminophen in a patient with normal liver function is 4000 mg/day. Patients who consume alcohol tolerate a much lower dose before liver toxicity develops. Patients with preexisting liver function compromise should avoid taking any acetaminophen-containing compounds.

2. Aspirin and nonsteroidal anti-inflammatory drugs should be avoided because of enhanced gastropathy in patients on chronic steroid therapy.

3. COX-2 inhibitors (Vioxx, Celebrex) are relatively safe to use.

21. How should the dentist adjust the use of narcotics and sedatives in patients with liver transplant?

1. Narcotics should be prescribed in reduced doses because of the concern over decreased drug metabolism. Meperidine (Demerol), codeine, and tramadol (Ultram) should be prescribed in reduced dose.

2. All sedatives and tranquilizers should be avoided, if possible, in patients with compromised hepatic clearance.

22. How should the dentist approach patients with heart transplant?

1. The dentist should be aware of the current status of the heart transplant. No dental procedures should be undertaken when there may be concern about cardiac rejection.

2. A recent cardiac evaluation from the patient's physicians should be available to ensure stability of the transplant.

3. The list of medications should be carefully reviewed.

4. Blood pressure should be determined before dental intervention.

23. How should the dentist modify the use of antibiotics in patients with cardiac transplant?

1. Penicillins and cephalosporins are generally safe to use.

2. Erythromycin preparations and macrolides should be avoided. These drugs interfere with metabolism of cyclosporine and Prograf by the cytochrome p450 system, and even a short course can markedly elevate drug levels and result in toxicity. Although Azithromycin (Zithromax) does not affect the cytochrome p450 system, it carries a labeling warning because it is classified as a macrolide.

3. Tetracycline, minocycline, and doxycycline are relatively safe to use.

4. Clindamycin (Cleocin) and metronidazole can be used judiciously.

24. How should the dentist modify the use of analgesics in patients with cardiac transplant?

1. Acetaminophen is safe to use.

2. Aspirin should be avoided because of enhanced gastropathy in patients on chronic steroid therapy.

3. Similarly, nonsteroidal anti-inflammatory drugs should be avoided.

4. COX-2 inhibitors are safe to use, provided that renal function is normal. Renal dysfunction is more frequent in these patients because of the nephrotoxicity of cyclosporine.

25. How should the dentist modify the use of narcotics and sedatives in patients with cardiac transplant?

1. Codeine, oxycodone, and hydroxycodone can be prescribed, but care should be exercised to minimize oversedation.

2. Sedatives should be used judiciously.

26. How should the dentist modify the use of analgesics in patients with lung transplant?

1. Acetaminophen is safe to use.

2. Aspirin should be avoided because of enhanced gastropathy in the patient on chronic steroid therapy.

3. Similarly, nonsteroidal anti-inflammatory drugs should be avoided.

4. COX-2 inhibitors are safe to use, provided that the renal function is normal. Renal dysfunction is more frequent in these patients because of the nephrotoxicity of cyclosporine.

27. How should the dentist modify the use of narcotics and sedatives in patients with lung transplant?

1. Codeine, oxycodone, and hydroxycodone can be prescribed, but care should be exercised to minimize oversedation.

2. Sedatives should be used judiciously.

29. SEIZURE DISORDERS

Robert C. Fazio, D.M.D., and Leslie S.T. Fang, M.D., Ph.D.

1. What is a seizure disorder?

Epilepsy is not a disease but rather a symptom complex, the result of diverse neuronal disturbances. Symptoms range from altered consciousness and motor activity to aberrant sensory phenomena and behavior.

2. How common are seizure disorders?

The incidence of seizure disorders is estimated at 0.5–2% of the general population.

3. How are seizure disorders classified?

Seizure disorders are generally classified as generalized or partial (focal) seizures. Generalized seizures often involve loss of consciousness, whereas focal seizures do not.

4. What are the most common forms of seizures?

The most common form of seizure is the generalized grand mal (tonic clonic) seizure. Of patients with seizure disorders, 90% have grand mal seizures at some phase of the disease, and 60% have this form of seizure exclusively. Patients have abrupt loss of consciousness and abnormal motor activities. Patients often have clonic contractions of muscles of the extremities, progressing to generalized muscular contractions. The episodes usually last about 2–5 minutes. During the grand mal seizure, patients may have urinary or fecal incontinence. After the seizure, the patient is usually quite lethargic and confused and is said to be in the postictal state.

5. What is the second most common form of seizures?

Petit mal seizures (absence spells) are the second most common form of seizures. Of all patients with seizures, 25% experience this form during some phase of their illness. Most patients with petit mal seizures also have grand mal seizures. Only 4% of patients have petit mal seizures exclusively. Petit mal seizures are characterized by a 10- to 30-second loss of consciousness, often without loss of motor tone and with little or no abnormal motor activity. Patients typically stop in the middle of activity and stare blankly or blink their eyes rapidly during the attack. Then they resume normal activity and usually do not have a postictal phase.

6. What is the third most common form of seizures?

The third most common form of seizure disorder is psychomotor seizures. These seizures are partial seizures, because there is usually no loss of consciousness. During a psychomotor seizure, the patient exhibits bizarre behavior, makes unintelligible sounds, and cannot communicate. The seizures usually last a few minutes, followed by a short period of confusion. As with petit mal, most patients with psychomotor seizures also have grand mal seizures. Only 6% of all patients with seizure disorders have psychomotor seizures exclusively.

7. What are the causes of seizures?

The physician usually classifies seizures into two categories: symptomatic or idiopathic. Patients with symptomatic seizures have an identifiable underlying disorder causing the seizures, whereas patients with idiopathic seizures do not have identifiable underlying disorders.

8. What are the common identifiable causes of seizures?

The common disorders include tumors, cerebrovascular accidents, and scars from head trauma. Other identifiable causes include high fevers in young children (febrile seizures), central nervous system infections (meningitis, encephalitis), excessive alcohol ingestion, and metabolic derangements such as hypoglycemia, hypocalcemia, uremia, hypernatremia, and hyponatremia.

Drugs, including cocaine, amphetamines, and excessive amount of theophylline, can cause seizures. In some instances, cerebral hypoperfusion due to cardiac arrhythmia may result in seizures.

9. How is the diagnosis of seizures usually made?
The most important clue is usually a detailed history from people who have witnessed the seizures. Witness reports are important because patients often have altered consciousness and their recall is likely to be compromised. The physician should ask about the presence of aura. From the history, the physician usually can determine whether the patient is having grand mal, petit mal, or psychomotor seizures.

10. What diagnostic tests are useful in the diagnosis of seizures?
Electroencephalogram (EEG) is usually the diagnostic test of choice. Abnormal EEG with epileptiform features (spikes or sharp waves) supports the diagnosis and may provide information about the type of seizure disorder. However, abnormal EEG alone is inadequate for the diagnosis of seizures in patients who are otherwise asymptomatic. Conversely, up to 20% of patients with seizure disorders have normal EEG between seizures. EEG, therefore, has to be interpreted with consideration of the clinical scenario.

Sleep EEG increases sensitivity for detection of partial complex seizures. In some instances, ambulatory EEG with monitoring of up to 72 hours increases the yield of abnormal activities.

11. What imaging studies are helpful in the diagnosis of seizures?
Cranial magnetic resonance imaging (MRI) with and without gadolinium contrast is sometimes helpful, particularly in detecting abnormalities in medial temporal region. Positron emission tomography (PET) and single photon emission computed tomography (SPECT) studies should be reserved for special instances in which examination of cerebral function is desired.

12. What is the most common drug used in seizure disorders?
By far the most common drug used in seizure disorders is phenytoin (Dilantin). It is the first-line drug for treatment of grand mal seizures.

13. What other drugs are used in grand mal seizures?
Carbamazepine (Tegretol), valproic acid (Depakote), phenobarbital, primidone (Mysoline), gabapentin (Neurontin), topiramate (Topamax), tiagabine (Gabitril), and felbamate (Felbatol) have been used for grand mal seizures.

14. What drugs are commonly used for petit mal seizures?
Dilantin is still an important drug because many patients with petit mal seizures progress to grand mal seizures at some phase of their illness. Other drugs include carbamazepine (Tegretol), valproic acid (Depakote), phenobarbital, primidone (Mysoline), gabapentin (Neurontin), topiramate (Topamax), oxycarbazepine (Trileptal), tiagabine (Gabitril), and felbamate (Felbatol).

15. What should the dentist be concerned about in the management of patients with a seizure disorder?
1. In patients with a history of poorly controlled seizure disorder, elective procedures should be deferred.
2. Patients with a seizure disorder are at risk for aspiration during a seizure. The dentist, therefore, should consider the possibility of a seizure during the dental procedure with aspiration of loose intraoral material.
3. A clinical approach that maximizes the ease of rapid removal of all dental instruments and aids must be taken. A rubber dam and a rubber dam clamp with an attached floss lead are preferable to the use of multiple cotton rolls.
4. In patients with seizure disorders, the choice of restorations also may be influenced by concern over possible aspiration during a seizure. In general, fixed, permanent, cemented restorations

are preferred over a removable partial denture. Unilateral "Nesbit-type" partial dentures should not be used.

5. When a partial or full denture is necessary, full palatal coverage with metal designs for the major connector are preferred over primarily plastic prostheses.

6. Attention also should be paid to the preparation of temporary restorations. Whereas all-acrylic, office-cured temporary bridges may normally suffice, the dentist may choose laboratory-processed, metal-reinforced bridges for patients with a seizure disorder.

16. What are the dental concerns in patients receiving phenytoin therapy?

Because phenytoin is the most commonly prescribed drug for seizure disorder, the dentist often must deal with complications of long-term phenytoin therapy. Patients receiving long-term Dilantin therapy deserve special attention, because they may develop gingival hyperplasia. The frequency of this complication is not well established, and reports have cited an incidence ranging from 25% to 85% of patients on long-term phenytoin therapy. A reasonable estimate is that 50% of adults on long-term treatment with phenytoin develop gingival hyperplasia. The incidence is higher in children.

17. How should dentists manage patients who develop gingival hyperplasia while taking phenytoin?

Phase I hygiene therapy, including oral hygiene instruction, scaling, root planing, and curettage, should be completed. The correction of defective restorations and caries is essential. The frequency of dental prophylaxis should be increased.

If these conservative means are inadequate for the control of gingival hyperplasia, consultation with the patient's physician should be undertaken to assess the possibility of discontinuing phenytoin. Only then should surgical excision be considered.

18. What considerations are important when the dentist discusses with the physician significant and refractory gingival hyperplasia in a patient taking phenytoin?

1. The frequency of clinically significant gingival hyperplasia is approximately 50% of patients taking phenytoin (higher for children).

2. Conservative dental measures to minimize the impact of the drug have been exhausted. The patient's dentition is at risk for progressive dental disease, including periodontal disease and caries.

3. The possibility of use of alternate agents in the management of the patient, such as barbiturates or carbamazepine, should be raised.

19. What is the second most common drug used in seizure disorder?

Carbamazepine (Tegretol) is probably the second most common drug used in seizure disorder.

20. What drugs are contraindicated in patients on carbamazepine therapy?

1. The use of propoxyphene (Darvocet) may create carbamazepine toxicity.

2. The use of certain macrolides (Biaxin and Dynabac) can raise the carbamazepine level and induce toxicity.

3. Use of carbamazepine can increase the rate of metabolism of doxycycline and render it ineffective.

21. Should tramadol (Ultram) be used in patients with seizure disorders?

Tramadol can decrease seizure threshold and precipitate seizures in a patient with an otherwise stable course and is contraindicated in patients with a seizure disorder.

22. How should a dentist approach the patient with a seizure in the dental office?

1. Some patients have an aura before the onset of seizures; they should be instructed to report any aura to the dentist. The dental procedure should be terminated immediately when the

patient reports an aura. The patient should be placed supine on the floor, preferably on a carpeted area away from hard surfaces and objects.

2. A seizure may occur without any prodrome in the dental chair. In such an instance, the patient should be left in the dental chair and placed in a supine position. Instruments should be removed from the area. The patient can be gently but not forcibly restrained to prevent injury.

3. If possible, part of a towel or a padded tongue blade can be placed between the teeth to prevent biting of the tongue and lips.

4. Extraordinary effort to introduce objects between the teeth should be avoided.

5. During a seizure, airway patency should be established by gently extending the patient's head.

6. Vital signs should be monitored carefully.

7. Most seizures last 2–5 minutes, followed by a postictal phase. No interventions are necessary except for conservative measures listed above.

8. On rare occasions, medications may be necessary to terminate a seizure (status epilepticus). If the seizure continues beyond 2 minutes, medical help should be sought, and arrangements should be made for emergency transport.

9. If medications are necessary, only trained medical personnel should administer the drug.

10. The drugs must be administered intravenously and can cause significant respiratory and cardiovascular depression.

11. For termination of seizures, the drug of choice is diazepam (Valium), 5–10 mg (1 or 2 ml of a 5-mg/ml solution), given slowly intravenously over a period of 1–2 minutes. Complications of the drug include respiratory depression, transient hypotension, and bradycardia. Intravenous diazepam should be reserved for patients in status epilepticus.

12. After the seizure, the patient is often lethargic and confused (postictal state) and should continue to be monitored. Usually the postictal state lasts for about 1 hour.

13. After a seizure, the patient should be discharged in the custody of a responsible person.

14. If there is a concern about possible complications such as aspiration during the seizure, the patient should be referred to the emergency department for further evaluation and management.

30. CEREBROVASCULAR DISEASE

Stephen T. Sonis, D.M.D., D.M.Sc.

1. Is cerebrovascular disease common in the United States?
Cerebrovascular disease is the third most common cause of death in the U.S., trailing only cancer and cardiac disease.

2. What forms of cerebrovascular disease are of most signficance to dentists?
Transient ischemic attacks (TIAs) and cerebrovascular accidents (CVAs) or strokes are probably the most important.

3. What is the difference in outcomes between a TIA and a CVA?
As opposed to CVAs, TIAs result in reversible neurologic disability.

4. Discuss the cause of cerebrovascular disease in under 30 seconds.
• The most significant cause is the formation of thrombi, which may embolize. Once a vessel is occluded, ischemia and damage result.
• Symptoms relate to ischemia.
• If the patient has a TIA, the thrombus is fragmented or dissolved so that normal function is restored.
• If ischemia persists, cerebral infarction occurs, and damage is permanent.
• The most important risk factor for cerebrovascular disease is atherosclerosis.

5. List risk factors for TIA and stroke other than atherosclerosis.
• Untreated hypertension
• Smoking
• Diabetes mellitus
• Hyperlipidemia
• Hypercholesterolemia
• Cardiac disease leading to emboli, such as defective heart valves or valvular prostheses
• Older age
• Use of oral contraceptives

6. Why is the medical evaluation of TIAs critical?
One-third of all patients with untreated TIA later develop a complete stroke, and 30% die within 5 years. Consequently, the physician must try to find a correctable cause.

7. Stroke patients can be categorized into what two categories?
Stroke patients can be categorized into those who are having a stroke (ongoing or evolving stroke) or those who have completed a stroke. Patients in the former category get progressively worse, as noted by their neurologic symptoms over the course of a few days. Aggressive intervention may reduce the ultimate effects of an evolving stroke. On the other hand, a completed stroke does not demonstrate any worsening of neurologic symptoms up to 3 days after the initial event.

8. What is the cornerstone of the medical management of cerebrovascular disease ? How is it accomplished?
Prevention is the cornerstone of management and may be accomplished in a number of ways:
• Treatment of hypertension
• Carotid endarterectomy
• Correction of atrial fibrillation

• Replacement of corrective heart valves
• Anticoagulant therapy
• Stress reduction

9. What are the major concerns for the dentist in treating patients with cerebrovascular disease?

• The history of significant cerebrovasular disease is a strong indicator of major-league atherosclerosis. Therefore, the patient is at risk for stroke and acute and chronic cardiac disease.
• Known causative factors for cerebrovascular disease may affect management in other ways. For example, subacute bacterial endocarditis prophylaxis is a concern in patients with a history of TIA, atrial fibrillation, and mitral stenosis.
• The relative stability of the cerebrovascular disease is important. Patients who have had recent TIAs or strokes (within 6–12 months) are at risk of exacerbation. Patients with repeated TIAs are at high risk.
• Patients who are taking anticoagulant therapy, such as warfarin, for prophylaxis require additional management.

10. What alterations should you make in prescribing an analgesic for patients with a history of stroke?

Nonnarcotic analgesics are preferred in this patient population.

31. CRANIOFACIAL NEUROLOGIC DISORDERS

Stephen T. Sonis, D.M.D., D.M.Sc.

1. Taste disorders are fairly common. What are the three major categories into which they can be grouped?
1. Ageusia, or absence of taste
2. Hypogeusia, or diminshed taste
3. Dysgeusia, or altered or distorted taste

2. Taste buds are what type of receptor? How many cells are typically found in each taste bud?
Taste buds are chemoreceptors, and each taste bud consists of about 50 cells.

3. Where are taste buds located?
Taste buds are located on the fungiform, foliate, and circumvalate lingual papillae as well as many other sites within the mouth, such as the palate, lips, and cheeks. In addition, taste buds are present in the pharynx, larynx, uvula, and upper esophagus.

4. Why is taste altered by drugs that modify cell proliferation?
The cells within taste buds typically turn over every 10 days. Consequently any therapy that modifies mitosis can modify the ability to taste.

5. The lingual taste buds are of major functional significance. Identify the location and innervation of the fungiform, foliate, and circumvalate papillae.
Fungiform papillae are located on the anterior two-thirds of the tongue and are innervated by the facial nerve.
Foliate papillae are located on the lateral borders of the tongue and are innervated by the glossopharyngeal nerve.
Circumvallate papillae are arranged in a V-shaped configuration on the posterior third of the tongue. They are also innervated by the glossopharyngeal nerve.

6. Which cranial nerves mediate taste from the tongue?
This is a giveaway if you read question 5: cranial nerves VII (facial) and IX (glossopharyngeal).

7. Why does nasal obstruction alter taste?
Taste depends on stimulation of both taste buds and olfactory nerves.

8. What is the most common local reason for alterations in taste?
Taste dysfunction most commonly results from local problems such as periodontal disease, infection, poor hygiene, or physical or chemical irritation. Other factors that affect taste are aging, xerostomia, and drugs that have a chemical interaction with the taste buds.

9. What systemic diseases may affect a patient's ability to taste?
Disorders of taste and smell are tightly linked. Although many diseases can affect these senses, they can be grouped into six major categories:
1. Neurologic or nervous disorders
2. Taste or smell disorders resulting from nutritional deficiences
3. Endocrine diseases
4. Local problems
5. Viral infections
6. Other diseases or conditions

10. The six categories in question 9 are much too vague. Give specific examples of each.

1. Nervous disorders
   - Bell's palsy
   - Damage to the chorda tympani
   - Familial dysautonomia
   - Head trauma
   - Multiple sclerosis
   - Raeder's paratrigeminal syndrome
2. Nutritional disorders and diseases affecting nutrition
   - Cancer
   - Chronic renal failure
   - Cirrhosis
   - Niacin deficiency
   - Thermal burn
   - Zinc deficiency
3. Endocrine disorders
   - Adrenocortical insufficiency
   - Congenital adrenal hyperplasia
   - Panhypopituitarism
   - Cushing's syndrome
   - Cretinism
   - Hypothyroidism
   - Diabetes mellitus
   - Gonadal dysgenesis
   - Pseudohypoparathyroidism
4. Local conditions
   - Facial hypoplasia
   - Sjögren's syndrome
   - Radiation therapy
5. Viral infections
   - Human immunodeficiency virus (HIV)
   - Herpes zoster
   - Acute viral hepatitis
   - Influenza
   - Mononucleosis
6. Other conditions
   - Cystic fibrosis
   - Hypertension
   - Laryngectomy

Adapted from Schiffman SS: Taste and smell in disease. N Engl J Med 308:1276, 1983.

11. List common drugs that can alter taste and smell.
- Metronidazole
- Local anesthetics
- Chlorpheniramine HCl
- Ampicillin
- Tetracyclines
- Anticancer drugs (e.g., methotrexate, doxorubicin)
- Thiouracil
- Carbimazole
- Sodium laryl sulfate (the stuff in toothpaste)
- Captopril
- Baclofen
- Levodopa
- Codeine
- Lithium
- Carbamazepine
- Amphetamines
- Oxyfedrine

12. What is glossodynia?
Glossodynia is a burning tongue and is a relatively common presenting symptom. Although most cases are due to local irritation, glossodynia may be a manifestation of an underlying systemic disease. In many cases, however, an underlying etiology is impossible to identify.

13. What three elements in the history of a patient with glossodynia may be especially helpful in making a diagnosis?
1. Nature of onset: mechanical or chemical irritation tends to have an acute onset, whereas glossodynia in a patient with atrophy of the tongue has a more chronic course.
2. Location of symptoms: localized pain is more likely to be of mechanical origin than generalized lingual discomfort.
3. Medical history: glossodynia may be an oral manifestation of a systemic disease.

14. What types of tongue lesions are most often associated with glossodynia due to local irritation?

Ulceration, erosion, or erythema of the tongue may be produced by local irritation; all cause discomfort.

15. Atrophy of the lingual papillae is often associated with glossodynia and may be a sign of an underlying systemic disease. Which systemic diseases may be associated with glossodynia due to papillary atrophy?
- Plummer-Vinson syndrome
- Pernicious anemia
- Celiac disease
- Iron-deficiency anemia
- Pellegra
- Diabetes mellitus
- Amyloidosis
- Multiple myeloma
- Carcinoma
- Metastases

16. What fungal infection is often associated with glossodynia?

Candidiasis may produce glossodynia. Clinically patients may present with a coated tongue due to surface necrosis overlying an eroded or atrophic base. Patients complain of burning or pain.

17. What congenital anomaly may be associated with glossodynia?

Although usually asymptomatic, geographic tongue with or without fissuring may be associated with glossodynia, particularly in response to acidic or salty foods.

18. True or false: The cause of most cases of glossodynia cannot be determined.

True. The cause of about 75% of cases cannot be elicited. The most likely cause of symptoms is neurologic or psychotropic.

19. Halitosis affects almost half of the population. How often is the mouth its source?

The mouth has been cited to be the source of halitosis in most cases. Volatile sulfur compounds (VSCs) of gram-negative bacterial origin have been identified as the offending agents.

20. What oral conditions are associated with halitosis?
- Xerostomia
- Periodontal disease
- Odontogenic infections
- Necrotic oral lesions such as aphthous stomatitis
- Oral cancer
- Faulty restorations or caries that contribute to the accumulation of debris

21. What nonoral diseases may produce halitosis?
- Respiratory diseases
- Sinus infections
- Diabetes mellitus
- Renal failure
- Hepatic failure
- Myelodysplatic diseases
- Gastrointestinal diseases

22. Define tic douloureux.

Tic douloureux, or idiopathic trigeminal neuralgia, is a condition that produces episodes of acute-onset, severe facial pain. The condition is most common among people of middle to old age. The discomfort associated with tic douloureux is initiated by contact with a facial or intraoral trigger zone. The pain is excrutiating but of short duration. The mandibular branch of the trigeminal nerve is most often involved. The cause of trigeminal neuralgia is unknown.

23. What condition should be suspected if trigeminal neuralgia is noted in a woman in her 20s?

Multiple sclerosis.

24. Is trigeminal neuralgia more common on the right side or left side? Why?

The right side is more often involved, but the reason is unknown.

25. Is trigeminal neuralgia more common in males or females?
Females.

26. How is the diagnosis of trigeminal neuralgia made?
Diagnosis usually is based on the clinical history. Blocking the trigger point with local anesthesia should prevent the onset of symptoms and confirm the diagnosis.

27. How is trigeminal neuralgia treated?
Carbamazepine (Tegretol) is probably the mainstay of treatment. The drug, which inhibits the action of polysnaptic reflexes, has been tested fairly extensively. Alternatively, baclofen, lamotrigine, phenytoin, and oxcobazepine are among other drugs that have been used. Surgical intervention is necessary in a minority of cases.

28. What are migraine headaches?
Migraine headaches are recurring vascular headaches that affect about 20–30% of adults. Migraines are most common in women, usually start in puberty, and then decrease in frequency and severity during older age. Two forms have been identified: classic migraines and common migraines. Patients with classic migraines often experience a prodrome that may include dizziness, spots before the eyes, and changes in vision. Migraines may involve the entire head (in two-thirds of cases) or be hemicranial.

29. Do other symptoms accompany the headaches of migraines?
Yes. Patients often experience gastrointestinal symptoms, including nausea, vomiting, and diarrhea.

30. What precipitating factors are associated with migraines?
• Head trauma   • Chocolate   • Exercise
• Alcohol   • Lack of sleep   • Stress
• Cigarette smoking • Family history   • Hormonal changes

31. What nerve is responsible for facial paralysis?
The seventh cranial nerve (facial nerve).

32. Paralysis of the facial nerve is most commonly associated with what condition?
Bell's palsy.

33. What is the most common cause of Bell's palsy?
Bell's palsy is most commonly associated with polyneuritis that is a sequela of viral infection. Paralysis is not always complete, and patients with partial facial nerve paralysis recover more quickly than patients with complete paralysis. About 80% of patients recover.

34. How can you induce iatrogenic Bell's palsy?
By misplacing a local anesthetic during an inferior alveolar block in which you placed drug into the body of the parotid gland, through which the facial nerve runs. If this happens, the most important step is to protect the patient's eye by keeping it shut with surgical tape until lid function returns.

32. OUTPATIENT PSYCHIATRIC DISEASE

Robert C. Fazio, D.M.D., and Leslie S.T. Fang, M.D., Ph.D.

1. Relative to dental care, what are the most important issues for the dentist treating a patient undergoing outpatient psychiatric therapy?
- Assessing patient compliance and the ability to sustain a prolonged dental treatment plan.
- The potential interaction between commonly used psychoactive drugs and the drugs usually prescribed by the dentist.
- The problem of drug-induced xerostomia and its dental management.

2. What are the dental management considerations?
The common psychoactive drugs are used to treat anxiety, depression, and substantial depression or psychoses. The dentist must evaluate the patient's ability to commit to a complex treatment plan, to follow up on appointments, and to fully understand his or her participation in active treatment.

3. Suggest an example of a problem with an outpatient psychiatric patient.
A patient who presents with complex periodontal and prosthetic problems typically becomes involved in a treatment plan of multiple scaling and root planings, the undertaking of complex oral hygiene measures, possible periodontal surgery, and follow-up prosthetics. The dentist must assess the patient's ability to maintain a continuity throughout care, including the commitment to oral hygiene and multiple scheduled appointments. In addition, the dentist must assess the ability of the patient to deal with the stress of the procedures and react appropriately to that trauma.

4. How should the dentist alter his or her treatment plan in the potentially uncooperative patient?
The cornerstone of treatment of the uncooperative patient may be as simple as palliative care; at the next level, it may involve simple Phase I periodontal therapy with more aggressive extraction of questionable and hopeless teeth. A prosthetic treatment plan that is limited to simple, removable appliances rather than more sophisticated fixed prostheses or implant dentistry may be indicated.

5. What are the major drug interactions for the dentist?
When reviewing the variety of outpatient medications used in outpatient psychiatry, the dentist must be aware of the following potential drug interactions or problems:
A potential interaction of these medications with the vasoconstrictors and local anesthesia. There is also interaction of psychiatric drugs with central nervous system depressants (narcotics) used for analgesia. Finally there is the potential complication of drug-induced xerostomia, increasing the risk of caries and periodontal pathology.

6. What are the major classes of drugs used in outpatient psychiatry?
Generally, the major drugs utilized are
- Benzodiazepines
- Phenothiazines
- Tricyclic antidepressants
- Selective serotonin reuptake inhibitors
- Monoamine oxidase inhibitors
- Other psychoactive medications and combination drugs

7. What are the most common benzodiazepines?

GENERIC NAME	TRADE NAME
Diazepam	Valium
Alprazolam	Xanax
Chlordiazepoxide	Librium
Lorazepam	Activan
Hydroxyzine	Atarax, Vistaril
Oxazepam	Serax

8. What are the major dental issues with the use of benzodiazepines?
- The use of these drugs as a premedication to reduce patient apprehension.
- The potential of these drugs to interact with central nervous system depressants (narcotics).
- Specific drug interactions that contraindicate use of the medication.
- Potential drug-induced xerostomia.

9. How are these drugs typically used for premedication?
The dentist often selects benzodiazepines as a premedication 1 hour prior to a scheduled appointment. The intended effect is to allay patient anxiety. The patient must be accompanied by another individual, since operating a motor vehicle while on these medications is contraindicated. The most commonly prescribed medications include 5–10 mm of diazepam (Valium) or 25–50 mg of hydroxyzine (Vistaril), taken orally. In addition to their antianxiety effects, these medications have analgesic effects additive to those of opioids.

10. Is there potential for benzodiazepines to interact with central nervous system depressants?
Benzodiazepines can potentiate narcotics. On the positive side, there is increased positive analgesic effect. On the negative side, there is potential enhanced central nervous system compromise. Caution is advised in the use of opioids for the patient taking benzodiazepines. Lower initial doses to assess potential drug interactions for the individual patient with additive doses later on is the recommended approach.

11. Are there any specific drug contraindications with the benzodiazepines?
The drug alprazolam (Xanax) contraindicates the use of the analgesia propoxyphene (Darvon and Darvocet). Benzodiazepine toxicity is a potential complication.

12. Is there a risk of drug-induced xerostomia with the benzodiazepines?
Although they are not usually a major problem, benzodiazepine use can induce chronic xerostomia in a very small percentage of patients. This is most common with hydroxyzine use but may occur across the drug category. The degree is relatively insignificant, however, compared to the severe xerostomia commonly induced by tricyclic antidepressants or the significant xerostomia produced by the phenothiazines. Specific dental management considerations are discussed under those drug categories.

13. What about the effects of clonazepam (Klonopin)?
Clonazepam is a benzodiazepine with a very different therapeutic indication. It is used for seizure disorders and also for panic attacks.

14. What are the common tricyclic antidepressants used for depression?

GENERIC NAME	TRADE NAME
Amitriptyline	Elavil
Imipramine	Tofranil

Cont'd. on next page

GENERIC NAME	TRADE NAME
Doxepin	Sinequan
Nortriptyline	Pamelor
Protriptyline	Vivactyl
Meprotiline	Ludiomil

15. What are the dental considerations for the use of the tricyclic antidepressants?
• The potential for severe drug-induced xerostomia.
• The potential for significant interaction with central nervous system depressants.
• The potential for significant interaction with vasoconstrictors in local anesthetics.

16. Is xerostomia a significant problem with tricyclic antidepressants?
Among all the psychoactive drugs utilized in the outpatient setting, tricyclic antidepressants carry the highest risk for drug induced xerostomia and with it an elevated risk for caries and dental disease. This is the major red flag in the category.

17. How should the dentist treat these patients?
First, the dentist should see these people on a stepped up recall program. A patient who might normally be seen twice a year for prophylaxis and examination may be best seen three or four times per year. The drugs in this category are probably the highest possible producers of xerostomia of all out-patient medications. The patient should be advised of the risks. Dietary counseling to avoid simple sugars and multiple meals should be instituted. Salivary stimulation with sucrose-free lemon drops or artificial saliva substitutes (e.g., carboxymethyl cellulose [Salivart], [Xerolube]) should be considered.

18. Is there any other protocol that the dentist should follow?
The dentist should strongly recommend a fluoride protocol. Minimally, 1.1% neutral sodium fluoride gel topically applied daily should be recommended. The suggested protocol for application should be full oral hygiene measures, i.e., toothbrush, floss, rubber-tip gingival massage, and water pik, followed by rebrushing the teeth using a 1.1% neutral fluoride gel (e.g., PreviDent). The patient should be instructed to spit out the excess but not to rinse out. Also, the patient should avoid any additional food or drink before bed.

19. What is the protocol for a patient who has already demonstrated significant caries risk?
For this patient, the dentist should strongly consider the fabrication of custom-made fluoride trays. This allows a 7-minute application per arch with significantly increased contact of the gel to the dentition. The only drawback is the cost of the trays.

20. Why not recommend an acidulated phosphate fluoride?
If the patient is to be recommended for routine fluoride use, it is strongly advisable to recommend a pH neutral gel. The acidulated phosphate fluorides have an acidic pH. These fluorides can potentially etch porcelain restorations in the mouth and compromise the aesthetics of those restorations. Constant use of an acidic gel can also irritate the gingiva and mucosa.

21. Is there drug therapy for xerostomia?
Pilocarpine (Salagen), 5 mg tid, can be prescribed. Side effects include excess sweating and rhinitis. The drug can also exacerbate chronic bronchitis and emphysema.

22. What is the potential for interaction between the tricyclic antidepressants and central nervous system depressants?
Tricyclic antidepressants enhance the potential central nervous system depressant effect of narcotic analgesics. Again, caution is recommended for initial dosing, and incremental doses of

narcotics should follow only after evaluation of the response of the patient to the lower initial doses. For example, first prescribe one acetaminophen with 30 mg codeine (Tylenol No. 3), and if the patient is not heavily sedated by this dose, two tablets every 4 hours may be prescribed later.

23. What is the potential for tricyclic antidepressants to interact with the vasoconstrictors of local anesthesia?

Several reports suggest the potential for hypertensive reactions (the acute elevation of blood pressure) as the result of interactions of dental vasoconstrictors with tricyclic antidepressants.

24. What is the specific recommendation?

In general, if the dentist chooses 2% xylocaine with 1:100,000 epinephrine, the dose should not exceed two Carpules for patients concomitantly utilizing tricyclic antidepressants. This may necessitate shorter appointments and multiple visits for a particular treatment plan.

25. What if the procedure is of necessity a longer procedure, for example, the removal of a defective, multiple unit fixed bridge, repreparation, and retemporization?

The dentist has several options. First, he or she may utilize repeat injections of local anesthetics without vasoconstrictors. Second, he or she may choose a long-acting local anesthetic such as bupivacaine (Marcaine) with decreased vasoconstrictor (1:200,000 epinephrine). The latter option would allow the utilization of four Carpules as a maximum dose.

26. How about the use of levonordefrin as a vasoconstrictor?

Levonordefrin is typically found in a 1:20,000 combination with mepivacaine (Carbocaine). Unfortunately, the potential for hypertensive reactions is significantly elevated for levonordefrin compared with epinephrine. The dentist should consider levonordefrin to be contraindicated for patients on tricyclic antidepressants. Estimates of the potential to induce hypertensive reactions are at least two- to three-fold more likely with levonordefrin.

27. What is the bottom line treatment plan recommendation for patients on tricyclic antidepressants?

- If the patient requires local anesthetic with vasoconstrictor, limit use to two Carpules of 2% lidocaine with 1:100,000 epinephrine; 4 Carpules of anesthetic with 1:200,000 epinephrine. Avoid the use of local anesthetics with 1:50,000 epinephrine. Local anesthetics with levonordefrin as a vasocontrictor are generally contraindicated.
- Recognize the risk for significant severe drug-induced xerostomia. Plan treatment accordingly for an anticaries protocol, including increased recall prophylaxes and examinations, increased bitewing radiograph surveys, and a fluoride protocol.
- Be aware that tricyclic antidepressants enhance the central nervous system depressant effects of narcotics. Therefore, titrate the patient dose at a lower level initially to assess that potential on an individual basis.

28. What are the common phenothiazines used for maniac depression psychoses?

GENERIC NAME	TRADE NAME
Chlorpromazine	Thorazine
Thioridazine	Mellaril
Trifluoperazine	Stelazine
Fluphenazine	Prolixin
Promazine	Sparine

29. What are the dental management considerations for patients on phenothiazines?

The major dental issues involved in treating patients on phenothiazines include an assessment of the following:

• The risk for interaction with vasoconstrictors and local anesthetics.
• The risk for drug-induced xerostomia.
• The risk for interactions with central nervous system depressants.

30. What about the phenothiazines and xerostomia?
Phenothiazines definitely can induce significant xerostomia in dental patients. The risk is not as significant as it is with tricyclic antidepressants but it is, nevertheless, a concern.

31. How should the dentist approach a patient on phenothiazines?
Again, as with the patient on tricyclic antidepressants, the dentist should assess the need to increase frequency of recall prophylaxes, bitewing radiograph examinations, and clinical caries examinations. The dentist should also consider a fluoride protocol for these patients.

32. Should the dentist make custom fluoride trays for these patients?
Although custom fluoride trays are more likely to be recommended for patients on tricyclic antidepressants, this is still a significant possibility for patients on phenothiazines. The dentist should consider custom fluoride trays for a patient with a significant history of previous caries predating the phenothiazine therapy, or a patient with a complex prosthetic treatment plan that would be severely compromised by single abutment caries in a multiple abutment splint.

33. What is the dental management for patient on phenothiazine therapy relative to narcotic analgesic selection?
Like the tricyclic antidepressants and the benzodiazepines, the phenothiazines can enhance the central nervous system depressant effects of narcotic analgesics. Again, the dentist should start with a lower dose of narcotic and titrate upward as the patient is assessed for interaction. A patient with significant sensorium reaction to lower-dose narcotic therapy should not have added doses prescribed.

34. Is there a potential for the phenothiazines to interact with vasoconstrictors?
The phenothiazines do have the potential to interact with vasoconstrictors. However, the interaction is quite different from that occurring with the tricyclic antidepressants.

35. How does the phenothiazine interaction with vasoconstrictors differ from tricyclic antidepressants?
Epinephrine and levonordefrin, when they interact with the tricyclic antidepressants, have the potential to create hypertensive reactions (an acute elevation of blood pressure). The effect is significant with both vasoconstrictors but most severe with levonordefrin. The phenothiazines, on the other hand, have the potential to interact with epinephrine in a reverse fashion, resulting in what is called "epinephrine reversal."

36. What is epinephrine reversal?
Epinephrine reversal is the potential for phenothiazines to reverse the normal epinephrine effects. For example, rather than prolonging anesthesia, when given with the phenothiazines epinephrine may shorten the duration of the local anesthetic. Rather than enhancing hemostasis, when combined with the phenothiazines it may induce vasodilation and excess bleeding in the setting of soft-tissue trauma.

37. How does epinephrine usually work?
The intraoral microscopic vasculature has alpha and beta receptors. The alpha receptors cause vasoconstriction. The beta receptors affect vasodilatation. Epinephrine has a dominant alpha effect. Therefore, when it is given alone, vasoconstriction dominates, delaying vascular uptake of local anesthetic, prolonging anesthesia, and improving hemostasis. Epinephrine, however, also has beta potential.

38. What is the beta potential?
Epinephrine can attach beta receptors and cause vasodilatation. The vasoconstrictive alpha effects of epinephrine, however, usually dominate the vasodilatory effects. Phenothiazines, among their other pharmacologic effects, are alpha blockers. If a phenothiazine blocks the attachment of epinephrine to alpha receptors, it has the potential to unmask the beta effects of epinephrine. The net effect, therefore, could be vasodilatation, more rapid uptake of local anesthetics, and a failure to effect hemostasis, namely, epinephrine reversal.

39. Are there other alpha-blocking agents that can potentially cause epinephrine reversal?
The most common alpha blockers used in medicine are medications used for hypertension.

GENERIC NAME	BRAND NAME
Prazosin	Minipres
Terazosin	Hytrin
Dioxazosin	Cardura

The latter two medications, terazosin (Hytrin) and dioxazosin (Cardura), are also commonly used to treat benign prostate hyperplasia in elderly men. Therefore, they are commonly used medications among dental patients.

40. When used as an alternative vasoconstrictor in local dental anesthesia, does levonordefrin have the same drug interaction with phenothiazines as other vasoconstrictors?
No, levonordefrin is purely an alpha-receptor drug with no beta-receptive capability. Therefore, there is no potential to unmask a vasodilatory effect.

41. What is the best dental protocol?
For patients who are receiving phenothiazines, the dentist should choose local anesthetics without vasoconstrictors, or if a vasoconstrictor is desirable, the dentist should limit himself or herself to a local anesthetic with levonordefrin as the vasoconstrictor. The potential for epinephrine reversal is then ruled out. The most common local anesthetic in this category would be 2% mepivacaine with 1:20,000 levonordefrin.

42. Are there dental considerations for patients receiving monoamine oxidase inhibitors?
Monoamine oxidase inhibitors have a potential life-threatening interaction with central nervous system depressants. All narcotic analgesics are strictly contraindicated in patients receiving these drugs.

43. What are the common monoamine oxidase inhibitors?

GENERIC NAME	TRADE NAME
Isocarboxazid	Marplan
Phenelzine sulfate	Nardil
Tranylcypromine sulfate	Parnate

44. It has been thought that epinephrine should never be used with monoamine oxidase inhibitors? Is this true?
Vasoconstrictors are not contraindicated for use in patients receiving monoamine oxidase inhibitors; there is no drug interaction in this circumstance. Other sympathomimetic agents, such as ephedrine in cold remedies, can be life-threatening to patients on monoamine oxidase inhibitors. However, the enzyme that breaks down epinephrine is unrelated to the monoamine oxidase inhibitor effect, and normal use of epinephrine in dental anesthesia can be utilized for patients on monoamine oxidase inhibitors. Even limitations of ephinephrine are not indicated.

45. Is xerostomia an issue with monoamine oxidase inhibitors?

Not unlike the benzodiazepines, monoamine oxidase inhibitors can cause xerostomia. However, it occurs much less frequently than the xerostomia induced by phenothiazines and it is less severe than the xerostomia induced by tricyclic antidepressants.

46. Many patients are using selective serotonin reuptake inhibitors (SSRIs) for depression. Are there dental management considerations with these medications?

Generally, there are not major problems with SSRIs and dental therapy. Tramadol (Ultram), a common analgesic used in dentistry, is contraindicated for all patients receiving SSRIs. The potential drug interaction is the induction of seizures.

47. What are the commonly prescribed SSRIs?

The commonly prescribed SSRIs are

GENERIC NAME	TRADE NAME
Fluoxetine	Prozac
Sertraline	Zoloft
Paroxetine	Paxil
Citalopram	Celexa

48. There are a variety of other psychoactive medications not among the benzodiazepines, phenothiazines, tricyclic antidepressants, SSRIs, and monoamine oxidase inhibitors. What are these medications and what are the dental considerations?

The list of psychoactive drugs is too long to definitively review each and every drug. Some isolated drugs worth mentioning are discussed below.

49. What are the dental considerations for patients on lithium carbonate?

Nonsteroidal anti-inflammatory drugs are commonly chosen by dentists for analgesics. They are contraindicated for patients who are receiving lithium. Lithium toxicity is a complication. In addition, the antibiotic metronidazole (Flagyl) and all tetracyclines can induce lithium toxicity.

50. Buspirone (Buspar) is among the top 100 drugs prescribed in this country for anxiety and depression. Are there dental considerations when patients are receiving this drug?

A significant number of patients receiving buspirone will have drug-induced xerostomia, and the appropriate caries and fluoride protocols are recommended.

51. The drug valproate/valproic acid (Depakote/Depakene) is utilized as a psychoactive medication for panic disorders, absence seizures, and bipolar disease. Are there dental considerations when patients are receiving this drug?

Valproic acid has several potential problems for the dentist. Nonsteroidal anti-inflammatory drugs such as ibuprofen (Motrin) or naproxen (Anaprox) are contraindicated. The dentist must rely on narcotic preparations with acetaminophen.

Valproic acid toxicity also has a potential interaction with the benzodiazepines, and these drugs are generally contraindicated as antianxiety medications.

Erythromycin therapy can also lead to valproic acid toxicity and is relatively contraindicated in patients taking Depakote or Kepakene.

Last, valproic acid can induce significant thrombocytopenia and thrombocytopathy (compromised platelet function and platelet numbers). Bleeding risk must be assessed for these patients prior to dental surgery. A bleeding time and platelet count assessment should be ordered.

33. ANTIBIOTICS AND ODONTOGENIC INFECTION

Robert C. Fazio, D.M.D., and Leslie S.T. Fang, M.D., Ph.D.

1. What is the role of antibiotics in odontogenic infection?

Antibiotics serve as a complement to débridement. Débriding the lesion is the single most important aspect of therapy for odontogenic infection. Infection of an endodontic source involves débriding the canals of active infection and necrotic tissue. Débridement of the periodontal lesion involves surgical curettage or flap surgical curettage debridement of the wound or both.

2. If antibiotic therapy is an adjunct to débridement, is it always necessary?

If a localized infection is fully débrided, an antibiotic may be unnecessary. The choice to use an antibiotic is twofold. First, the clinician must estimate whether the antibiotic will complement the débridement to the level that it will increase the success rate. Second, will the antibiotic decrease the chance that the infection will spread.

3. What is the significance of a spreading infection?

A spreading infection increases the risk to the patient of systemic impact. This could range from extraoral swelling to fistulization, fever, airway compromise, brain abscess, and other distal seeding of infection.

4. When is a spreading infection more likely to occur?

Spreading infection is more likely to occur in an immunocompromised host. Most commonly, this would involve the treatment of infection in a patient who has diabetes mellitus or who is concurrently on prednisone for a variety of systemic conditions. It might also involve the patient undergoing chemotherapy. The very young and the very old, infants and the elderly, are also more likely to be at risk for spreading infection.

5. How should a spreading infection be treated?

A spreading infection mandates not only débridement but also the selection of an adjunctive antibiotic.

6. In general, what are the treatment goals in the therapy of odontogenic infection?

The treatment goals for the dentist are to minimize the risk of infection spread and ultimately to eliminate the infection.

7. How does the dentist choose a particular antibiotic?

As in the selection of all drugs, selecting and prescribing an antibiotic involves assessment of the benefits of the drug against the risks involved in administering it.

8. What are the benefits?

The fundamental benefit of prescribing an appropriate antibiotic is that the predominant microbiota causing the infection are susceptible to that antibiotic. Generally, a bactericidal drug is preferable to a bacteriostatic one, since the latter depends on the active immune system of the patient to make the antibiotic effective.

9. What are the risks involved in the prescription of antibiotics?

The risks involved in the prescription of antibiotics are the potential for unwanted adverse effects or allergic reactions. These include adverse effects attributed to the drug itself or adverse drug interactions with other medications the patient is receiving.

10. Does the level of infection at the time of presentation of the infection dictate antibiotic choice?

When presented with a spreading infection, the clinician should choose an antibiotic with the broadest possible spectrum of susceptible microbiota. Such drugs may be significantly more costly or may carry an increased potential for side effects. These risks are justified, however, when the margin for error for systemic complications has been reduced.

11. What would be the most common example of matching choice of antibiotic to the level of infection?

The first drug of choice in the treatment of localized odontogenic infection is a penicillin. Amoxicillin, 875 mg bid, has an excellent spectrum of susceptible organisms and has a very high safety profile. If the patient has a spreading infection at the initial appointment, the clinician would want to prescribe an antibiotic with a broad spectrum of susceptible microbiota. An antibiotic that fits these criteria is Augmentin, a combination of amoxicillin and a second drug, clavulanate acid. The usual dose is 875 mg bid. This drug has an extended spectrum of susceptible microbiota and therefore provides a more likely rapid resolution of the infection. With the prescription of Augmentin, however, there is an increased risk of diarrhea, complicating the course of the antibiotic when compared with that same risk for amoxicillin alone.

12. What is meant by "extended spectrum, susceptible microbiota"?

Dentistry in particular and medicine in general are faced with an increasing number of strains of organisms that have become resistant to antibiotic therapy. The number of organisms isolated from the subgingival flora that are resistant to either amoxicillin or tetracycline has doubled in the last 10 years.

13. What are these resistant strains?

Most of the oral organisms with increasing resistance to antibiotic therapy are specific strains of gram-negative anaerobic rods or gram-positive anaerobic cocci. There has also been a marked increase in *Staphylococcus* species appearing in oral infection. When choosing an antibiotic with an extended spectrum of susceptible microbiota, one should select an antibiotic effective against the anaerobic rods and cocci and *Staphylococcus* species.

14. What are the causes of failure of an odontogenic infection to respond to treatment?

The clinician must first assess the possibility of inadequate débridement as the cause of the failure of the infection to respond. Second, the possibility of resistant microbiota should be considered. A third consideration is noncompliance on the part of the patient, i.e., failure of the patient to take the medication at the proper intervals or to take the medication at all. Fourth is a previously undiagnosed severe systemic problem that is unmasked by the nonresponding odontogenic infection.

15. If penicillin is the first drug of choice, why not prescribe Penicillin VK at a dose of 500 mg qid?

Penicillin VK at a dose of 500 mg qid is an appropriate drug to use. However, amoxicillin at a dose of 875 mg bid is a better choice. First, the compliance of the patient significantly increases with once or twice a day compared to three or four times a day dosing. Second, although amoxicillin and Penicillin VK have similar spectra, amoxicillin is slightly more effective against several of the newer isolates of resistant anaerobes.

16. What if the patient is allergic to penicillin or is otherwise intolerant to the drugs?

Conventional alternatives to penicillin usually include the selection of either a tetracycline or an erythromycin.

17. What is the best choice of tetracycline?

All of the tetracycline preparations have similar antibacterial properties. Therefore, there is no advantage at this level. The most compelling differentiation among the tetracyclines relates to potential patient compliance. Tetracycline hydrochloride in a therapeutic dose is prescribed as a 250-mg tablet taken four times a day. In addition, it is unstable with food and therefore needs to be taken 1 hour before or 2 hours after meals. If taken with meals, proper absorption will not occur and therapeutic levels will be inadequate. The preferred drug is doxycycline in 100-mg tablets, prescribed as one tablet bid. The twice a day dosing ensures better patient compliance. Minocycline is a similar alternative. Doxycycline is preferred because even at 100 mg/day there is a therapeutic benefit.

18. What are the contraindications to use of tetracycline?
Tetracycline is contraindicated in the pregnant patient, in the breast feeding patient and in the patient receiving Coumadin. Patients on the common antiseizure disorder medications, including phenytoin (Dilantin), barbiturates, and carbamazepine (Tegretol), have accelerated degradation of tetracycline, which could result in a subtherapeutic levels. This is, therefore, a relative contraindication. Patients on birth control pills may have a breakthrough pregnancy while on broad-spectrum antibiotics and must be advised to use alternative birth control measures. Renal failure is a contraindication to the use of tetracycline, except for doxycycline. Doxycycline is metabolized in the liver and can be used in the patient with renal failure. The most common clinical situation that the clinician will encounter is the patient with diabetes mellitus and renal failure.

19. What are the major issues with prescribing erythromycins?
The two most important issues in the use of erythromycins include gastrointestinal toxicity affecting compliance and decreasing effectiveness against many of the strains of bacteria involved in oral infection.

20. What are the basic distinctions among the erythromycins?
The erythromycins belong to the group of antibiotics referred to as the macrolide antibiotics. Conventional erythromycin includes erythromycin stearate as the erythromycin base; enteric-coated erythromycin (E-Mycin), delayed released capsule erythromycin (ERYC) and erythromycin ethylsuccinate (EES). These drugs share a similar spectrum of bacterial sensitivity. They do not cover *Staphylococcus* species and increasingly bacteria involvement in odontogenic infection are resistant.

21. How do the erythromycins differ with regard to gastrointestinal toxicity?
Erythromycin stearate has the highest gastrointestinal toxicity. A significant number of patients discontinue or interrupt therapy when taking this drug for this reason. In addition, it is unstable with food and must be taken 1 hour before or 2 hours after meals, increasing the difficulty of compliance. Enteric-coated erythromycin (E-Mycin) is kinder to the stomach but still a potential problem. Both erythromycin stearate and enteric-coated erythromycin are prescribed as 250 mg qid. Delayed release capsule erythromycin (ERYC) comes in 250-mg capsules but has an extended half-life and is prescribed as two tablets bid. The total dose, 1 g, is the same as that for erythromycin stearate and enteric-coated erythromycin but it is divided into a two-dose schedule, which increases patient compliance. In addition, this preparation has less effect on the stomach and, therefore, is much better tolerated, also furthering compliance. Erythromycin ethylsuccinate is prescribed in 400-mg capsules but they are bioequivalent to a 250-mg capsule of the other basic erythromycin preparations. It is prescribed as 400 mg qid and produces a gastrointestinal upset pattern similar to that of enteric-coated erythromycin. In summary, the preferred drug in this category would be ERYC 250 mg,. two tablets bid.

22. How about more recent erythromycins?
Three recent additions to this category include azithromycin (Zithromax), clarithromycin (Biaxin), and dirithromycin (Dynabac).

23. What are the advantages of these medications?
First, they are generally much kinder to the stomach with significantly fewer gastrointestinal complications. This increases patient compliance. Second, they have an extended spectrum coverage for more gram-positive and gram-negative anaerobes and for *Staphylococcus* species.

24. How do we choose among them?
Azithromycin (Zithromax) and clarithromycin (Biaxin) are commonly used, dirithromycin (Dynabac) less so. Clarithromycin is prescribed as 250-mg or 500-mg tablets bid . Dirithromycin is made in 250-mg tablets and is prescribed as two tablets once daily. Azithromycin comes in 250-mg tablets and is prescribed as two tablets the first day and one tablet a day for days 2 through 5.

25. How does azithromycin differ from the other compounds?
Like other antibiotics, clarithromycin and dirithromycin are at subtherapeutic levels in the body shortly after discontinuing the medication. Azithromycin, on the other hand, is given for 5 days but still has therapeutic levels of the medication in the body at day 9 or day 10.

26. Are there relative advantages among the three?
Azithromycin clearly has the superior compliance profile. The patient takes medication for 5 days and ends up with a 10-day course. All are similar in gastrointestinal complications and extended spectrum microbiota sensitivity and all are, therefore, superior to the conventional erythromycins.

27. What are the contraindications for erythromycin therapy?
Most macrolide antibiotics are processed by the cytochrome p450 enzyme system in the liver. This series of enzymes, which degrade most erythromycins, also metabolize several other drugs. The clinician should view this system of enzymes as a low capacity system. Therefore, when a patient is receiving multiple drugs processed by the cytochrome p450 system, toxic levels of one may accumulate as the other is preferentially metabolized. This is particularly true for the macrolide antibiotics.

28. What complications can ensue?
This depends on the second medication being taken by the patient but may include serious cardiovascular complications including life-threatening arrhythmias.

29. What are two outstanding examples of such complications?
Three drugs have recently been removed from the marketplace: terfenadine (Seldane) and astemizole (Hismanal), used for allergic rhinitis, and cisapride (Propulsid), used for heartburn, are both metabolized by the cytochrome p450 enzyme system and have both been associated with life-threatening arrhythmias when administered concurrently with macrolide antibiotics.

30. What other drugs interact in a similar way with the macrolide antibiotics and with what complications?
Astemizole (Hismanal)—arrhythmias
Theophylline (Slobid, Theo-Dur)—arrhythmias
Digoxin (Lanoxin)—arrhythmias
Disopyramide (Norpace)—arrhythmias
Midazolam (Versed)—toxicity
Cyclosporine (Neoral, Sandimmune)—renal failure
Warfarin (Coumadin)—increased prothrombin time
Buspirone (Buspar)—toxicity
Carbamazepine (Tegretol)—toxicity
Simvastatin (Zocor)—myositis
Lovastatin (Mevacor)—myositis

31. Are any of the macrolide antibiotics safe when prescribed with these medications?

Azithromycin is not processed by the cytochrome p450 system and, therefore, should not interact at this level with other medications processed by this system. Because of its inclusion in the macrolide antibiotic category, however, the manufacturer warns about "potential interactions" and advises monitoring drug levels. From a practical standpoint for the clinician in an outpatient setting, alternative drugs, when available, should be considered. However, the safety margin of azithromycin is clearly superior to that of the other macrolide antibiotics.

32. When should the clinician use doxycycline (Vibramycin) or azithromycin (Zithromax)?

For the patient who is allergic to penicillin or is intolerant of penicillin for localized or spreading infections, respectively.

33. If the patient has a localized infection and is intolerant of or allergic to amoxicillin, what is recommended?

Doxycycline, 100 mg bid for 7 to 10 days.

34. For the patient with a spreading infection who is allergic to or intolerant of penicillin, what is recommended?

Azithromycin (Zithromax), 250 mg two tablets day 1 and one tablet days 2 through days 5.

35. Is there a more convenient way of writing a prescription for azithromycin?

Yes, azithromycin, 250 mg "dispense a Z-pack sig. as directed." The patient receives a card containing the six pills of azithromycin in a push-out cellophane individually wrapped container. Directions for taking the pills are quite clear.

36. Is there any fundamental difference between azithromycin (Zithromax) and clarithromycin (Biaxin)?

Azithromycin has an extended half-life requiring only 5 days of therapy for a 10-day dose. Clarithromycin requires 10-day dosing. Azithromycin is not processed by the p450 system, whereas clarithromycin is. Therefore, clarithromycin carries all of the risks of drug interactions of other macrolide antibiotics. Azithromycin is a pregnancy category B drug; clarithromycin is a pregnancy category C drug.

37. Why not use azithromycin for the penicillin-allergic patient with a localized infection?

Although azithromycin has an extended spectrum of antibacterial activity, including coverage for *Staphylococcus*, it is an expensive medication compared with doxycycline. The latter should be more than sufficient for localized infection. Azithromycin should be reserved for the treatment of a spreading infection, a refractory infection, or for an immunocompromised patient (for example, a patient with diabetes or a patient receiving prednisone therapy.)

38. Summarize the advantages of azithromycin.

Azithromycin has the highest possible compliance level (5-day dosage for 10 days of therapy). It has an extended spectrum antibacterial profile, including *Staphylococcus* and anaerobes. The drug is pregnancy category B and is stable in food. It is not processed by the cytochrome p450 system of enzymes significantly, thus limiting drug interactions compared with other macrolides.

39. Should clindamycin (Cleocin) be part of the clinician's armamentarium?

Yes, clindamycin shares the benefits of azithromycin in that it has extended spectrum coverage for multiple anaerobes and also covers *Staphylococcus*. Its advantages over azithromycin are that there is no issue of interaction with cytochrome p450 enzyme metabolized drugs whatsoever, and it is significantly less costly. The major disadvantage of clindamycin is an increased risk of pseudomembranous colitis and potential compliance problems with the qid dosing schedule.

40. What is pseudomembranous colitis?
Pseudomembranous colitis is the result of suppression of the gastrointestinal microflora, which allows the emergence of the organism *Clostridium difficile*. Initially, this causes significant diarrhea. If the diarrhea persists, electrolyte imbalances and severe, potentially fatal sequelae can emerge. Most often, when the drug is discontinued the diarrhea stops, but these patients must be monitored closely.

41. When should a dentist refer a patient for possible pseudomembranous colitis evaluation?
If a dentist has prescribed clindamycin (Cleocin) and the patient still has persistent, severe diarrhea 48 hours after the discontinuation of the drug, the patient needs to be referred to a physician. The treatment of pseudomembranous colitis usually involves the prescription of the antibiotic metronidazole (Flagyl) or vancomycin (Vancocin). A physician will confirm the diagnosis using a specific test for *Clostridia difficile*.

42. How big a problem is this?
While initial concerns regarding pseudomembranous colitis related to clindamycin (Cleocin) administration were overstated, the antibiotic still carries a significant warning box in the *Physicians' Desk Reference*. Generally the drug should be reserved for more serious infections when other antibiotics are inappropriate. It is notable that any antibiotic can cause pseudomembranous colitis. However, statistically, it is most common with clindamycin.

43. When should a dentist use clindamycin (Cleocin?)
As a first drug of choice for localized infection, Cleocin is probably inappropriate. If, however, a localized infection does not respond to either penicillin or doxycycline administered to the penicillin-allergic patient, the dentist must consider resistant organisms as a possible diagnosis. After inadequate débridement and noncompliance on the patient's part have been ruled out, the patient can be considered for a course of clindamycin (Cleocin), 150–300 mg qid. The drug can also be used as a back-up for more serious infections that do not respond to amoxicillin + clavulanate (Augmentin) or azithromycin, as noted above. Clindamycin (Cleocin) can be considered as a first-line drug in the setting of an infection that is spreading and one in which Augmentin or azithromycin is an inappropriate choice.

44. If pseudomembranous colitis is a side effect of clindamycin (Cleocin), why does the American Heart Association recommend it as a first option for subacute bacterial endocarditis prophylaxis in the penicillin-allergic patient?
The risk of pseudomembranous colitis is significant for multiple day dosage. There has only been one case report in the international literature of pseudomembranous colitis resulting from a single dose. The issue, therefore, is length of course of the antibiotic.

45. Which patients should not receive a prescription for clindamycin (Cleocin)?
Any patient with a previous history of intolerance of or allergy to clindamycin should not receive it. Any patient with a history of diarrhea in response to antibiotic use or a history of gastrointestinal disorders with diarrhea as a prominent finding should probably be given an alternate choice of antibiotic.

46. Which medical conditions are relative contraindications to clindamycin?
A patient with irritable bowel syndrome or inflammatory bowel disease often has diarrhea as a dominant symptom. These patients are not candidates for clindamycin.

47. Where do the use of cephalosporins fit in treatment of odontogenic infection?
First-generation cephalosporins, for example cephalexin (Keflex), have a antibiotic spectrums similar to Penicillin VK or amoxicillin in that they are effective against *Streptococcus viridans* species often found in isolates of odontogenic infection. The first-generation cephalosporins

have the advantage of covering *Staphylococcus* species as well. The first-generation cephalosporins are probably not as effective against routine *Streptococcus viridans* identified in odontogenic infections and do not cover the extended spectrum or commonly resistant strains of anaerobic rods and cocci. Therefore, their only possible advantage over amoxicillin is when *Staphylococcus* species are involved.

48. Indicate when *Staphylococcus* species should be considered in treatment of odontogenic infection.

The two most common situations would be an oral injury with trauma to the lip and contamination of the epidermal wound. Antibiotic coverage following such trauma is prophylactic in nature but needs to take into consideration the possibility of staphylococcal contamination from the skin into the oral wound. The second instance involving the presence of *Staphylococcus* is in at risk infections of prosthetic joints. *Staphylococcus* accounts for two thirds of the infections of prosthetic joints attributable to on an oral source for which the first-generation cephalosporins are the recommended prophylaxis.

49. What dose of cephalexin (Keflex) is appropriate?

In most clinical situations, a loading dose of 2 g of cephalexin, followed by 500 mg qid, would be appropriate to treat oral wounds contaminated by skin microbiota. Prophylaxis for prosthetic hip joints, when cephalexin is utilized, is a 2-g single dose 1 hour before procedure.

50. How about the second generation cephalosporins?

The most commonly prescribed second-generation cephalosporins are cefuroxime (Ceftin) and loracarbef (Lorabid). These drugs have an extended microbiota spectrum similar to that of augmentin (amoxicillin + clavulanate), azithromycin (Zithromax), and clindamycin (Cleocin) and are effective against *Staphylococcus* species and the extended spectrum anaerobes.

51. How are they prescribed?

Cefuroxime (Ceftin) is given as 250–500 mg bid, loracarbef (Lorabid) as 200–400 mg bid 1 hour before or 2 hours after meals.

52. Can you use cephalosporins in the patient who is allergic to penicillin?

In the outpatient setting of the dental office, it is inappropriate to prescribe cephalosporins. Approximately 8% of the patients who are allergic to penicillin are also allergic to cephalosporins.

53. Is metronidazole (Flagyl) suitable for the treatment of odontogenic infections?

Metronidazole is not appropriate for the treatment of an acute odontogenic infection. Metronidazole covers only gram-negative anaerobic rods and does not impact on the *Streptococcus viridans* species, the species most commonly isolated in odontogenic infections.

54. Is there a role for metronidazole in the treatment of odontogenic infections?

Metronidazole can be used in a piggy-back fashion in addition to a first-line drug to provide an enhanced gram-negative anaerobic rod coverage. An example would be in the patient who was started on amoxicillin, 875 mg bid, for a localized infection and who has not responded well after 48 to 72 hours. The clinician's option is to discontinue the oral amoxicillin and go to a back-up drug for resistant strains (for example, clindamycin) or have the patient continue with the amoxicillin and add on a similar dose of metronidazole.

55. What are examples of these dosages.

If the patient is taking amoxicillin, 875 mg bid, a reasonable add-on drug would be metronidazole, 500 mg bid. If the patient is taking amoxicillin, 500 mg tid, it would be appropriate to add metronidazole, 500 mg tid. A similar regimen would be appropriate if the patient is not responsive to doxycycline therapy bid.

56. Is metronidazole ever used to treat dental infections?

Yes, but only in the chronic infection of rapidly progressive periodontitis, often after specific culture data demonstrate the susceptibility of the isolated strains to metronidazole. Some clinicians also use metronidazole alone to treat acute necrotizing ulcerative gingivitis.

57. What are the common side effects and contraindications of metronidazole?

The most common adverse effect of metronidazole is alcohol intolerance. Severe gastrointestinal side effects can result if a patient ingests alcoholic beverages while taking metronidazole. A metallic taste during therapy may also be a significant side effect. Other more severe reactions, such as peripheral neuropathy, are rare. Metronidazole significantly enhances the effects of Coumadin and is relatively contraindicated for patients on Coumadin. If it is prescribed, prothrombin times must be monitored. Antacids, as they do with tetracyclines, decrease the metronidazole effect by decreasing its absorption. Therefore, patients who are regularly using antacids should be given an alternate medication. Metronidazole also can possibly decrease the metabolism of carbamazepine (Tegretol). Tegretol toxicity is, therefore, possible when taken with metronidazole. Similarly, metronidazole can decrease the metabolism of phenytoin (Dilantin) and can result in phenytoin's toxicity.

Metronidazole may decrease contraceptive drug effectiveness; thereby contributing to breakthrough pregnancies. In the patient on chronic steroid therapy, a decreased metronidazole effect may result from increased metabolism.

Metronidazole prescribed for a patient taking cyclosporine may result in cyclosporine toxicity and, therefore, is relatively contraindicated.

58. What are the contraindications for the use of cephalosporins?

Cephalosporins can cause cyclosporine toxicity (i.e., renal failure) when administered to patients receiving cyclosporine and are relatively contraindicated, therefore, in patients receiving this drug for immunosuppressive maintenance of organ transplants.

59. Are fluoroquinolones used in the treatment of odontogenic infection?

Generally, quinolones are not utilized for the treatment of odontogenic infections. The spectrum of susceptible organisms, however, is consistent with their use. Most often, ciprofloxacin (Cipro) is used in the treatment of rapidly progressive periodontitis in which documented culture data demonstrate the susceptibility of the active organisms. In this setting, most often ciprofloxacin is prescribed at a 500-mg bid dose. With most culture programs, the ciprofloxacin is used as a substitute for amoxicillin if the organisms have demonstrated amoxicillin susceptibility but when the patient is allergic to penicillin.

60. What are the adverse effects and contraindications of ciprofloxacin?

First, the patient must be advised to monitor his or her use of caffeine. Ciprofloxacin blocks caffeine metabolism and can result in caffeine toxicity.

Ciprofloxacin is also contraindicated in patients under age 18. There are documented adverse effects of this drug on cartilage development in immature joints.

Like tetracycline and metronidazole, quinolone effectiveness is decreased by concurrent administration of antacids.

Ciprofloxacin causes an increased anticoagulant effect of warfarin (Coumadin) and is relatively contraindicated with that drug. If it is utilized, the patient's prothrombin time must be monitored closely.

Fluoroquinolones can cause cyclosporine toxicity with coadministration. Nephrotoxicity is the most common complication.

Quinolones adversely affect the metabolism of phenytoin (Dilantin), with variable effects on the latter.

Quinolones can result in theophylline toxicity with coadministration. Significant cardiac arrhythmias may result.

61. Are there any other reasons for failure of an odontogenic infection to respond to antibiotic therapy?

As noted above, the most common cause of failure is inadequate debridement of the lesion. This is followed by noncompliance of the patient, resulting in inadequate dosing. The third cause is failure of odontogenic infections to respond to treatment of resistant organisms. Last, the clinician must consider the existence of an overriding, previously undiagnosed debilitating systemic disease.

62. What examples of systemic disease may alter the patient's response to the treatment of odontogenic infection?

The most common situation would be the presence of previously undiagnosed diabetes mellitus (see Chapter 10). Fifty percent of the adult diabetics in the population are not aware that they are diabetic. With poor glucose metabolism comes a susceptibility to infection and a slow response rate. Patients who have a history of diabetes mellitus in their families are two and one half times more likely to be diabetic themselves. The clinician should review this possibility in patients whose disease does not respond to conventional treatment.

Rarer conditions include undiagnosed leukemia with compromised white blood cell function that prohibits adequate response to antibiotic therapy.

63. What are the most common antibiotics used today in the treatment of odontogenic infection when the maximal spectrum of antibiotic microbiota is desired?

In the setting of a spreading infection or in a significant infection in a medically compromised host, the following maximal spectrum oral antibiotics should be considered in the treatment of odontogenic infection.

- Amoxicillin-clavulanate (Augmentin), 875 mg bid for 10 days
- Azithromycin (Zithromax), 500 mg day 1, 250 mg for day 2 to 5
- Clindamycin (Cleocin), 150–300 mg tid for 10 days
- Cefuroxime (Ceftin), 250–500 mg bid for 10 days
- Loracarbef (Lorabid), 200–400 mg bid 1 hour before or 2 hours after meals for 10 days

64. Summarize your approach to selecting an antibiotic in the treatment of odontogenic infection.

If the infection is a localized infection, the first decision must be whether an antibiotic is necessary. Will débridement of the wound alone adequately treat the infection? If an antibiotic is part of the regimen, the first choice would be amoxicillin, 875 mg bid, usually for a 7-day course. For patients allergic to penicillin, doxycycline (Vibramycin), 100 mg bid for 7 days, would be an appropriate alternative. In the setting of suspected resistant organisms in those patients not responding to the initial antibiotic dose, clindamycin (Cleocin) is an alternative at 150 mg tid. Another alternative is to piggyback a metronidazole dosage in addition to the initial medication when the patient fails to respond after 48 to 72 hours.

65. What is the protocol for a patient with a spreading infection?

The selection of an antibiotic with a maximal spectrum to include coverage for staphylococcal species and for extended spectrum gram-positive and gram-negative anaerobes. Generally, the first choice drug is Augmentin, 875 mg bid. For those patients allergic to penicillin, azithromycin (Zithromax), prescribed in a Z-pack of 250 mg two tablets day 1 and one tablet days 2 through 5, would be prescribed.

Alternate choices might include clindamycin, 150 to 300 mg bid, cefuroxime 250–500 mg bid, and loracarbef 200 to 400 mg bid.

34. HIV INFECTION AND SEXUALLY TRANSMITTED DISEASES

Stephen T. Sonis, D.M.D., D.M.Sc.

HIV INFECTION

1. What does HIV stand for?
Human immunodeficiency virus

2. Since HIV and acquired immunodeficiency syndrome (AIDS) were first reported in 1981, how many cases have been recorded in the United States? How many people have died of AIDS?
Since the infection was first described in 1981, there have been over one million cases in the US. Of patients with the infection, almost half (400,00) have died. Fortunately, the prognosis of patients infected with HIV has improved since the introduction of highly active antiretroviral therapies in 1996.

3. What are the primary targets for HIV?
The main targets for the virus are cells expressing the CD4 membrane receptor, such as T4-helper lymphocytes, macrophages, and monocytes.

4. HIV causes immunosuppression in the host. How does this happen?
Viral replication occurs within the CD4 cell, leading to its destruction and loss of function. As a result the number of CD4 cells declines, and the patient becomes at high risk for opportunistic infections.

5. How is the status of an infected patient monitored?
CD4+ lymphocyte counts and viral load are the most predictable indicators of how the disease will progress.

6. How is HIV most commonly transmitted?
Sexual transmission accounts for the majority of cases. Although the disease has historically been seen in homosexual males, heterosexual transmission now accounts for most of the new cases. Needle sharing among intravenous drug abusers also accounts for a significant number of infections. Early in the history of HIV infection, transmission through therapeutic blood and blood products was not uncommon.

7. How many documented cases of HIV have resulted from occupational exposure of dentists, dental hygienists, or dental assistants?
None.

8. Are there certain populations at particular risk for HIV infection?
Although African Americans account for only 13% of the US population, more than half of new HIV cases occur in this population. Hispanics also seem to be at higher risk of contracting the disease. Thirty percent of new infections now occur in women, mostly through sexual transmission.

9. Briefly describe the incubation period for HIV infection.
Since the virus can remain dormant in lymphocytes for long periods of time, the incubation period is lengthy, averaging about 10 years from initial infection to the appearance of clinical signs of the disease. During the incubation period, the host is infectious.

10. What serologic tests are available for HIV infection? How are they used?

TEST	PURPOSE
ELISA	Screening
Western blot	Confirmation
Polymerase chain reaction	Identification of viral genome

11. Many medications used to treat HIV have side effects or adverse reactions that impact on dental management or cause oral mucosal lesions. Describe the possible dental consequences of the following: abacavir, flycytosine, foscarnet, ganciclovir, hydroxyurea, interferon, lopinavir, pentamidine, rifampin, ritonavir, saquinavir, trimethoprim-sulfamethoxazole (SMZ/TMP), dideoxycytidine, and zidovudine.

- Abacavir — Oral ulceration
- Flycotsine — Myelosuppression
- Foscarnet — Oral ulceration and myelosuppression
- Ganciclovir — Myelosuppression
- Hydroxyurea — Oral ulceration
- Interferon — Xerostomia, metallic taste, myelosuppression
- Lopinavir — Ulceration, xerostomia
- Pentamidine — Metallic taste
- Rifampin — Salivary discoloration
- Ritonavir — Perioral paresthesia
- Saquinavir — Paresthesia, neutropenia, thrombocytopenia
- TMP/SMZP — Myelosuppression, oral ulceration, glossitis
- Dideoxycytidine — Myelosuppression, oral ulceration
- Zidovudine — Neutropenia

12. What are the oral manifestations of HIV infection?

Many but not all of the oral manifestations of HIV infection are associated with opportunistic infections.

- Hairy leukoplakia caused by the Epstein-Barr virus
- Candidiasis
- Herpes zoster infection
- Human papilloma virus infection
- Herpes labialis or intraoral herpes simplex virus infection
- Aphthous-like ulcers
- Acute necrotizing ulcerative gingivitis
- HIV-related periodontitis
- Palatal petechiae secondary to thrombocytopenia
- Kaposi's sarcoma
- B-cell lymphoma
- Salivary gland enlargement

13. Nonhealing ulcers may occur in patients with HIV. What is the differential diagnosis? How would the dentist make a definitive diagnosis?

Ulcers in patients with HIV may be the consequence of major aphthous stomatitis, infection, or malignancy. Among the infections causing soft tissue ulceration in this patient population are tuberculosis, herpes simplex virus type I, and cytomegalovirus. Ulceration may also occur in neutropenic HIV patients. The most definitive means of diagnosis is biopsy.

14. What is the clinical presentation of Kaposi's sarcoma in the mouth?

Kaposi's sarcoma is a cancer that is frequently associated with AIDS. Its presentation in the mouth is often unimpressive. Lesions may appear as bluish-black asymptomatic macules. More aggressive lesions may be raised and, if they involve the gingiva, hyperplastic. Bone lesions may produce swelling of the overlying soft tissue that mimics a periapical abscess. Biopsy is required for definitive diagnosis.

15. Patients with AIDS are at increased risk of B-cell lymphoma. Describe the clinical presentation of this type of tumor.

B-cell lymphomas usually present as a rapidly enlarging soft-tissue mass. The overlying mucosa is usually intact. The tumors are firm on palpation—the tissue is like fish flesh in consistency—but lack the rock-hard feeling of squamous cell carcinomas. Biopsy is mandatory for diagnosis.

16. What is the first thing the dentist should do if he or she stuck the hand with a sharp instrument?

Wash the area thoroughly with soap and water.

17. Name some of the sequelae of AIDS that can impact on the dental management of patients.

Anemia, thrombocytopenia, and leukopenia are all possible sequelae of AIDS that would markedly impact on dental management.

18. The CD4 cell count is probably the best way to gauge the state of a patient's immunosuppression. Would you be concerned if your patient's CD4 count was 275 cells/mm³?

Yes, you should be. The normal CD4 count is >600 cells/mm³. Patients with counts below 400 cells/mm³ may manifest opportunistic infections and a patient with only 275 cells/mm³ would be at significant risk of infection.

19. Is there a good summary of the oral manifestations and dental management of HIV-infected patients?

Yes. The American Academy of Oral Medicine has an excellent publication on the subject. It, and other AAOM publications are available from the Executive Secretary, 2910 Lightfoot Drive, Baltimore, MD 21209.

SEXUALLY TRANSMITTED DISEASES

20. Is the incidence of gonorrhea increasing or decreasing in the U.S.?

Although the rate of gonorrhea has been decreasing since a peak in 1975, probably as a consequence of prevention and educational programs, in 2000, over 6000 new cases per week were reported. The frequency of gonorrhea among young people remains high, especially between the ages of 15 and 19 years. Other risk factors for infection include multiple or casual sexual contacts, sexual activity related to drug use, and low socioeconomic status.

21. What is the causative organism of gonorrhea?

Neisseria gonorrhoeae.

22. What is the most common anatomic site of infection for gonorrhea?

The urethra.

23. What is the risk that a man will develop gonorrhea after exposure to infection in a sexual partner?

25–50%.

24. Describe the clinical course of gonorrhea.

A purulent urethritis developes in men after an incubation period of 2–14 days. The infection may spread to contiguous tissues, including the prostate, seminal vesicles, and epididymis.

Women also may develop urethritis, although it tends to be mild. Infection also may spread in women and cause pelvic inflammatory disease.

25. Are all cases of gonorrhea symptomatic?
No. In women, most cases are asymptomatic; asymptomatic cases are rare in men.

26. What are the most common symptoms of gonorrhea?
The most common symptoms of gonorrhea are severe dysuria and the presence of a creamy white, purulent urethral discharge.

27. What laboratory test is most commonly used to diagnose gonorrhea?
Gram stain of the discharge typically demonstrates neutrophils containing gram-negative diplococci in 93% of symptomatic men. Cultures also may be used but may not be as sensitive because of the fragility of the organism.

28. What is the most common treatment regimen for uncomplicated gonococcal infection?
Ceftriaxone given as an initial single injection, followed by doxyclycline or tetracycline for 1 week is the treatment of choice. Because men are symptomatic, they seek care and get treated. Their female partners should be identified (often they are asymptomatic) and also treated.

29. Do gonococcal infections ever affect the mouth?
Oral gonococcal infections are not uncommon and are seen in about 20% of homosexual men and in women who practice fellatio.

30. Describe the clinical course of oral gonorrhea.
Lesions tend to be aysmptomatic and occur within 1 week of genital contact. The gingiva are the most frequent site of oral gonorrhea and typically manifest a necrotizing ulcerative gingivitis. Unlike conventional acute necrotizing ulcerative ginginvitis (Chapter 33), the necrotizing gingivitis of oral gonorrhea is often seen in conjunction with mucosal manifestations of the infection, which typically are seen in the oropharynx as diffuse erythema.

31. What three characteristic lesions (Hutchinsonian triad) are associated with congenital syphilis?
1. Interstitial keratitis
2. Eighth nerve involvement
3. Deformed central incisors (notched and screwdriver-shaped)

32. Describe the three phases of syphilis, and explain the oral manifestations associated with each.
Primary syphilis occurs shortly after contact transmission (around 3 weeks). The oral lesion associated with primary syphilis, called a chancre, presents as an indurated ulcer most often of the lip, tongue, or tonsils. It is often associated with lymphadenopathy and usually disappears spontaneously in about 4 weeks.

Secondary syphilis. Raised, grayish-white areas overlying an inflamed, erythematous base constitute the oral lesions associated with secondary syphilis. These lesions are called mucous patches and may be seen on the tongue, buccal mucosa, tonsil, pharynx, and lips. They also may cause angular cheilitis.

Tertiary syphilis. The oral manifestations of tertiary syphilis have been reported to be the most common of the three stages and consist of two findings: gumma and luetic tongue. Gumma presents as a destructive ulceration, most often involving the hard palate. Luetic tongue presents with marked atrophy. It is viewed as a precancerous lesion.

33. Which stage of syphilis is most infectious?
The second stage.

34. Can herpes simplex type 2 (genital herpes) affect the mouth?

Oral-genital contact may result in oral herpes simplex type 2 (HSV-2). The clinical presentation is similar to HSV-1 (see Chapter 35).

35. VIRAL INFECTIONS

Stephen T. Sonis, D.M.D., D.M.Sc.

1. Viral invasion of cells and the production of new viral particles occur in a six-stage process. What are the stages?
1. Attachment of the viral particle to the cell surface.
2. Viral penetration of the cell.
3. Viral uncoating or the functional release of nucleic acid.
4. Replication of the nucleic acids.
5. Reconstitution or assembly of the viral particle.
6. Viral particle release from the cell.

2. Does viral invasion destroy the infected cell?
Viral invasion does not destroy the infected cell by itself. Host cell destruction is dependent on the mode of viral release from the cell, the effect of the virus on cell metabolism, and the release of viral toxins.

3. What are the two major forms of viral infection based on the extent of involvement?
• Viral infections may be confined to the entry site, such as respiratory infections.
• Viral infections may be systemic, such as measles.

4. Which has a shorter incubation period, local or systemic viral infection?
Local infections have a shorter incubation period, a duration of immunity that is less, and there is no hematogenous spread of the virus.

5. Are viral infections of the mouth common or rare?
Viral infections are among the most common causes of oral lesions.

6. Are there common features among the symptoms of acute viral infections that affect the mouth?
Yes, oral mucosal changes are similar and consist of crops of vesicles or of ruptured small ulcers. A nonspecific coating of the tongue may be present. Patients usually give a history suggesting viremia such as fever, malaise, myalgia, upper respiratory symptoms, or anorexia. Typically, pain associated with the lesions is what prompts the patient to visit the dentist.

7. How is the diagnosis of virally associated oral lesions typically made?
The diagnosis is usually made based on clinical appearance and history. Among patients who are at risk for significant sequelae such as bone marrow transplant recipients, cancer patients receiving myeloablative therapy, or solid organ transplant recipients for whom a rapid definitive diagnosis is critical and who may have lesions associated with uncommon viruses, culture is desirable.

8. What group of viruses accounts for most oral infections?
Members of the human herpesvirus group are the most common viruses to cause oral disease. These include herpes simplex types 1 and 2, the varicella-zoster virus, the Epstein-Barr virus, and cytomegalovirus. Newer forms of the group, human herpesviruses 6, 7, and 8, may have roles in the etiology of infections in immunocompromised patients.

9. What two forms of oral disease are produced by infections of herpes simplex virus-1 (HSV-1)?
HSV-1 is the etiologic agent for primary herpetic gingivostomatitis and secondary or recurrent herpes infection.

10. Describe the clinical course and the appearance of the oral manifestations associated with primary herpes infections.

Primary herpetic gingivostomatitis occurs following the patient's first infection with HSV-1. Consequently, it is most common in children and adolescents, although it may be seen in young adults as well. Patients initially develop a typical viral prodrome consisting of lethargy, malaise, arthralgia and myalgia, anorexia, and chills that is usually accompanied by fever. About 1 to 2 days later, diffuse vesicular lesions appear throughout the mouth, commonly on the movable mucosa. These rapidly rupture, forming crops of small, very painful ulcers. An acute gingivitis accompanies the vesicular lesions. The tongue is coated. Patients are uncomfortable and febrile.

11. Is there any oral condition that can be confused with primary gingivostomatitis?

Because of its acute onset and predilection for younger patients, acute necrotizing ulcerative gingivitis may be confused with primary gingivostomatitis. However, there are major differences in the course and presentation of the two conditions:

- HSV-1 is associated with a prodrome, whereas acute necrotizing ulcerative gingivitis has an explosive onset with no early signs.
- HSV-1 results in mucosal vesicle and ulcer formation in addition to an acute gingivitis. There are no mucosal lesions associated with acute necrotizing ulcerative gingivitis.
- The gingival architecture is unaffected by HSV-1. The papillae and marginal gingiva demonstrate necrosis and a consequent alteration in their normal configuration in acute necrotizing ulcerative gingivitis.
- Patients with HSV-1 are generally more systemically ill than those with acute necrotizing ulcerative gingivitis.

12. How can the diagnosis of herpes infection be confirmed?

The diagnosis of HSV-1 infection can be confirmed by obtaining a viral culture (usually unnecessary) or by obtaining a serum sample during the acute phase of the disease and a second sample 6 weeks later. The second sample, called the convalescent sample, demonstrates a rise in antibody titer if an infection has occurred.

13. What is normally seen in a cytologic smear obtained from a lesion caused by an acute HSV-1 infection?

- Multinucleated giant cells (Tzank cells)
- Viral inclusion bodies

14. Do all individuals infected with HSV-1 for the first time develop symptomatic disease?

No, in fact it has been reported that only 12% of children who have antibodies to the virus actually remember being sick.

15. What are the histologic features associated with the epithelium from HSV-1-induced oral lesions?

- Acantholysis
- Nuclear clearing
- Nuclear enlargement (ballooning degeneration)
- Nuclear fragmentation
- Chromatin condensation around the edge of the nucleus
- Fusion of adjacent epithelial cells to form giant cells

16. What is the usual treatment for an otherwise healthy patient who has primary gingivostomatitis?

- Bedrest
- Fluids (if the patient can not take anything by mouth, intravenous support may be indicated)
- Acetaminophen (Tylenol) (avoid aspirin in children)
- Pain control—topical mouth rinses may help

17. What signs and symptoms would suggest that your patient is dehydrated?
- Modified state of consciousness
- Low blood pressure
- Decreased skin turgor
- Rapid pulse
- Pale or gray skin color
- Reduced urine output
- Dry mouth

18. What autoimmune disease may occur following acute HSV-1 infections?
Erythema multiforme may occur about 6 weeks after the primary infection.

19. What are the common names for recurrent HSV-1 infections?
Herpes labialis, secondary herpes infections, cold sores

20. What is the etiology of recurrent HSV-1 infection?
During the acute infection, the virus infects the sensory nerves and colonizes the trigeminal ganglion, which goes into a dormant state. Upon activation, the virus travels to the skin or mucosa to induce the lesions associated with recurrent infection.

21. What factors have been reported to be associated with reactivation of HSV-1 infection?
- Exposure to sun
- Local trauma
- Menstrual cycle
- Other infections
- Stress
- Eczema
- Pregnancy
- Immunodeficiency
- Gastrointestinal disorders
- Food and medication intolerance

22. What is the recurrence frequency among patients who get secondary HSV infections?
Twenty-five percent of patients affected by secondary HSV infections have one or more episodes per month.

23. What is the clinical course and appearance of herpes labialis?
Clinically, herpes labialis presents as small, single, or multiple vesicular lesions that typically occur at the corners of the mouth, at the mucocutaneous junction of the lips, or under the nose. Patients with recurrent disease are often able to predict the appearance of lesions as they experience a prodromal period during which they describe tingling, itchiness, or drawing in the area. Painful vesicle formation usually follows about 24 hours later. Some patients experience mild flulike symptoms with lymphadenopathy. After a couple of days, the vesicles rupture and form ulcers, which then crust over. Lesions usually resolve spontaneously in about a week to 10 days.

24. Are the lesions of herpes labialis infectious?
The viral titer is highest during the first 2 days of the infection, but sufficient viral titers are present through the crusting stage so that the infection may be transmitted by contact. Before the routine use of gloves by dental professionals, herpetic skin infections following contact with infected patients were not uncommon.

25. What are the skin lesions caused by HSV-1 infection called?
Herpetic whitlow.

26. What can be done to treat routine secondary herpes labialis?
Only one topical antiviral medication is approved for the treatment of secondary herpes. Penciclovir (Denavir) is a cream that contains the antiviral agent penciclovir. The drug inhibits herpes viral DNA synthesis and, therefore, its replication. It is recommended for the treatment of lesions of the lips and face but not lesions on mucosal surfaces. Denavir is supplied in 1.5-g tubes and should be put on lesions every 2 hours while the patient is awake for 4 days. The earlier the patient starts using the drug, the better.

27. How effective is Denavir?

It is not a cure-all. In studies of over 3000 patients, half of whom received Denavir and the remainder placebo, Denavir reduced the duration of lesion pain by one half day (12 hours). From a cost-benefit standpoint, that translates to about $2.50 of cost per hour of relief.

28. Is there any place for acyclovir in the treatment of HSV-1?

Acyclovir is effective for primary or recurrent herpes infections in immunocompromised patients. For cancer patients who are being treated with myeloablative chemotherapy, acyclovir is best administered intravenously.

29. What clinical conditions are caused by the varicella-zoster virus?

The varicella-zoster virus is responsible for two conditions that may affect the mouth: chickenpox and herpes zoster (shingles).

30. What is the difference between chickenpox and herpes zoster infection?

Chickenpox is the result of primary infection with the virus, whereas herpes zoster represents secondary infection. Consequently, chickenpox is most commonly seen in children and herpes zoster in adults.

31. What is the clinical appearance of the skin lesions associated with chickenpox and where do they typically first appear?

The skin lesions of chickenpox go through four stages:
1. Erythematous macules
2. Vesicle
3. Pustule
4. Crusting

The lesions are characteristically itchy and begin on the trunk, often in areas of clothing-induced friction, such as the waist, and on the face. Involvement of the extremities follows. Mouth lesions may occur earlier than skin lesions.

32. Describe the oral appearance of chickenpox.

The oral lesions of chickenpox are similar to those of other viral infections and consist of vesicles that rupture to form small ulcers. As in primary HSV-1 infections, a nonspecific gingivitis may also occur. The most common locations for lesions are the palate and buccal mucosa, although the tongue may also be involved. Lesions typically last about a week.

33. How is chickenpox typically spread?

Saliva, nasal droplets, and direct contact with lesions.

34. Following exposure to the virus, how long does it take for chickenpox to develop?

Symptoms usually begin between 11 and 20 days after exposure.

35. What is herpes zoster?

Herpes zoster is a painful viral infection of the posterior root ganglion caused by the varicella-zoster virus. Herpes zoster may affect any branch of the trigeminal nerve, resulting in involvement of the mouth or face.

36. What is the most common presenting symptom of herpes zoster infection?

Extreme unilateral pain.

37. What is the clinical course of herpes zoster infections?

About 3 to 5 days after patients note severe pain, crops of small vesicles that are unilateral and usually linear in distribution appear. These generally rupture, leaving ulcers that go on to healing in about 1 to 2 weeks.

38. How common is herpes zoster infection?
Herpes zoster is pretty common and occurs in about 10 to 20% of individuals over their life-time. It is especially common in immunocompromised patients such as those undergoing cancer therapy, solid organ transplants, or with human immunodeficiency viral infection.

39. How often do patients have recurrent lesions caused by herpes zoster?
Recurrent infections are rare.

40. What are potential complications of herpes zoster infection?
• Neuralgia
• Facial paralysis
• Corneal scarring

41. Is there anything that can be used to treat herpes zoster?
Acyclovir tablets, 800 mg/day, have been shown to be an effective intervention for herpes zoster.

42. What is herpangina?
Herpangina is a viral disease that affects the mouth. It is caused by the group A coxsackie-virus and is most common in children under the age of 4 years.

43. Herpangina typically demonstrates seasonal variation in frequency. When is it most commonly seen?
Summer.

44. What are the typical initial clinical manifestations of herpangina?
• Usually the acute onset of a high fever (> 100°F or 38°C).
• The patient may also complain of sore throat, dysphagia, and flulike symptoms, including malaise, myalgia, and runny nose. Nausea, vomiting, and headache may also occur.
• The predominant clinical lesions of herpangina occur in the mouth and are multiple, small, oval vesicular lesions often surrounded by erythema. The distribution of the oral lesions is usually posterior, affecting the soft palate and oropharynx. In fact, it is unusual to find le-sions in the anterior two thirds of the mouth.
• Multiple vesicles are usually present. They often rupture, forming small, painful ulcers.

45. Does lymphadenopathy occur in patients with herpangina?
Although it is not a consistent finding, lymphadenopathy may occur in patients with herpangina.

46. How long do the acute symptoms of herpangina last?
The acute symptoms of herpangina typically are present for about 3 days. The lesions heal in about a week to 10 days.

47. What is the treatment for herpangina?
Palliation: Bedrest, fluids, analgesics, soft diet, and topical palliative rinses.

48. What are some examples of topical palliative rinses that could be used for a patient with herpangina?
• Viscous lidocaine
• A 50/50 suspension of diphenhydramine (Benadryl) and loperamide (Kaopectate).

49. Since patients with herpangina often have fever and pain, an antipyretic and analgesic can be administered. Are there any drugs that you would specifically avoid? Why?
Salicylates have been associated with Reye's syndrome, a condition that produces an acute, noninflammatory encephalopathy in children. Consequently, it is best to avoid the use of aspirin in kids.

50. What other diseases can be confused with herpangina?
- Other viral infections
- Streptococcal or bacterial pharyngitis
- Aphthous stomatitis

51. What is the most effective way to make a diagnosis of herpangina?
Usually history and clinical appearance and the age of the patient provide enough information to make diagnosis of herpangina. However, if a bacterial pharyngitis is a possibility, a bacterial culture should be performed.

52. Are there other coxsackievirus infections that affect the mouth?
Hand, foot, and mouth disease is a relatively rare infection caused by a group A coxsackievirus. Although the disease follows a course similar to that of herpangina, patients also develop lesions on the palms and soles. Typically, these lesions are small, ovoid, erythematous macules. Lesions last for a couple of weeks. Treatment is palliative.

53. What oral lesion is associated with the Epstein-Barr virus?
The Epstein-Barr virus is associated with hairy leukoplakia seen in patients with human immunodeficiency virus.

36. FUNGAL INFECTIONS

Stephen T. Sonis, D.M.D., D.M.Sc.

1. Are oral fungal infections common?

No; most are associated with an underlying systemic condition, especially those in which immunosuppression occurs. Thus, patients with solid organ transplants who are immunosuppressed; patients with acquired immunodeficiency syndrome, anemia, diabetes, uremia, or leukemia; and patients receiving cancer therapy are all at risk. In addition, patients who have conditions that modify the normal oral environment are at increased risk of fungal infections. Among these individuals are patients with xerostomia and patients who have taken broad-spectrum antibiotics.

2. Upon what is the diagnosis of oral fungal infections most often based?
* History
* Clinical appearance
* Culture
* Potassium hydroxide preparation
* Biopsy

3. What is the most common fungal infection to affect the mouth?
Oral candidiasis, caused by *Candida albicans*. It is classified into acute and chronic forms.

4. Are there are age predilections for candidiasis?
Patients at either age extreme are affected, probably because of the status of their immune systems.

5. What is the typical clinical presentation of oral candidiasis?
* Pseudomembranous candidiasis is the most typical clinical presentation of the infection. Patients present with white, cottage cheesy–looking raised lesions, most often of the tongue or palate. The lesions can be scraped off, leaving a painful, raw, often bleeding base. This type of candidiasis is known as thrush.
* Hyperplastic candidiasis is less common. Lesions appear as areas of leukoplakia at the corners of the mouth or on the cheeks. Unlike the pseudomembranous forms, these lesions cannot be scraped off.
* Erythematous candidiasis is most often present on the dorsal surface or edges of the tongue and on the palate. The degree of mucosal erythema may be variable. Symptomatically, patients with this form of candidiasis often complain of a burning mouth.
* Angular cheilitis may be caused by candidiasis.

6. What does a smear or biopsy from an infected area of candidiasis demonstrate?
Fungal hyphae can be seen in both types of specimens. In addition, a biopsy specimen also demonstrates epithelial proliferation in response to the infection.

7. How do you do a potassium hydroxide (KOH) preparation for candidiasis?
* Take a sample from the lesion and smear it onto a glass slide.
* Add a few of drops of a 10% solution of potassium hydroxide.
* Look under the microscope for fungal forms.

8. Name three drugs that can be used for the treatment of oral candidiasis.
1. Nystatin suspension
2. Clotrimazole
3. Fluconazole

9. How is nystatin typically administered for the treatment of oral candidiasis?
Nystatin is a thick, yellow, cherry-tasting suspension that is usually administered by having the patient swish and then swallow between 200,000 U and 400,000 U three or four times a day.

10. How is clotrimazole administered?
Clotrimazole (Mycelex) is dispensed as 10-mg troches. Patients should be instructed to let one melt on their tongues five times per day for 2 weeks.

11. Is there a difference in efficacy or cost between nystatin and clotrimazole?
They cost and work just about the same.

12. How does fluconazole differ from nystatin and clotrimazole?
Fluconazole (Diflucan) is a relatively new antifungal agent that is more potent than either nystatin or clotrimazole. Fluconazole is typically administered as a 100-mg tablet—two tablets to start and then once daily for 2 weeks.

13. What are the advantages and disadvantages of using fluconazole to treat oral candidiasis?
• Major advantages are its efficacy and ease of dosing (once daily compared with multiple dosings).
• Disadvantages are cost and potential toxicities.

14. What toxicity would you most likely be concerned about in a patient for whom you prescribed fluconazole?
Hepatoxicity.

15. What would be a reasonable approach to the treatment of candidiasis in a 25-year-old, healthy female who has been using tetracycline?
Start with either nystatin oral suspension or clotrimazole troches.

16. Give three examples of patients for whom fluconazole would be the treatment of choice for oral candidiasis.
   1. A patient who has persistent oral candidiasis even after treatment with clotrimazole for 2 weeks.
   2. A patient who is receiving myelosuppressive chemotherapy for the treatment of cancer and has diffuse oral candidiasis.
   3. A patient with human immunodeficiency virus who has significant oral candidiasis and difficulty swallowing.

17. What deep fungal infections can be seen in the mouth?
• Mucormycosis   • Sporotrichosis
• Histoplasmosis   • Blastomycosis
• Aspergillosis   • Coccidioidomycosis
• Cryptococcosis

18. In general, how do deep fungal infections appear in the mouth? How would you make a diagnosis?
Virtually all the deep fungal infections present as some form of nonhealing ulceration. Clinically, they are difficult to distinguish from a malignancy. The diagnostic procedure of choice is biopsy.

19. How common are deep fungal infections of the mouth?
They are pretty rare.

20. What is histoplasmosis?
Histoplasmosis is a deep fungal infection that may produce ulcerative, nodular, or proliferative oral lesions. The infection is caused by the fungus *Histoplasma capsulatum*, which is endemic to certain areas in the Americas and Southeast Asia. In the US, it is most common in the Mississippi River Valley.

21. How common is histoplasmosis?
There are about half a million cases per year in the US, although most are subclinical or restricted to the respiratory tract. About 5% are disseminated and may have oral involvement. The infection is more common in men than women and is seen exclusively in patients over the age of 20 years.

22. What is the mode of infection of histoplasmosis?
The organism is found in soil spores and spread by birds. The spores enter the body via the respiratory tract.

23. What are the nonoral clinical manifestations of histoplasmosis?
Since most infections involve the respiratory tract, typical symptoms include cough and dyspnea. Patients may also experience weight loss.

24. What are the oral manifestations of histoplasmosis?
• Painful ulcers
• Nodular lesions
• Vegetative lesions
Lesions may occur anywhere in the mouth but are most common on the oropharynx, palate, buccal mucosa, or tongue. Patients may have a mix of lesion types.

25. What drug is typically used for the treatment of histoplasmosis? What is its most common toxicity?
Amphotericin B is the drug most commonly used to treat histoplasmosis. It is highly nephrotoxic.

26. What is mucormycosis?
Mucormycosis is a rare invasive fungal infection that was first described with oral involvement in diabetic patients. It is now seen in immunocompromised patients such as those with acquired immunodeficiency syndrome or cancer patients receiving myeloablative chemotherapy. The infection is caused by organisms of the order Mucorales, especially of the genuses *Mucor* and *Rhizopus*.

27. Where are the organisms that cause mucormycosis typically found?
Both causative organisms associated with mucormycosis are common inhabitants of soil and decaying vegetable matter and are usually nonpathogenic in healthy individuals.

28. What is the typical clinical course of mucormycosis?
The disease is typically rhinocerebral. Organisms that normally reside in the nose produce infection that is invasive. The infection can affect the brain, lungs, and gastrointestinal tract. If untreated, the infection is fatal. Treatment is aimed at eradicating the infection with amphotericin B and correction of underlying systemic pathology.

29. What are the perioral and oral manifestations of mucormycosis?
• Nonhealing, progressive necrotic ulceration. Ulcer margins may be blackish.
• Facial swelling
• Proptosis

30. What histologic stain is helpful in making a diagnosis of mucormycosis?
Periodic acid–Schiff stain with biopsy is diagnostic.

31. What is aspergillosis?
Aspergillosis is a deep fungal infection that is most common in immunocompromised patients. *Aspergillus fumigatus* is the organism responsible for most infections, but it is nonpathogenic in normal individuals. Aspergillosis is caused by airborne spores. Patients with leukemia are among those most commonly affected.

32. What are the most common head and neck manifestations of aspergillosis?
Infection of the paranasal and maxillary sinuses.

33. How is a diagnosis of aspergillosis made?
• Culture
• Radiographs
• Clinical history and presentation

34. How is aspergillosis typically treated?
• Débridement and drainage
• Antifungal medication

35. What is North American blastomycosis?
Blastomycosis is another deep fungal infection and is generally transmitted by the respiratory route. Blastomycosis has three clinical forms: pulmonary, cutaneous, and systemic. Oral or nasal lesions occur in 25% of cases and consist of nonhealing ulcers. Lymphadenopathy is common. Biopsy is required for diagnosis.

36. Is there a gender or age predilection for blastomycosis?
Males between 40 and 60 years old.

37. In what region of the United States would you expect to find the highest frequency of coccidioidomycosis?
Coccidioidomycosis is caused by *Coccidioides immitis*, a spore and soil inhabitant that usually causes a self-limiting upper respiratory infection. Infections are most common in the southwestern part of the United States. Rarely, primarily in immunocompromised patients, the infection becomes disseminated, leading to a progressive and fatal outcome if untreated.

38. What are the head and neck manifestations of disseminated coccidioidomycosis?
Patients may develop nonhealing skin ulcerations of the face that resemble squamous cell carcinomas. These are reported to be most common in the nasolabial fold area. Intraorally, patients may have purplish nodular lesions.

37. ULCERS

Stephen T. Sonis, D.M.D., D.M.Sc.

1. What diseases can cause ulcers in the mouth?

- Aphthous stomatitis
- Trauma
- Syphilis
- Tuberculosis
- Cancer
- Neutropenia
- Viral stomatitis
- Deep fungal infections
- Human immunodeficiency viral infection

2. What is the most common oral mucosal disease in North America?

Recurrent aphthous stomatitis (RAS) is the most common oral mucosal disease in North America, with prevalences reported of up to 66% among professional (including dental) students. The overall prevalence is 20%.

3. What are the clinical features of RAS?

- One or more painful ulcers that usually last from 7 to 10 days.
- Ulcers are present on the "movable mucosa" and rarely seen on the hard palate, gingiva, or dorsal tongue.
- Frequency of recurrence is variable from days to months.

4. What are the different forms of RAS?

There are three forms of RAS:
- Minor RAS
- Major RAS
- Herpetiform ulcers

5. Which is the most common form of RAS?

Over half of patients (54%) who get RAS develop the minor type. The next most common form is major aphthous (22%). The herpetiform type of RAS is only seen in 4% of patients. There are another 20% who fall into an "intermediate" category—somewhere between major and minor RAS.

6. What is the typical clinical course of minor RAS?

Patients with minor aphthous typically develop lesions every few months. They may experience a prodromal stage during which they note localized burning or itching of the mucosa a day or two before an actual ulcer develops. The ulcers that appear in minor RAS are usually oval, with a diameter of a centimeter or less. Despite their small size, they are very uncomfortable and especially bothersome if they occur on the lateral borders of the tongue, which is continually being traumatized. The center of the ulcer is yellowish-gray in color and is surrounded by an erythematous ring. The ulcers usually last about 7 to 10 days with maximum discomfort for about half that time. Patients may note lymphadenopathy. When the ulcers heal, there is no scarring.

7. How does the course of major aphthous stomatitis differ from that of minor RAS?

As the name implies, major aphthous is more severe than minor RAS. The ulcers are bigger, usually in the range of 1 to 3 cm, deeper, and occur more often. Unlike the ulcers of minor aphthous, the lesions of major RAS tend to be more long lasting and may be present for a month or more. It is not unusual for sufferers of major aphthous to have continuous ulcers some place in their mouths continually. When lesions do heal, they may leave a scar.

8. Is herpetiform RAS caused by a virus?
Herpetiform RAS is not caused by a virus but its clinical appearance, crops or clusters of small (1–3 mm) ulcers, is viral in appearance. However, unlike most oral viruses, the distribution of lesions is still predominantly on the movable mucosa. There seems to be a slight gender predilection for the herpetiform type of RAS in women.

9. At what age does RAS typically begin?
Although RAS is most often described as starting during puberty or adolescence, about 1% of children in developed countries have been reported to have the condition. The frequency is higher in selected groups of children. Interestingly, rich kids are more likely to have RAS than poor kids. RAS in young children is almost always of the minor type.

10. What systemic conditions have been associated with the onset of aphthous stomatitis?
Although most patients with RAS have no underlying systemic disease, it has been associated with a number of systemic conditions. These include:
* Behçet's syndrome
* Vitamin B deficiencies (in particular vitamin B_{12})
* Folic acid deficiencies
* Human immunodeficiency virus infection
* Agranulocytosis
* Cyclic neutropenia
* Crohn's disease and other inflammatory bowel disease
* Periodic fever syndrome

11. What is the effect of cigarette smoking on RAS?
Smoking actually seems to favorably impact on the course and prevalence of RAS. On the other hand, the use of smokeless tobacco seems to result in an increase in the incidence of RAS.

12. What is the most consistent symptom of patients with RAS?
Pain is the thing that patients with RAS complain of most frequently.

13. Can stress be a cause of RAS?
Although the results of a number of studies suggest that psychological stress can result in RAS, this association is controversial. Interestingly, some of the most supportive studies of stress as a cause of aphthous were done in dental students. For the most part the use of antianxiety medications does not seem to be beneficial in reducing the frequency with which aphthous ulcers develop.

14. Is there any evidence to support a genetic basis for RAS?
It is possible but unlikely. Familial tendencies for RAS have been observed. Patients with a strong family history of RAS seem to develop the condition at a younger age than individuals in whom there is no family history. Although this could be due to a genetic relationship, it might also be a result of individuals living in the same environment and eating similar foods. While certain HLA types have been reported to be associated with RAS the evidence to support an underlying genetic basis for the disease is weak.

15. In the study of oral immunology, a lot of space is devoted to aphthous stomatitis. What are the reasons for this?
There are a lot of data to support an immunopathogenic basis for RAS, including the following:
* Patients with RAS may have increased levels of peripheral blood CD8+ and reduced CD4+ lymphocytes. This reversal of the norm in CD4 and CD8 ratios is more dramatic in patients with severe RAS.
* The ulcerative phase of RAS is associated with the appearance of cytotoxic T cells in mucosa.

- Adhesion molecules in the submucosa may lead to the aggregation of lymphocytes.
- Increased T-cell receptor-γδ⁺ cells are seen in patients with active RAS compared with patients with inactive RAS or patients who do not develop the condition.
- Increased tumor necrosis factor-alpha (TNF-α) is seen in patients with the condition.

16. How is a diagnosis of aphthous typically made?
Almost all cases of minor RAS can be diagnosed based on the history of recurrent lesions and the clinical appearance of the ulcers. Since the ulcers of major aphthous tend to stick around longer than 2 weeks, a biopsy is indicated to confirm the diagnosis. Herpetiform aphthous is relatively rare and may be confused with a viral infection. Consequently, the diagnosis is based on history and clinical appearance, but a negative viral culture might be beneficial to help make the diagnosis.

17. If you did biopsy an ulcer in a patient with RAS, what would you see?
The histologic appearance of aphthous is nonspecific. You would see an ulcer below which there would be an inflammatory cell infiltrate. T lymphocytes would be the most common cell type, although mast cells, neutrophils, and macrophages would be present. Vasodilation of the underlying small blood vessels is common.

18. What is Behçet's disease? According to the International Study Group, what are the criteria for its diagnosis?
Behçet's disease is a multisystem disease that includes aphthous stomatitis as one its primary features. The etiology of Behçet's disease is complicated and probably includes a combination of immune dysregulation, inflammatory cytokines, and possibly viral or bacterial microbes.
The criteria for the diagnosis, as described by the International Study Group, include the following:
- Recurrent aphthous stomatitis that occurs at least three times per year.
- Plus two of the following:
  - Recurrent genital ulceration
  - Eye lesions
  - Skin lesions
  - Positive pathergy test

19. What is a positive pathergy test?
Pathergy is the occurrence of a pustular lesion 24 hours after a needle stick. It isn't all that helpful in making a diagnosis of Behçet's disease.

20. When should you consider ordering a blood test in a patient with recurrent oral ulcers? What tests would you order?
Most patients with occasional recurrent oral ulcers do not require anything more than a clinical assessment to make a diagnosis. However, if the patient has major RAS or if the ulcers are increasingly frequent or severe or do not behave normally, it makes sense to rule out a vitamin B_{12} or folic acid deficiency. If there is periodicity to the onset of lesions, particularly with fever, cyclic neutropenia needs to be excluded by obtaining a white blood cell and differential white blood cell count during periods of ulcer formation.

21. What topical medications are available for the treatment of aphthous stomatitis?
Treatment for aphthous stomatitis depends on the severity and extent of the disease. For patients with mild, occasional ulcers, a topical analgesic like benzocaine in Orabase may palliate the discomfort of the lesions effectively. Amlexanox gel is available by prescription and when applied topically, reduces the duration of ulcers. Topical steroids may be helpful in reducing local inflammation and pain. Triamcinolone acetonide (Kenalog) in Orabase is readily available but is variable in its efficacy. Fluocinonide gel (0.05%) or clobetasol propionate (0.05%) applied to ulcers three times per day is often effective. For patients who have ulcers in areas that are difficult

to access for ointment or gel placement, dexamethasone (Decadron) suspension (0.5 mg/5 ml) can be used as a rinse or gargle three times daily.

22. What if topical medications don't work? Are there systemic medications to treat significant aphthous?

Systemic steroid therapy (prednisone) or thalidomide may be used to treat severe cases of aphthous. Since both of these medications have potentially significant side effects, the decision to use them should be made carefully. Recently, pentoxifylline has been suggested to be of benefit in the management of RAS.

23. Are traumatic ulcers of the oral mucosa common?

Very common. With all the motion of the masticatory mucosa over and around the teeth, the presence of sharp edges on restorations or prostheses, and hard and sharp foods and very hot food, traumatic ulcers of the oral mucosa are frequent. They generally occur within a couple of days of injury. Frequently the patient can identify the event that led to the lesion. In the case of toothbrush trauma, the ulcers are often linear. In fact, almost all linear ulcers are of mechanical origin. Traumatic ulcers usually last about a week and then resolve spontaneously. The clinical appearance of traumatic ulcers is similar to that described above for aphthous lesions.

24. Can chemicals cause mucosal ulcerations?

Some chemicals can cause burns that result in ulcer formation. Probably the most common is aspirin. Patients may place aspirin on the mucosa opposite a painful tooth. Not only does the aspirin fail to help the toothache, but the acetylsalicylic acid can burn the underlying mucosa and cause additional discomfort.

25. Do malignancies of the mouth manifest as ulcers?

Nonhealing ulcers are one of the commonest presentations of oral cancers. These are usually squamous cell carcinomas, but other types of tumors such as lymphomas may also appear as ulcers. Unlike the more common types of oral ulcers, malignant lesions are usually painless, growing and do not heal spontaneously. Consequently, biopsy of any ulcer that is present in the mouth for more than 2 weeks is mandatory.

26. What infectious diseases can cause oral ulcers?

• Human immunodeficiency viral infection
• Syphilis
• Tuberculosis
• Viral infections
• Mucormycosis

27. Are ulcers the primary lesions that result from viral infections?

No, viral lesions usually produce vesicular or blistering eruptions. However, by the time that they are seen, the vesicles have probably ruptured, leaving the patient with crops of small painful ulcers.

28. What stage of syphilis is associated with oral ulcers?

Oral ulcers may occur with two stages of syphilis.

Syphilis has a three-stage clinical presentation. The primary lesion of syphilis, the chancre, appears about 3 weeks after infection and may result in the formation of a painless ulcer with raised borders. Clinically, chancres often resemble early cancers. Chancres associated with the mouth are usually found on the tongue, lips or corners of the mouth and are loaded with the causative spirochete of the disease, *Treponema pallidum*. Consequently, they are markedly infectious.

The tertiary lesion of syphilis is called a gumma. The gumma does not need to appear at the site of infection and usually does not appear for 2 or more years. Gummas only occur in about

50% of patients who are primarily infected, and lesions of the mouth are rare. When they do occur, they appear as nonhealing painless ulcers.

29. What does tuberculosis look like in the mouth? How do you make a diagnosis?

Oral lesions associated with tuberculosis are rare and are usually caused by undiagnosed primary pulmonary infections. Even though the incidence of tuberculosis is on the rise as a consequence of human immunodeficiency viral infection, the frequency of oral lesions associated with this infection has not increased. Oral tuberculosis infection results in the formation of a nondescript, nonhealing ulcer with undermined borders. There is little surface inflammation, although the base of the ulcer is granulomatous. The lesions have been described as stellar or starlike in shape. Biopsy is the key to diagnosis.

30. What is acute necrotizing ulcerative gingivitis?

Acute necrotizing ulcerative gingivitis (ANUG) is a fusospirochetal infection of the gingiva. It was formerly called trench mouth because of its frequency among soldiers during World War I, and it was thought to be contagious (it is not). It is the only periodontal infection in which the gingiva is invaded by bacteria.

31. What is Vincent's infection?

Vincent's infection is another former name for ANUG. Vincent was the name of one of the individuals who first documented the condition.

32. What are the clinical characteristics of ANUG?

• Sudden onset of localized or diffuse gingival pain
• Acute gingival bleeding
• Bad taste and fetor oris
• 50% of patients experience systemic manifestations of infection, including malaise, fever, and lymphadenopathy

33. Who typically gets ANUG?

ANUG is most common in young adults in their early twenties. It is often seen in college student populations around examination time.

34. Does ANUG have a unique clinical appearance?

The clinical appearance of ANUG is characterized by
• Localized or generalized areas of papillary and marginal necrosis that usually start interproximally and then spread laterally
• The areas of necrosis produce a pseudomembrane that overlies an inflammatory base
• Loss of the interdental papilla causes a "punched-out" appearance. There is usually cratering interproximally.
• The tissue is friable and bleeds easily.
• The patient feels like "the pits."

35. What microorganisms have been associated with ANUG?

ANUG is thought to be caused by a fusospirochetal complex that includes
• *Fusobacterium fusiformis*   • Streptococci
• *Vibrio* organisms   • Diplococci
• *Treponema vincentii*   • Filamentous forms

36. How is ANUG treated?

Although some texts suggest débridement with scaling and root planing as the initial treatment for ANUG, most patients are so sensitive that such an approach is unrealistic. The goal of primary treatment should be a reduction in the bacterial load that is causing the condition.

Fortunately, the bacteria that cause ANUG are penicillin-sensitive. Consequently, initial treatment should consist of a loading dose of penicillin (1 g) to start, followed by 500 mg four times per day for a week. Gentle débridement of the infected area can be performed using peroxide-soaked cotton pellets. Chlorhexidine irrigation also can be prescribed. Once the lesion has quieted down, more definitive débridement can be performed. Patients typically respond to antibiotic therapy in a day.

37. Should I be concerned if my patient has recurrent ANUG?
Yes. While most cases of ANUG are of local etiology, some systemic conditions predispose to ANUG-like changes in the gingiva. Among the most common are neutropenia and human immunodeficiency virus infection. If a patient presents with recurrent ANUG regardless of the response to antibiotic, additional diagnostic follow-up is warranted.

38. What is NOMA?
NOMA, also called gangrenous stomatitis or cancrum oris, is an acute gangrenous process of oral origin resulting in severe destruction of the oral mucosa that perforates the face. The disease is rare and is primarily limited to nutritionally-deficient children in Western Africa, although it has been reported in severely immunocomprised patients elsewhere.

39. What is the etiology of NOMA?
It is believed that the bacterial etiology of NOMA is similar to that of ANUG and consists primarily of a fusospirochetal complex. In fact, most cases of NOMA start as necrotizing gingivitis. However, both gram-negative organisms and herpessimplex virus have been isolated from lesions of NOMA.

40. What is the outcome of NOMA and how is it treated?
If untreated, NOMA results in progressive and severe facial disfigurement. With the advent of antibiotics, however, especially penicillin, the morbidity and mortality associated with the condition have improved.

41. What fungal infections cause ulcerative lesions in the mouth?
Histoplasmosis and phycomycosis (mucormycosis) both can cause oral ulcers.

42. Where is the organism that causes histoplasmosis found? How is it spread? What is its natural history? How common is it?
- Histoplasmosis caused by the fungus *Histoplasma capsulatum.*
- *Histoplasma capsulatum* is endemic in certain parts of the world.
- In the US, the Mississippi Valley Region is its most common location.
- The organism is found in spores in soil and is spread by birds.
- Spores enter the body through the respiratory tract and localize to the lung.
- There are an estimated 500,000 new cases in US annually. Most are subclinical or involve only the respiratory tract.
- 5% of patients have disseminated infection, and this group may have oral involvement.

43. What are the clinical manifestations of histoplasmosis?
- Cough
- Dyspnea
- Weight loss

44. What are the oral manifestations of histoplasmosis?
The oral manifestations of histoplasmosis may be varied and include
- Painful ulcerations
- Nodules
- Vegetative processes

Patients usually have more than one type of oral lesions. Ulcers may vary in depth and appearance. Lesions can occur anywhere in the mouth but are most common on the oropharynx, buccal mucosa, tongue, and palate. The clinical appearance is similar to that of epidermoid carcinoma.

45. How are the oral lesions of histoplasmosis diagnosed?
Biopsy is mandatory for the diagnosis of histoplasmosis, as the lesions clinically resemble carcinoma. Organisms are specifically stained with Gomori's methenamine silver. Although a skin test for histoplasmosis may be helpful in assisting in the diagnosis, it is dependent on when the patient was infected. Cultures of smears of lesions often result in false-negative results.

46. What drug is used to treat histoplasmosis?
Amphotericin B.

47. What are the oral manifestations of mucormycosis?
The typical oral appearance of mucormycosis is of a nonhealing progressive ulcer. Underlying bone destruction may occur. Tissue destruction is the result of vessel thrombosis. Facial swelling, proptosis and eye and facial symptoms may be noted in patients with extensions of the infection into the orbits, sinuses, nasal cavity, or cranium.

48. Which patients are at risk for oral mucormycosis?
Historically, oral mucomycosis has been reported in patients with poorly controlled diabetes mellitus. More recently it has been reported in bone marrow transplant recipients, or patients receiving chemotherapy who are neutropenic and patients who are immunosuppressed by diseases such as acquired immunodeficiency syndrome.

49. Name the most common intraoral location for the following ulcerative conditions:
- **Aphthous stomatitis**   • **Neutropenic ulcer**
- **Chancre of primary syphilis**   • **Deep fungal infections**
- **Tuberculosis**   • **Viral stomatitis**
- **Carcinoma**
- Aphthous stomatitis—usually on the mucosal surface. No gingival involvement, rarely palatal involvement.
- Chancre of primary syphilis—lip, tongue, tonsils
- Tuberculosis—tongue, tonsils, soft palate
- Carcinoma—anywhere. Most often base of tongue, lower lip, floor of mouth
- Neutropenic ulcer—usually begins on attached gingiva, then spreads to any surface
- Viral stomatitis—nonspecific; depends on virus
- Deep fungal infections—oropharynx, buccal mucosa, tongue, palate

38. WHITE LESIONS

Stephen T. Sonis, D.M.D., D.M.Sc.

1. What are the two basic causes of white lesions in the mouth?
• Hyperkeratosis
• Necrosis

2. What causes the white coloration of necrotic lesions in the mouth?
The white coloration is caused by the collection of dead cells, bacteria, and debris on the tissue surface.

3. What causes the white coloration of keratotic lesions?
The coloration of keratotic lesions is attributable to the presence of excess keratin.

4. What are the diagnostic steps in evaluating a white lesion in the mouth?
• The initial diagnostic step in evaluating white lesions is aimed at differentiating between necrotic and keratotic lesions. Since most necrotic lesions are associated with some form of injury, a thorough history often reveals the cause.
• Necrotic lesions are usually painful, whereas keratotic lesions are most often asymptomatic.
• The surface of necrotic white lesions can usually be scraped off with a moistened tongue blade. No amount of scraping will modify a keratotic lesion.
• Definitive diagnosis of a keratotic lesion is made by biopsy.

5. What are the two most common causes of necrotic white lesions in the mouth?
• Burns
• Candidiasis

6. What is the clinical appearance of a burn of the oral mucosa?
Clinically, burns of the mouth appear as areas of white necrotic tissue overlying a connective tissue or mucosal base, depending on the depth of the burn. The white appearance of the lesion is caused in large part by epithelial sloughing.

7. What are the more common causes of burns in the mouth?
• Electrical burns may occur in children who chew on wires. Typically, these burns involve the corners of the mouth and the lips and tongue.
• Chemical burns are common and may be caused by a variety of agents, including astringent mouthwashes such as undiluted hydrogen peroxide, aspirin placed on the mucosa (usually in the mucobuccal fold opposite a painful tooth), or sodium hypochlorite used in irrigation for endodontic procedures.
• Thermal burns are most commonly caused by hot, sticky foods such as cheese.

8. What is the most common fungal infection to occur in the mouth?
Candidiasis, which is caused by *Candida albicans.*

9. Does candidiasis show an age predilection? Who is at risk for infection?
Candidiasis is most common in patients at either age extreme. In newborns, the infection is called thrush. It is also more frequently found in immunosuppressed patients such as individuals talking steroids or with acquired immunodeficiency syndrome, among neutropenic patients such as those receiving cancer chemotherapy, and in debilitated patients such as those with diabetes. Prolonged antibiotic use also enhances the likelihood of developing infection.

10. Does oral candidiasis always present in the same way?
Clinically, candidiasis has a range of presentations. Patients may be totally asymptomatic or may complain of burning, especially of the tongue. Some individuals feel like their mouths are coated. Pseudomembranous candidiasis, the type of infection that causes white lesions, appears as white, curdy, raised patches that have been likened to cottage cheese in appearance. The borders of the lesions are often erythematous. The white necrotic coating overlies a raw base that usually bleeds easily on provocation.

11. What are the most common drugs used to treat candidiasis?
• Nystatin suspension
• Clotrimazole troches
• Fluconazole (Diflucan) capsules

12. What is the difference in the way the various antifungal therapies are administered?
Nystatin suspension is typically administered as a swish and swallow liquid. Clotrimazole (Mycelex) troches dissolve in a patient's mouth. Diflucan is taken as a pill.

13. Is there any difference in price between nystatin, clotrimazole, and fluconazole?
Nystatin and clotrimazole are about the same price. Fluconazole, however, is markedly more expensive.

14. How would a prescription for nystatin read?
Nystatin oral suspension, 200,000 U–400,000 U, tid or qid for 10 days.

15. How is clotrimazole (Mycelex) dispensed?
Clotrimazole is dispensed in 10-mg troches with instructions to dissolve one troche in the mouth five times per day for 2 weeks.

16. Is amphotericin B ever indicated for treatment of candidiasis?
Because of its profound potential for systemic toxicity, amphotericin B is limited to the treatment of systemic, esophageal, or pulmonary candidal infections, particularly in immunocompromised patients.

17. What is the major toxicity associated with amphotericin B?
Amphotericin, typically administered intravenously, has often been dubbed "amphoterrible." Shaking chills, hypotension, nausea, vomiting, headache, tachypnea, and fever often accompany its use. Renal toxicity may be dramatic. Consequently, the use of amphotericin is limited to patients with life-threatening fungal infections.

18. How can you effectively treat candidiasis in a patient who wears full dentures?
Dentures often act as a carriage for *Candida*. Treatment of palatal candidiasis is most easily done using nystatin (Mycostatin) ointment that the patient can apply as a denture liner. The denture should be soaked in diluted bleach to eliminate fungi and then washed well before use.

19. What is leukoplakia?
Leukoplakia simply means "white plaque." The term has erroneously been used to imply malignant changes.

20. What is the differential diagnosis of oral keratotic white lesions?
• Hyperkeratosis   • White sponge nevus
• Carcinoma   • Lupus erythematosus
• Lichen planus

21. The simplest white lesions that affect the mouth are those caused by increased production of keratin. What is the most common cause of this reaction?

Chronic irritation of the oral mucosa is the most common cause of mucosal hyperkeratosis. Areas of hyperkeratosis caused by chronic irritation may occur anywhere in the mouth but are most common on the buccal mucosa and on the lateral borders of the tongue. Frequently they are bilateral and represent a bite line.

22. What is the treatment of choice for bite-line hyperkeratosis?

No treatment is required.

23. What causes localized areas of hyperkeratosis?

Localized areas of hyperkeratosis are usually associated with a specific source of irritation such as a partial denture clasp, a fractured restoration, or a sharp cusp or tooth edge. These lesions may have an element of inflammation associated with them. Patients with white keratotic lesions associated with a specific irritant should be treated. First, the irritant should be eliminated. Two weeks later, the site should be re-evaluated. If the white lesion persists, it should be biopsied to rule out a diagnosis of dysplasia or carcinoma.

24. Does tobacco use cause hyperkeratosis?

Yes, especially cigar and pipe smoking. In both cases, hyperkeratosis is most often seen on the hard palate. In some cases, the minor salivary glands become inflamed, giving a speckled, erythematous, petechiae-like appearance that contrasts with the white of the keratosis. This condition is so linked to tobacco use that it is referred to as nicotinic stomatitis.

25. Should you be concerned about leukoplakia?

Since about 7% of cases of leukoplakia demonstrate histologic evidence of dysplasia or carcinoma, the dentist cannot be complacent about the condition. If the condition appears to be the consequence of local irritation, the source should be eliminated and the patient re-evaluated in a couple of weeks. If the lesion remains, it should be biopsied.

26. What is lichen planus?

Lichen planus is an inflammatory autoimmune condition that may result in both mouth and skin lesions. It is possible to have one without the other. The condition is among the most common diseases of the oral mucosa and affects about 1% of the adult population in the United States. Histologically, lesions of lichen planus are characterized by an extensive submucosal T-cell and mast cell infiltrate.

27. Since some patients may have both skin and mouth lesions of lichen planus, it's important to know what the skin lesions look like. Describe them.

Lichen planus of the skin is most common on the flexor surfaces of the arms or legs, such as the inner aspect of the elbow or wrist. The lesions are usually bilateral and appear as an itchy, purplish, papular rash in which the papules are either individual or contiguous. Close examination demonstrates raised, discrete polygonal papules that form plaques when contiguous.

28. What is the epidemiology of lichen planus?

Lichen planus is a disease of middle-aged adults. A female predilection of about 2:1 has been suggested.

29. What causes lichen planus?

The etiology of lichen planus is not fully understood. The histologic finding of an intense subepithelial lymphocytic infiltrate and its similarity in appearance to the oral manifestations of graft-versus-host disease have suggested an autoimmune etiology. It is clear that certain medications are capable of eliciting a lichenoid reaction in the mouths of some patients that could be the result of a cell-mediated immune response directed against drug-induced mucosal antigens. Stress has frequently been mentioned as a cause for the condition, but sound evidence supporting its etiologic role is lacking.

30. Name eight drugs that have been reported to cause lichenoid lesions in the mouth (lichenoid stomatitis).

1. Chlorpropamide
2. Tolazamide
3. Hydroxyurea
4. Gold

5. Alpha-methyldopa
6. Propranolol
7. Carbamazepine
8. Phenytoin

31. How does lichen planus appear in the mouth?
Oral lichen planus has three clinical manifestations:
• A hyperkeratotic or reticulated form
• An erosive form
• A bullous form

32. Describe the clinical appearance and symptoms of the keratotic or reticulated form of oral lichen planus.
The keratotic form of oral lichen planus is the most common form and often occurs in conjunction with the other two types. When it is present alone, the keratotic form is usually asymptomatic. Patients may, however, complain of a rough feeling to their mucosa. Keratotic lesions of lichen planus are most common on the buccal mucosa (80%) and tongue (65%). The lesions present in a unique and characteristic lacey, reticulated pattern that forms a striated network of contiguous, raised, white papules called Wickham's striae. The lesions are usually bilateral.

33. What is the best way to diagnose the keratotic, reticulated form of lichen planus?
Clinical examination is usually sufficient, although if there is any evidence of inflammation a confirmatory biopsy is prudent.

34. What is the clinical course of lichen planus?
Lichen planus generally runs a chronic and benign course, with periods of exacerbation and remission.

35. This chapter deals with white lesions and does not discuss the erosive or bullous forms of lichen planus. What chapter deals with them?
Chapter 39.

36. What is lupus erythematosus?
Lupus erythematosus is a relatively common autoimmune disease. The disease has three forms: systemic lupus erythematosus (SLE), chronic cutaneous lupus erythematosus (CCLE), and subacute cutaneous lupus erythematosus. The forms are very dissimilar and, in fact, may represent different diseases. SLE is a serious systemic illness that is markedly more common in women than men. Typically its onset occurs early in the third decade of life. In contrast, CCLE has only a slight predilection for females and occurs at an older age than SLE. Although it is clear that lupus erythematosus is an autoimmune disease, its exact cause is unknown. Genetic and environmental factors, including chemicals, hair dyes, drugs, foods, and infectious agents have been implicated in its etiology.

37. What are the common nonoral clinical features of SLE?

Arthritis and joint pain	91% frequency
Fever	83% frequency
Skin involvement	71% frequency

Adenopathy	58% frequency
Anemia	56% frequency
Myalgia	48% frequency
Nephritis	46% frequency
Pleurisy	45% frequency
Central nervous system symptoms	25% frequency

38. How often do oral lesions occur in patients with SLE?
Oral lesions occur in about 40% of cases.

39. How does lupus erythematosus appear in the mouth?
One of the presentations of lupus erythematosus, especially of CCLE, is mucosal hyperkeratosis. However, lupus erythematosus (including SLE) can present in the mouth as ulcers or vesiculobullous lesions with erythema and may even look like lichen planus. Lesions are typically seen on the palate, buccal mucosa, and gingiva but can also be seen on the floor of the mouth.

40. What would be included in your differential diagnosis for the oral manifestations of SLE?
• Lichen planus
• Carcinoma
• Chronic cutaneous lupus erythematosus

41. Are there any skin lesions that could give you a clue that the patient might have lupus erythematosus?
Forty to fifty percent of patients with SLE develop a "butterfly" rash on their faces. The rash involves both cheeks and spreads from one side to the other across the nose in a butterfly pattern.

42. How is lupus erythematosus diagnosed?
Patients with lupus erythematosus develop an autoantibody directed at the nuclear components of damaged cells. This antibody, called an antinuclear antibody, forms the basis for a blood test for the disease.

43. Is lupus erythematosus the only condition that is associated with a positive antinuclear antibody test?
No, other diseases can result in a positive antinuclear antibody test. These include:
• Rheumatoid arthritis   • Mixed connective tissue disease
• Systemic sclerosis   • Chronic hepatitis
• Polymyositis   • Infectious mononucleosis
• Dermatomyositis   • Certain drug reactions

44. Name seven drugs that are associated with a positive antinuclear antibody test.
1. Procainamide   5. Sulphasalazine
2. Isoniazid   6. Methyldopa
3. Chlorpromazine   7. Quinidine
4. D-penicillamine

45. Other than mouth lesions, what are other common gastrointestinal manifestations of SLE?
Gastrointestinal manifestations of SLE occur in about half of patients with the disease and include
• Esophagitis   • Abdominal pain
• Esophageal ulceration   • Diarrhea
• Esophageal dysmotility   • Pancreatitis

46. What is the frequency of kidney involvement in patients with SLE?

Almost all patients with SLE demonstrate histologic evidence of renal disease.

47. Is SLE a serious disease?

SLE is a multisystem condition. Its prognosis varies, but 5% of patients with the condition die within 5 years of diagnosis, usually because of renal failure. Twenty-five percent of patients with the condition succumb within 15 years of diagnosis.

48. How is SLE treated?

- Minimization of ultraviolet light exposure
- Systemic corticosteroid therapy
- Antimalarial agents
- Cytotoxic drugs such as azathioprine and cyclophosphamide

49. What is white sponge nevus?

White sponge nevus is a benign, genetically inherited keratotic condition that affects the mouth and other mucosal surfaces. In contrast to other keratotic oral white lesions, because it is inherited, it is seen in children.

50. What are the clinical presentation and course of white sponge nevus?

The condition is completely asymptomatic. Patients present with areas of bilateral, raised, spongy hyperkeratosis usually of the buccal mucosa. No treatment is required, and diagnosis is based on the age of onset, family history, and clinical appearance.

39. VESICULOBULLOUS DISEASES AND AUTOIMMUNITY

Stephen T. Sonis, D.M.D., D.M.Sc.

1. What is a vesicle?

Vesicles are small, fluid-filled, blisters on the mucosa that are usually ovoid. They generally do not exceed 0.5 cm in diameter. In the case of viral diseases, vesicles occur in clusters; in other diseases they may occur singularly. Since vesicles become painful after they rupture, the clinician usually sees them as oval, open, erosive lesions.

2. What is a bulla?

Bullae resemble vesicles in appearance but are larger in size and scope. Bullae may occur singularly or coalesce to form large areas of involvement. After they rupture, the edges of the roof of the bulla may be still be visible.

3. What are the major vesiculobullous or blistering diseases that effect the mouth?
- Pemphigus vulgaris
- Mucous membrane pemphigoid
- Bullous and erosive lichen planus
- Erythema multiforme
- Certain drug eruptions

4. What is the pathobiologic etiology of most oral blistering diseases?

Although the specific cause of oral blistering diseases varies, autoimmunity is thought to be the triggering event leading to pathology.

5. Are all autoimmune diseases systemic?

Autoimmune disease may be considered to be either systemic or organ-specific. In the case of systemic autoimmune diseases, multiple organs or tissues are typically involved. Systemic lupus erythematosus is an example of a systemic autoimmune disease. Virtually all cases of oral blistering disease represent organ-specific autoimmune diseases and affect the mouth and/or skin.

6. How are autoimmune diseases diagnosed?
- History
- Clinical examination
- Biopsy with immunohistochemical studies
- Sometimes serologic testing

7. Are autoimmune diseases common?

Not individually, but if lumped together they affect about 5% of the population of Western countries.

8. What are some of the triggers of autoimmune reactions?
- Environmental factors
- Infectious agents
- Drugs
- Some food substances
- Loss of regulatory cells

9. What is pemphigus vulgaris?

Pemphigus vulgaris is the most serious of the oral blistering diseases. It causes severe, chronic, progressive vesiculobullous lesions of the oral mucosa and skin that result in epithelial sloughing. If left untreated, it is fatal.

10. Describe the demographics and etiology of pemphigus vulgaris.
- Rare.
- Usually seen in adults in the fourth and fifth decades of life.

213

- No gender predilection.
- Noted most often in individuals of Mediterranean or Middle Eastern background.
- Appears to have a strong genetic predisposition.
- Autoimmune etiology is suggested by the presence of lesion antibodies localized in the intercellular spaces of the epithelium (antidesmosomal).

11. What specific genetic alterations are associated with pemphigus vulgaris?
It appears that specific alterations in the hypervariable region of the beta-1 chain of HLA class II genes confer susceptibility to pemphigus vulgaris. Such alterations are linked to DRB1*0402, a subtype of HLA DR4.

12. What is unique about the histopathologic appearance of pemphigus vulgaris?
The presence of antidesmosomal antibodies results in the destruction of the substance that cements epithelial cells together. As a result, intraepithelial separation of the stratum germinativum from the underlying stratum spinosum occurs, resulting in acantholysis.

13. Is oral involvement common in patients with pemphigus vulgaris?
Almost all patients with pemphigus vulgaris present with oral lesions or develop them during the course of their illness. At the time of diagnosis, the mouth is involved in 70% of cases and is the only site of presentation in 50%. As is the case with many diseases, early diagnosis affects the intensity of treatment and its outcome.

14. Describe the clinical features of the oral lesions of pemphigus vulgaris.
- Any area of the mouth may be involved but most commonly lesions are found on the posterior buccal mucosa and gingiva. They appear as a desquamative gingivitis.
- In severe cases, virtually all of the oral mucosa may be involved.
- Development of oral lesions can be stimulated by trauma.
- Vesiculobullous lesions appear at different stages of development, regression, and healing.
- Bulla production can be initiated by rubbing the mucosa with a finger or thumb (Nikolsky's sign).

15. What is the best way to diagnose pemphigus vulgaris?
Biopsy is the best way to diagnose pemphigus. If the disease is suspected, pathologic evaluation should include both routine histologic and immunohistologic examinations.

16. What is the prognosis for patients with untreated pemphigus vulgaris?
If left untreated, pemphigus vulgaris is a fatal disease.

17. What are the treatment options for patients with pemphigus vulgaris?
Immunosuppressive therapy with steroids has historically been the mainstay of treatment. However, a variety of other immunosuppressive drugs have been reported to be effective, including azathioprine, cyclosporine, cyclophosphamide, dapsone, and gold. Intravenous gamma globulin has also been found to offer a treatment option in some cases.

18. What is pemphigoid?
Pemphigoid is an autoimmune disease in which antibodies directed against the basement membrane adhesion complex cause separation of the epithelium from the underlying connective tissue, resulting in a subepithelial blister.

19. What forms of pemphigoid affect the mouth?
Two forms of pemphigoid affect the oral mucosa—mucous membrane pemphigoid and bullous pemphigoid.

20. What is cicatricial pemphigoid?
Another name for mucous membrane pemphigoid.

21. Which form of pemphigoid most commonly affects the oral mucosa?
Virtually all patients with mucous membrane pemphigoid have oral lesions. In contrast, bullous pemphigoid primarily affects the skin and rarely causes oral lesions.

22. Is there a gender predilection for mucous membrane pemphigoid?
Yes, females appear to be at higher risk than males.

23. What is the most common age of onset of mucous membrane pemphigoid?
Although 60 years is the mean age of onset, the disease can be seen in younger adults and has been reported rarely in children.

24. Describe the clinical features of mucous membrane pemphigoid.
• Oral cavity most common site.
• Although lesions are initially blisters, they become erosive.
• The gingiva is almost always affected.
• The gingival manifestation is a desquamative gingivitis.
• Lesions may be aggravated by removable prostheses.
• Lesions are very painful.
• Secondary surface infection is common.
• A patient may have diseases at different stages simultaneously.
• The course is chronic and long lasting.

25. What is the best way to diagnose mucous membrane pemphigoid?
Biopsy for routine histologic examination and immunofluoresence testing.

26. What is the second most common site for mucous membrane pemphigoid?
The second most common anatomic site for mucous membrane pemphigoid is the conjunctiva. Conjunctival lesions may precede oral lesions, but usually occur simultaneously. The conjunctiva appear red and swollen. The development of lesions can lead to adhesions in the eyelid and eyeball areas called symblepharon. If untreated, these may lead to blindness.

27. What is the best way to treat the oral lesions of mucous membrane pemphigoid?
Unfortunately, nothing works 100% of the time. Topical steroids may be effective in managing mild cases of mucous membrane pemphigoid. A short course of systemic steroids can usually control more severe cases. Typically, an initial course of daily prednisone is followed by alternate-day treatment. Since corticosteroid therapy brings the risk of multiple short- and long-term side effects, alternative types of treatment are desirable. Intravenous immunoglobulin therapy seems to hold a great deal of promise in the control and treatment of pemphigoid.

28. How often are oral lesions present in patients with bullous pemphigoid?
Unlike mucous membrane pemphigoid, the skin is the primary site for lesions of bullous pemphigoid. Less than 20% of patients with bullous pemphigoid have oral lesions. If a patient does develop mouth lesions, these inevitably occur after skin lesions are already present.

29. Even though rare, oral lesions do occasionally occur in patients with bullous pemphigoid. What is the most common site in the mouth for these lesions?
The gingiva; oral lesions of bullous pemphigoid most commonly appear as a desquamative gingivitis.

30. Lichen planus was included in the chapter on white lesions of the mouth. Why is it included in this chapter as well?

In addition to presenting as a white, keratotic lesion, lichen planus may also appear in an erosive or bullous form. In fact, because the latter forms are usually symptomatic, it is more likely that a patient will seek professional care for erosive or bullous lichen planus.

31. How does erosive lichen planus appear?

Patients with erosive lichen planus frequently have painful desquamative gingivitis. Clinically, there is sloughing of the epithelium that leaves an erythematous, painful base that may bleed. Usually, the reticular form of lichen planus can be found somewhere else in the mouth or at the margins of the erosive lesions. Because the gingiva are often involved, erosive lichen planus is sometimes misdiagnosed as conventional gingivitis.

32. How does bullous lichen planus look?

Patients with bullous lichen planus have true mucosal blistering disease. Lesions may be present on the buccal mucosa or lateral borders of the tongue. Frequently, the bullae are ruptured by the time the patient is seen, and lesions are ulcerative, with the remnants of the blister roof visible. As in erosive lichen planus, it is common to find evidence of the striated keratotic form of lichen planus at the borders of the bullae or in other areas of the mouth.

33. What is the best way to diagnose a lesion suspected of being lichen planus?

Biopsy. If you cannot clinically rule out the other blistering diseases, then immunofluorescence testing should be included with conventional histologic evaluation.

34. How is lichen planus treated?

Almost all cases of lichen planus respond well to moderate to strong topical steroid therapy. A short course of systemic steroids can be considered for patients who have severe disease that needs to be brought under control.

35. What is erythema multiforme?

Erythema multiforme is an acute mucocutaneous disease that is thought to be a consequence of an immune complex formation resulting in a dramatic inflammatory reaction. Although it is typically classified as one of the vesiculobullous diseases, its clinical presentation is varied.

36. What are the clinical course and presentation of erythema multiforme?

Unlike the other oral vesiculobullous diseases that tend toward smoldering, chronic conditions, erythema multiforme usually has an explosive onset. Patients may have dramatic blistering of the oral and/or labial mucosa, often with hemorrhage. However, the severity of oral lesions is variable. Despite the dramatic nature of the clinical presentation, the disease is self-limiting and usually resolves on its own in about 2 weeks.

37. Can skin lesions occur in patients with erythema multiforme?

Yes. When they do occur they have a unique bulls-eye or target appearance in which a central area of necrosis is surrounded by an erythematous ring.

38. What causes erythema multiforme?

The cause of erythema multiforme is not fully understood. It has been relatively commonly reported following infection caused by herpes virus in which cases erythema multiforme occurs about 6 weeks after the infection. Erythema multiforme has also been reported to be a sequela of other infections caused by mycoplasma or fungi. In addition, it has been associated with administration of a long list of drugs, the common feature of which is to elicit the production of cross-reacting antibodies.

39. What drugs have been connected with the onset of erythema multiforme?
- Analgesics, including aspirin, codeine, and nonsteroid anti-inflammatory drugs.
- Antibiotics, including chloramphenicol, ciprofloxacin, clindamycin, penicillin, sulfon-amide, and tetracycline.
- Anticonvulsants, including carbamazepine and phenytoin.
- Antituberculosis agents, including isoniazid and rifampin.
- Antidiabetic drugs such as chloropropamide and tolbutamide.
- Antineoplastic agents, including alkylating agents and methotrexate.
- Antihypertensive drugs, including diltiazem, hydralazine, minoxidil, and verapamil.
- Antirheumatics such as gold and phenylbutazone.
- Psychopharmacologic agents and sedatives, including barbiturates, glutethimide, lithium, meprobamate, and methaqualone.

40. Is the patient population at risk for erythema multiforme the same as for the other oral blistering diseases?

No; erythema multiforme occurs in a younger population, typically in young adults, although children may also develop the condition.

41. How is erythema multiforme best diagnosed?

Most cases of erythema multiforme can be diagnosed clinically based on past history, acute onset, age of the patient, and appearance of the lesions. Biopsy is typically not needed for diagnosis.

42. How is erythema multiforme typically treated?

Some controversy surrounds the best treatment for erythema multiforme. Although systemic steroids were used to treat the condition in the past, current thinking suggests that supportive care is best. This should include pain medication and ensuring that the patient is well hydrated.

40. PIGMENTED LESIONS
Stephen T. Sonis, D.M.D., D.M.Sc.

1. What are three sources of endogenous pigmentation seen in oral lesions?
1. Melanin
2. Bilirubin
3. Iron

2. Of endogenous sources of mucosal pigmentation, which is the most common?
Melanin

3. Name three sources of exogenous mucosal pigmentation.
1. Deposits of foreign material
2. Chromophilic bacteria or fungi
3. Heavy metal deposition

4. Are vascular lesions considered to be true pigmented lesions?
No, while they do cause discoloration of the mucosa, they are not truly pigmented. The easiest way to differentiate between a true pigmented lesion and one of vascular origin is to determine if the lesion blanches when pressed. A lesion caused by pigment deposition does not blanch.

5. Pigmented oral lesions caused by melanin deposition may be classified into four groups. Name them.
1. Normal variations of melanin deposition
2. Pigmented nevi
3. Melanoma
4. Endocrine and metabolic disorders

6. Name four metabolic or endocrine diseases that may cause abnormal melanin deposition of the oral mucosa.
1. Addison's disease
2. Peutz-Jeghers syndrome
3. McCune-Albright syndrome
4. Von Recklinghausen's disease

7. What is Addison's disease?
Addison's disease is primary adrenal insufficiency that is most often caused by autoimmune destruction (80% of cases). Tuberculosis is the second leading cause, but Addison's disease may also result from surgery, tumor, radiation, sarcoidosis, infarction and other infections. In all cases inadequate amounts of adrenal corticosteroids are produced. Symptoms generally do not occur unless there is at least a 90% loss of adrenal function.

8. What are the signs and symptoms of Addison's disease?
- Progressive debilitating illness
- Malaise
- Weakness
- Anorexia
- Nausea
- Vomiting
- Weight loss
- Fatigue
- Salt craving
- Orthostatic hypotension
- Cutaneous and mucosal pigmentation

219

9. Describe the course and appearance of mucosal pigmentation seen in a patient with Addison's disease.
Oral pigmentation is an early sign of Addison's disease. Typically bluish-black or dark-brown areas appear on the buccal or labial mucosa. Gingival pigmentation may also be seen. There is no unique pattern to the pigmentation. Hyperpigmentation of skin may also be noted.

10. What is Peutz-Jeghers syndrome?
Peutz-Jeghers syndrome is an inherited disorder that is characterized by intestinal polyposis and perioral pigmentation. The intestinal changes do not usually undergo malignant transformation but may result in other forms of intestinal disease that are symptomatic. Women with the syndrome appear to be at increased risk for ovarian cancer.

11. Describe the perioral lesions associated with Peutz-Jehger's syndrome.
The perioral lesions associated with Peutz-Jehger's syndrome are multiple, flat, discrete, melanotic spots around the mouth and on the lips. The intraoral mucosa may also be affected.

12. List the features of McCune-Albright syndrome?
• Unilateral polyostotic fibrous dysplasia
• Areas of unilateral pigmentation
• Endocrine dysfunction

13. What area of the mouth most often demonstrates hyperpigmentation associated with McCune-Albright syndrome?
The lips

14. What tumor type is associated with von Recklinghausen's disease?
Neurofibroma

15. What are the pigmented lesions that accompany the tumors of von Recklinghausen's disease called, and where do they occur in and around the mouth?
Café-au-lait spots are seen on the lips, periorally, and, rarely, on the buccal mucosa.

16. What percentage of neurofibromas in a patient with von Recklinghausen's disease undergo malignant transformation?
5 to 10%

17. What serum bilirubin levels are associated with a clinical state of jaundice?
Higher than 1.5 mg/dl

18. List the common causes of jaundice in adults.
• Biliary tract obstruction by   • Hepatocellular carcinoma
  gallstones or tumor   • Hepatitis
• Congestive heart failure   • Cirrhosis

19. What changes in color are associated with jaundice?
Yellowish coloration of the skin, sclerae, and oral mucosa is seen. The most common sites for oral manifestations of jaundice are the ventral surface of the tongue, the buccal mucosa, and the soft palate.

20. Hemochromatosis is an iron storage disease in which excess amounts of iron are deposited in body tissues. It is sometimes termed bronze diabetes. What are the clinical signs of the condition?
• Hepatomegaly   • Cardiac disease
• Diabetes   • Hypogonadism
• Arthropathy   • Hyperpigmentation

21. What are the causes of hemochromatosis?
- Patient's inability to control iron absorption
- A manifestation of an erythropoietic disorder
- Alcoholism
- Excessive iron intake

22. What are the oral manifestations of hemochromatosis and how often do they occur?
About 10 to 15% of patients with the condition demonstrate bluish-black areas of pigmentation of the oral mucosa.

23. Melanomas of the skin are on the increase. Are intraoral melanomas common?
Oral melanoma is rare. When it does occur, it seems to be slightly more common in men than in women, with a peak incidence of between 40 and 60 years of age. Most cases involve the palate and maxillary gingiva.

24. What is the clinical presentation of an intraoral melanoma?
Intraoral melanomas may have a variety of appearances. Usually, they are deeply pigmented (dark-brown to bluish-black) and slightly raised or nodular. The nonpigmented form appears red. Most lesions have been present for some time, as the rate of growth may be slow initially.

25. Do melanomas metastasize?
Melanomas frequently metastasize to regional lymph nodes, liver, bone, and lungs, often early in their course.

26. What is an amalgam tattoo?
Small bits of amalgam can sometimes find their way into the mucosa adjacent to a treated tooth. The material becomes impregnated into the tissue and results in a flat, bluish-black lesion.

27. What is the treatment for an amalgam tattoo?
No treatment is required.

28. A young patient presents with pigmentation of the marginal gingiva. What are the concerns?
Lead toxicity. High systemic levels of lead and bismuth result in the deposition of metallic pigmentation in the marginal gingiva and the clinical appearance of a lead line. Such bluish-black pigmentation is asymptomatic, bilateral, and involves both the maxilla and mandible equally.

29. What is black hairy tongue?
The papillae on the dorsal surface of the tongue may become discolored as the result of an overproliferation of melanogenic bacteria. This may occur following a course of antibiotic, particularly those of the tetracycline class. Hyperplasia and discoloration of the lingual papillae may also occur following pipe, cigar or heavy cigarette smoking, the ingestion of certain foods or as consequence of candidiasis. The color of the discoloration is not limited to black and may be brown, green, white, or yellow. Bismuth salts also cause pigmentation of the tongue. This type of pigmentation is most commonly caused by the use of Pepto-Bismol (bismuth subsalicylate).

41. ORAL CANCER

Stephen T. Sonis, D.M.D., D.M.Sc.

1. How common is cancer of the oral cavity?
The frequency of oral cancer is not uniform throughout the world's population. For example, while oral cancer is the seventh most common cancer among African-Americans and twelfth among the US white population, it is the most common cancer in certain parts of India, Southeast Asia, and the Bas-Rhin region of France. There will be about 30,000 new cases of cancer in the United States this year, about 3% of all new cancers. About 8500 people will succumb to the condition.

2. Is the frequency of oral cancer uniform throughout the United States?
No. Among US males, there is a higher frequency of disease in the northern urban regions. In US females, oral cancer is found most often among those residing in the south and along the Pacific and Florida coasts.

3. How does the frequency of oral cancer compare with that of other types of cancers?
The frequency of oral cancer is much lower than that of the big four (colorectal, breast, lung, and prostate). There are about 138,000 new cases of colorectal cancer, 170,000 new cases of lung cancer, 183,000 new cases of breast cancer, and 245,000 new cases of prostate cancer annually. However, the frequency of oral cancer is greater than many other forms of the disease, including cancers of the stomach, cervix, pancreas, and ovary as well as the leukemias, Hodgkin's disease, and multiple myeloma.

4. How does the mortality rate of oral cancer compare to that of other cancers?
Despite the easy access of the mouth to physical examination, which should lead to early diagnosis and treatment, more people die of oral cancer than die of cancers of the larynx or cervix or of melanoma. The 5-year survival rate for cancers of the mouth and pharynx is only 55% for whites in the US and even lower (37%) for African-Americans.

5. Incidence and mortality statistics do not really describe the impact of oral cancer on a patient's life. What other things are affected by the disease?
Since surgery is included in the treatment of many oral cancers, the patient's appearance, ability to eat and speak, control secretions, and be accepted by family, friends, and colleagues are often affected. Early diagnosis impacts on both the extent of therapy and survival.

6. When we talk about mouth cancer, to which histologic diagnosis are we usually referring?
Ninety percent of cancers of the mouth are squamous cell or epidermoid carcinomas.

7. List eight factors that may affect the incidence of oral cancer.
- Age
- Gender
- Race
- Geographic location
- Nutrition
- Tobacco use
- Alcohol use

8. What is the most common age for the onset of oral cancer?
The rate of oral cancer rises with age. The median age for diagnosis of oral cancer in the US is 63 years.

9. Compare the differences in the 5-year survival rate between US white and African-American males and females for cancers of the tongue, pharynx, and other sites in the mouth.
- Tongue: white males 43%, white females 49% versus African-American males 24%, African-American females 35%

• Pharynx: white males 30%, white females 36% versus African-American males 18%, African-American females 28%
• Other mouth sites: white males 52%, white females 62% versus African-American males 36%, African-American females 47%

10. Secondary primary cancers occur frequently in patients with oral cancer. What percent of patients can be expected to develop a second primary cancer of the mouth or adjacent sites within 4 years of the original diagnosis? After 10 or more years?
• 11% of patients with an oral cancer were reported to develop a second primary tumor of the mouth or adjacent site within 3.4 years of their original diagnosis.
• 24% of patients who survived at least 10 years after their original diagnosis developed a second primary cancer.

11. What is the major risk factor in the development of oral cancer?
Without question, tobacco use is the most significant risk factor for oral cancer. For example, the relative oral cancer risk for men smoking a moderate amount of cigarettes (defined as 20 to 39 cigarettes per day for 20 or more years) is 2.8 times that of nonsmokers. Men who smoke heavily (>2 packs per day for 20 or more years) are 4.4 times more likely to develop mouth cancer than nonsmokers. The effect is even more dramatic in women. Light smoking women (1 to 19 cigarettes per day for 20 or more years) are at three times the risk of nonsmokers; moderate female smokers have a risk 4.4 times that of nonsmokers; and heavy women smokers are more than 10 times likely to develop mouth cancer than nonsmokers.

12. Do forms of tobacco use, other than cigarettes, also increase the risk of oral cancer?
Both pipe and cigar use double the risk of oral cancer. Smokeless tobacco, such as chewing tobacco and snuff, is a well-established cause of oral cancer. Studies in women who used snuff placed between the cheek and gingiva showed an increased risk of oral cancer of 4.2 compared to that of nonusers. For long-term snuff users, the risk was 50 times that of nonusers.

13. To what extent does alcohol consumption influence the risk of oral cancer?
There is conclusive evidence that alcohol consumption increases the risk of oral cancer. Heavy drinkers are nine times more likely to develop oral cancer than nondrinkers.

14. Does the type of alcohol consumed influence the risk of oral cancer?
Only limited data are available to answer this question. However, it certainly appears that beer and hard liquor are equally potent as etiologic agents for oral cancer.

15. Compare the relative risk for oral cancer based on alcohol consumption for American males and females.

NUMBER OF DRINKS/WEEK	MALES' RISK	FEMALES' RISK
<1	1.0	1.0
1–4	1.2	1.2
5–14	1.7	1.3
15–29	3.3	2.3
30+	8.8	9.1

From Blot et al 1988

16. Does the combination of tobacco and alcohol use increase the risk of oral cancer compared to that for each one alone?
Yes. About 75% of oral cancers are attributable to cigarette and alcohol use. Their combined use markedly increases the risk. For example, a heavy smoker (2+ packs per day) who drinks an

average of three beers per day is more than 20 times likely to develop oral cancer than a non-smoker and nondrinker. Even someone who has one or two drinks per day and smokes 1 to 2 packs per day increases his or her risk of oral cancer by more than four times.

17. How does diet affect the risk for oral cancer?
Whereas an increased risk of oral cancer is seen with some nutritional deficiencies, the risk of oral cancer decreases with the consumption of fruit and raw vegetables. In fact, eating fruit seems to be protective. For example, people who go bananas for fruit have a risk ratio that is 0.4 that of the meat and potato crowd.

18. What is the evidence to suggest that poor oral hygiene may increase the risk of oral cancer?
While the risk of oral cancer has been reported to be higher in denture wearers, a study by Winn found that there was a two- to three-fold risk of oral cancer among individuals who had lost 10 or more teeth whether they were denture wearers or not. A similar finding was noted among Brazilians. These data have been interpreted as suggesting that poor oral hygiene leading to tooth loss, and not denture use, is a risk factor for oral cancer.

19. Over 40% of Americans use mouthwash regularly. Does it have any effect on the risk for oral cancer?
This is an unresolved issue. There have been long-term case-controlled studies suggesting a relationship between the use of mouthwashes and an increase of oral cancer, particularly among nonsmokers and nondrinkers. The risk of oral cancer was greatest for those using mouthwashes in which the alcohol content was high. More studies are needed to definitively answer this question.

20. Name seven occupations for which there are studies to suggest an association with an increase risk of oral cancer.
1. Bartender
2. Brewery worker
3. Insulation worker
4. Electronics industry worker
5. Leather worker
6. Woodworker
7. Nickel refinery worker

21. Is the risk for head and neck cancer greater, less than, or equal for patients who smoke marijuana compared with those who smoke tobacco?
Smoking marijuana is more risky than smoking cigarettes for head and neck cancer. The reason is probably that marijuana smoke has a higher tar burden (four times) than tobacco and contains markedly more hydrocarbons and benzpyrene than cigarette smoke.

22. Provide evidence to suggest a role for genetic, viral, and immunologic factors in the development of oral cancer.
- A familial tendency for oral cancer, its association with certain syndromes, and its relationship to specific genetic polymorphisms suggests a potential genetic component in its development. Point mutations in the p53 gene have been associated with oral cancer development.
- Herpes simplex virus, Epstein-Barr virus, and papillomavirus have all been mentioned as having a causative role in oral cancer.
- Chronically immunosuppressed patients, such as renal transplant recipients and patients with graft-versus-host disease are at increased risk for oral cancer.

23. What is the role of the dentist in dealing with head and neck cancer?
- Diagnosis
- Managing and minimizing undesirable side effects of treatment
- Reconstruction and rehabilitation

24. How does oral cancer present clinically?
- Ulceration (endophytic)
- Leukoplakia (white patch)
- Erythroplasia (red and white patch)
- Exophytic lesion (mass-forming)
- Scirrhous carcinoma

25. What is the clinical appearance of an ulcer that is an oral squamous cell carcinoma?
Oral carcinoma may appear as a nonhealing, painless, expanding ulcer on any mucosal surface. The borders of the ulcer are usually slightly raised, firm, and indurated. The base of the ulcer may look pebbly or smooth or it may be necrotic.

26. What is the clinical appearance of leukoplakia that is a squamous cell carcinoma?
It is almost impossible to differentiate malignant from benign leukoplakia. The cancerous lesion appears as a white, nonscrapable, asymptomatic plaque that may be slightly raised. In the case of erythroplasia, erythematous islands may be interspersed in a sea of keratosis.

27. What is the clinical appearance of verrucous carcinoma in the mouth?
Verrucous carcinomas present as asymptomatic exophytic growths with a pebbly, papillary lesion atop a stalklike base.

28. How does a scirrhous carcinoma appear in the mouth?
Scirrhous carcinoma is a lesion in which the majority of the tumor is submerged beneath the tissue. Only a portion may actually be visible. Since the tumor most commonly occurs in the floor of the mouth, its spread to the lingual musculature may result in a restriction in lingual motion that is often what brings the patient to the dentist.

29. What are the most common clinical presentations of oral cancer?
Ulceration and leukoplakia

30. What aspects of the physical examination are most important in the diagnosis of oral cancer?
- Direct visualization
- Palpation

31. List the distribution of oral carcinoma from most frequent to least frequent.
- Lower lip, 38%
- Tongue, 22%
- Floor of mouth, 17%
- Gingiva, 6%
- Palate, 5.5%
- Tonsil, 5%
- Upper lip, 4%
- Buccal mucosa, 2%
- Uvula, 0.5%

32. Name three causes of cancer of the lower lip.
1. Pipe smoking
2. Cigarette smoking
3. Actinic rays from the sun

33. What is the most common location for cancers of the tongue?
The most common location for cancers of the tongue is on the lateral or ventral edge of the posterior tongue.

34. How common is the posterior third or base of the tongue as a site of lingual carcinoma?
One quarter of tongue cancers are found in the posterior third or base of the tongue. Since these lesions often metastasize, it is important to detect them early. Clinical examination of the base of the tongue that includes palpation is necessary, as these tumors are often difficult to see.

35. How does carcinoma in the floor of the mouth appear clinically?

Carcinoma of the floor of the mouth may appear in a variety of forms including ulceration, a mass or papillary enlargement or erythroplakia. Progressive lesions may involve the tongue or mandible. If the tongue is involved, its mobility may be limited. On palpation, tumors feel rock-hard because of their dense cellularity.

36. How do squamous cell carcinomas of the mouth spread?

Oral cancers spread by local invasion and metastasize via lymph channels to regional nodes. Distant metastases are rare.

37. What is the most common technique for the diagnosis of a suspected oral cancer?

Biopsy remains the most common and definitive technique for the diagnosis of oral lesions. Biopsies should be incisional rather than excisional so as not to obscure the extent of the tumor.

38. Does cytologic analysis have a role in the diagnosis of oral cancer?

Historically, the use of cytologic smears for the diagnosis of oral cancer has not been popular because of a high false negative rate (false-negative rate = the number of cancers that are missed by this technique, which is 15%). Recently, a new technique for cytologic sampling and interpretation has become available that appears to be more sensitive. Its acceptance among pathologists and clinicians will probably require more data and time.

39. What is the role of toluidine blue in the diagnosis of oral cancer?

The purported specificity for toluidine blue dye for mucosal cancers has led to its application as a screening tool. However, a high-false negative rate has limited its use.

40. Since oral cancers are in an anatomic site that is easy to examine, the prognosis for treated lesions must be excellent. Is that statement true or false? Support your answer.

False. You would think that a site as accessible for examination as the mouth would lead to early diagnosis and treatment. Unfortunately, many health care providers are not aggressive in their clinical examination of the mouth. That, coupled with the fact that oral cancers are usually asymptomatic, often delays diagnosis, which adversely affects prognosis.

For example, the 5-year survival rates for advanced cancers of the tongue is 20%, and for cancers of the floor of the mouth it is 18%.

41. Do early detection and treatment really impact on outcome?

Although the 5-year survival rate for advanced cancers of the tongue is only 20%, it is 65% for more localized tumors. The difference in survival rates for early and advanced floor of mouth cancers is even more dramatic. The 5-year survival rate is excellent for early tumors (78%). It plummets to only 18% for advanced lesions.

42. What factors influence the prognosis of oral cancers?

- Size
- Location
- Extent
- Nodal involvement

43. What is tumor staging? What is its value?

Tumor staging provides a uniform system to describe the extent of a lesion and its projected clinical behavior. The system by which carcinomas are clinically defined is called staging. Staging allows everyone involved in a patient's care to understand the magnitude of the disease and its prognosis.

44. How is staging of oral cancers done?

The staging of oral cancers involves three parameters: the size and extent of the tumor, the presence and extent of lymph node involvement, and the presence or absence of metastases. The system that was developed in 1942 is thus called the TNM system for tumor, nodes, and metastases.

Tumor size (T) is graded on a scale of 0 to 3 based on the following:
    T0   No evidence of primary tumor
    T1   Tumor equal to or less than 2 cm in greatest dimension
    T2   Tumor > 2 cm but equal to or less than 4 cm in greatest dimension
    T3   Tumor > 4 cm in greatest dimension
Regional lymph nodes
    N0   No clinically palpable lymph nodes and metastases not suspected
    N1   Clinically palpable cervical lymph nodes that are not fixed on the same side as the
          tumor
    N2   Clinically palpable contralateral or bilateral cervical lymph nodes that are not fixed
    N3   Clinically palpable lymph nodes that are fixed
Distant metastases
    MO   No distant metastases
    M1   Clinical or radiographic evidence of metastases other than cervical nodes
Tumors are staged on a I to IV scale based on the extent of the tumor as graded by the TNM
system.

45. Define the four stages for oral cancers based on the TNM system.
    • Stage I   T1 N0 M0
    • Stage II   T2 N0 M0
    • Stage III   T3 N0 M0 or any tumor size with N1 M0
    • Stage IV   Any tumor with N2 or N3 or any T or N with M1

46. Give some examples of the relationship between staging and prognosis.
    Overall 5-year survival rates for patients with cancers of the tongue by stage:
    • Stage I   65%
    • Stage II   53%
    • Stage III   29%
    • Stage IV   20%
    Overall 5-year survival for patients with cancers of the floor of the mouth by stage:
    • Stage I   78%
    • Stage II   65%
    • Stage III   43%
    • Stage IV   18%

47. What are the current therapeutic approaches for oral cancer?
    • Definitive surgery
    • Definitive radiation therapy
    • Surgery with planned postoperative radiation therapy
    • Definitive radiation with surgery only for salvage or recurrence
    • Palliation with chemotherapy or radiation therapy
    • Radiation therapy with concomitant chemotherapy

**48. What is the standard method of treatment for small primary tumors that do not have
regional metastases?**
    Surgical resection of the tumor with wide margins or radiation therapy is the standard forms
of therapy.

**49. What is the usual method of treatment for advanced oral cancers in which there is
nodal involvement?**
    These more extensive tumors (stage III or stage IV) are treated with a combination of surgery
and radiation. Recently, the use of concomitant chemotherapy with other forms of treatment has
produced promising results.

50. What are the objectives of surgical treatment of oral cancer?
 • Tumor resection with wide margins.
 • Resection of bone that has tumor involvement.
 • Removal of lymph nodes into which the tumor has spread.

51. What are the advantages and disadvantages of surgical treatment of tumors?
 • Advantages are that surgical treatment is tumor-specific and that histologic verification of tumor resection and margins can be ascertained in most cases.
 • The major disadvantages to surgical tumor resection are its cosmetic and functional consequences.

52. Name three forms of surgery that can be used to treat oral cancers.
 1. Conventional surgery using a scalpel and blade.
 2. Cryosurgery in which liquid nitrogen is used to freeze the tumor.
 3. Laser surgery which causes thermal lysis of the tumor.

53. What factors affect the radiosensitivity of an oral cancer?
The more exposed the tumor, the more radiosensitive it generally is. The inclusion of tumor in bone reduces its radiosensitivity.

54. What is the standard course of radiation therapy for patients with cancers of the head and neck?
The standard regimen in the United States is 180 to 200 cGy given daily for 5 days per week for 6 to 8 weeks.

55. What are the local side effects from radiation therapy for oral cancer?
 • Mucositis   • Radiation caries
 • Xerostomia   • Osteoradionecrosis

56. What is mucositis?
Mucositis is a common, painful, and dose-interrupting side effect from therapy of head and neck radiation and many forms of cancer chemotherapy. In its most dramatic form, it produces large, confluent ulcers of the oral mucosa that prohibit normal function and often require parenteral opiates for symptom control.

57. How significant a problem is mucositis?
From a patient's perspective, mucositis is the most commonly cited bothersome toxicity of patients undergoing aggressive forms of chemotherapy. It is mentioned more often than other toxicities such as nausea, vomiting, diarrhea, and lethargy. From a cost standpoint, the presence of mucositis increases the length of hospital stays, antibiotic and analgesic use, and cost. In patients who are neutropenic because of chemotherapy, the ulcers that develop with mucositis serve as a portal of entry for oral bacteria getting into the systemic circulation. About 40% of patients who receive chemotherapy develop some form of mucositis. Virtually all patients who are irradiated for head and neck cancer develop the condition.

58. What are the clinical stages of mucositis?
 • Erythema   • Erosion
 • Hyperkeratosis   • Ulceration and pseudomembrane formation

59. When does mucositis begin in a patient being irradiated for head and neck cancer?
Significant mucositis usually begins when the patient has received a total cumulative dose of about 20 cGy of radiation.

60. How long does radiation-induced mucositis last?

Mucositis usually heals spontaneously in about 2 to 3 weeks following the cessation of therapy.

61. Is there any predictable prophylaxis or treatment for radiation-induced mucositis?

Unfortunately not. Palliative mouth rinses can be used. Pilocarpine, which has been developed to treat radiation-induced xerostomia, may be of benefit. A number of drugs are under development and will, it is hoped, be available in the near future.

62. Why do patients who receive radiation to the head and neck develop xerostomia?

Shortly after the initiation of external beam radiation, fibroblast proliferation is noted in the interlobular areas of the salivary glands. This follows the appearance of lymphocytes and plasma cells and precedes an eventual progressive degeneration of the acinar epithelium. There is increasing fibrosis of both the interlocular and interlocular areas. Serous portions of the glands tend to be most involved. Thus the parotid gland is most affected and stops producing serous saliva.

63. Is there any treatment for radiation-induced xerostomia?

Two drugs are currently approved for the treatment of radiation-induced mucositis: pilocarpine and amifostine.

64. Differentiate between the mechanisms of action of pilocarpine and amifostine relative to radiation-induced xerostomia.

Pilocarpine is a cholinergic, parasympathomimetic agent that produces postganglionic parasympathetic stimulation to increase exocrine gland secretion. Pilocarpine does this by stimulating the salivary gland nerve supply, which results in the release of acretylcholine. In contrast, amifostine is a free-radical scavenger. Since free radicals play an important role in radiation-mediated injury, eliminating them has a mechanistic beneficial effect.

65. What is osteoradionecrosis?

Osteoradionecrosis is a chronic infection of bone that may occur as a sequela to radiation therapy. It occurs when radiation produces an increased risk of infection secondary to fibrotic thickening of the blood vessels, localized replacement of the marrow with connective tissues, and a lack of new bone formation. Patients with osteoradionecrosis present with a festering, foul-smelling wound involving the soft tissue and underlying bone.

66. What is the most common intraoral site for osteoradionecrosis?

Ninety percent of cases occur in the mandible.

67. How common is osteoradionecrosis of the mouth?

There is a wide range in the reported incidence of osteoradionecrosis. Some reports place the frequency as high as 35% of patients receiving radiation to the head and neck, whereas others are as low as 4%.

68. What are the risk factors for osteoradionecrosis?

- Anatomic site of the tumor
  - Patients receiving radiation to tumors anatomically related to the mandible are twice as likely to develop osteoradionecrosis as are patients who have tumors adjacent to bone. Osteoradionecrosis of the maxilla is rare.
- Dose of radiation
  - There is a nonlinear relationship between dose of radiation and the incidence of osteoradionecrosis. The risk of developing osteoradionecrosis at 80 cGy is twice as much as that for irradiation doses of 50 cGy.
- Dental status of the patient
  - Patients with dental disease are more likely to develop osteoradionecrosis than are patients without dental disease. Similarly, patients with good oral hygiene have a lessened risk.
  - Patients with denture sores are at increased risk of developing osteoradionecrosis.

69. Elimination of chronically infected teeth before head and neck radiation is a good strategy to reduce the risk of osteoradionecrosis. When is the best time to extract teeth?

It is generally agreed that extractions are best performed at least 2 weeks prior to the start of radiation therapy.

70. How is osteoradionecrosis treated?

A conservative approach consisting of long-term antibiotic therapy (penicillin), local irrigation, and excellent hygiene works in many cases. In particularly stubborn instances, surgical débridement may be required. Hyperbaric oxygen therapy mask may be helpful.

71. What should be done if a patient requires an extraction during radiation therapy?

In general, extractions during radiation therapy should be limited to symptomatic or infected teeth. If endodontics can be performed, it is more desirable than extraction. However, if extraction is necessary, it should be done using antibiotic prophylaxis with as atraumatic a technique as possible. Minimal soft-tissue manipulation is desirable. The placement of a denture is contraindicated for a year.

42. BENIGN TUMORS

Stephen T. Sonis, D.M.D., D.M.Sc.

1. What are some of the common features of benign tumors of the oral mucosa?
- Generally raised
- Well-circumscribed borders
- Freely movable
- Surface usually intact

2. What is the most satisfactory method for diagnosis of a benign mucosal tumor?
Excisional biopsy

3. List the benign tumors that are found on the oral mucosa.
- Pyogenic granuloma/pregnancy tumor
- Fibroma
- Papilloma
- Giant cell granuloma
- Myoma
- Lipoma
- Congenital epulis
- Epulis fissurata
- Mucocyst
- Ranula
- Neurofibroma
- Schwannoma (neurinoma)
- Neuroma
- Keratoacanthoma
- Myoblastoma
- Hemangioma
- Lymphangioma

4. Describe the clinical and histologic features of a pyogenic granuloma.
- Pyogenic granulomas are the result of proliferation of vascular granulation tissue in response to local mucosal irritation.
- Lesions appear as a raised mass, which, because of its vascularity, is bluish-red in coloration. The base may be pedunculated. Gingival lesions bleed easily when provoked.
- Most common location is the gingiva but can occur on cheeks, tongue, and lips.
- Size is variable from millimeters to a couple of centimeters.

5. What are pregnancy tumors?
Pregnancy tumors are no different than pyogenic granulomas. As the name implies, these lesions occur during pregnancy and are the consequence of an exuberant vascular response to local irritation. They are typically seen interproximally and bleed on provocation.

6. What is the clinical appearance of a pregnancy tumor?
Pregnancy tumors appear as raised, reddish, smooth-surfaced masses between teeth. Their size varies. When they occur, they typically arise rapidly after the first trimester. Patients with pre-existing gingival inflammation are at higher risk for developing pregnancy tumors than are patients in periodontal health.

7. What is the treatment for pyogenic granuloma?
Excision is curative. If a pregnancy tumor is asymptomatic, it may be prudent to wait until the pregnancy is concluded before excision is performed, as spontaneous resolution might occur.

8. What are the histologic features of pyogenic granuloma or pregnancy tumor?
- Loose, edematous connective tissue packed with many thin-walled blood vessels resembling granulation tissue. The vessels may be filled with blood.
- Overlying mucosa may be intact or ulcerated.
- Amount of inflammatory infiltrate varies.

233

9. What is a fibroma?
Fibromas are benign tumors consisting of dense collections of fibrous connective tissue. In most cases they represent a local response to chronic irritation. Fibromas are the most common benign tumors of the oral mucosa.

10. Describe the clinical appearance of a fibroma.
Fibromas appear as firm, well-defined, raised masses. The overlying mucosa is typically normal, although ulceration may be present if the tumor is subject to trauma from biting or a sharp restoration. Fibromas are generally asymptomatic. The most common location for fibromas is the buccal mucosa. The tongue and lip are also frequent sites.

11. What are the gender and age predilections for fibromas?
Women are twice as likely as men to have fibromas; fibromas are most common between the ages of 40 and 60 years.

12. What is the treatment of choice for fibromas?
Excisional biopsy.

13. What is the clinical presentation of a papilloma?
Papillomas appear as firm, white, exophytic, cauliflower-like lesions extruding from the mucosa, often on a stalk. The surface is rough, usually pebbled, and may be wartlike. Papillomas vary in size. They are most common on the buccal and labial mucosa, tongue, and gingiva.

14. Are papillomas limited to any age group?
Papillomas may be seen at any age but are most common between the ages of 30 and 50 years.

15. Why is an excisional biopsy especially important in a patient with a suspected papilloma?
Clinically, a benign papilloma is indistinguishable from a papillary carcinoma. Consequently, histologic diagnosis is mandatory.

16. What are the clinical course and appearance of a peripheral giant cell granuloma?
• Rapid onset
• Large, smooth-surfaced, purple-red to red, pedunculated mass of the attached gingiva
• Seems to originate from deep inside the tissue
• Starts on either the buccal or lingual aspect of the gingiva but grows to overwhelm and bury the teeth.
• Bleeds on provocation

17. What is the etiology of peripheral giant cell granulomas?
Although the cause is unknown, giant cell granulomas are thought to represent a local tissue reaction to trauma or irritation.

18. What is the treatment for peripheral giant cell granuloma?
Excisional biopsy with curettage of the underlying base, since recurrence has been reported in about 10% of cases.

19. Which endocrine disorder would you consider ruling out in a patient with peripheral giant cell disorder?
Hyperparathyroidism, since lesions of similar appearance have been reported in patients with this condition.

20. What are lipomas?
Lipomas are benign tumors of fat tissue. Although they occur relatively commonly under the skin, they are rare in the mouth. Lipomas appear as asymptomatic, soft, pedunculated mucosal

masses with a yellowish coloration beneath a normal, intact surface. Histologically, lipomas are composed almost entirely of adipose tissue.

21. What are the most common intraoral sites for lipomas?
The most common intraoral locations for lipomas are the buccal or lingual mucosa. Less frequently, they involve the floor of the mouth or gingiva.

22. The optimum treatment for lipomas is (multiple choice):
  • **Incisional biopsy**
  • **Excisional biopsy**
  • **Cautery**
  • **Curettage**
  • **They're very slow growing, so watch and wait**
Answer: Excisional biopsy

23. What is an epulis fissurata?
Epulis fissurata is a mass of hyperplastic tissue that most often arises as a result of denture flange irritation in the mucobuccal fold. Consequently, these tumor-like masses are most often present at the margins of alveolar mucosa and an edentulous ridge. Epulis fissurata may occur soon after placement of a new denture or later, when after alveolar ridge resorption occurs, the denture is no longer stable.
Clinically, epulis fissurata appears as an elevated mass of tissue, often with linear folds. The overlying mucosa may look mildly erythematous. Pain occurs, if mucosal ulceration is present. The size of the tumor is variable.

24. What is the treatment for epulis fissurata?
  • Excisional biopsy
  • Correction of the denture

25. A 25-year-old patient presents with a bluish, domed, round, tender swelling of the mandibular labial mucosa. You think the lesion is a mucocele. Why?
Mucoceles are either extravasation or retention cysts of the minor salivary glands that usually arise on the mandibular labial mucosa following trauma or irritation. They are most commonly noted in young adults and may recur. The smooth, raised, domed appearance on the mandibular labial mucosa is common (53.6% of mucoceles occur in this location).

26. What would you recommend for treatment for your patient with the mucocele?
  • Excisional biopsy of the lesion, including the underlying minor salivary gland
  • Elimination of any sources of mucosal irritation

27. Where in the mouth would you most likely encounter a ranula?
Ranulas are large retention cysts that occur in the floor of the mouth. The name is derived from the blue-purple-pink vascular surface appearance of the cyst, which resembles the belly of a frog. Ranulas usually arise from the ducts of the sublingual glands but may also be associated with the submandibular duct.

28. At what age do ranulas typically occur?
Ranulas may occur at any age.

29. What is the treatment for a ranula?
The recommended treatment is marsupialization, a procedure in which the dome of the cyst is removed.

30. What is von Recklinghausen's disease?
von Recklinghausen's disease is a condition in which neurofibromas present as multiple lesions, usually of the skin. The condition usually has its onset in childhood. There is no gender predilection. In addition to their presence on the skin, neurofibromas may appear on the mucosa of the tongue; gingiva and lips also may be involved. Neurofibromatosis is an inherited disorder, although about one half of patients have no family history. Lesions are often accompanied by deep brownish pigmentation called café-au-lait spots.

31. Describe the clinical appearance of the neurofibromas seen in von Recklinghausen's disease.
Lesions may appear as multiple raised masses that have a dull consistency or as flabby folds of tissue.

32. Why might you want to follow a patient with von Recklinghausen's disease?
The neurofibromas have a potential for malignant transformation. Consequently, any change in their appearance or course should be cause for concern and biopsy.

33. Is there an effective treatment for neurofibromatosis?
Unfortunately, not. Large, symptomatic, or unsightly lesions may be excised. Laser and dermabrasion have also been used.

34. What movie portrays a patient with von Recklinghausen's disease?
The Elephant Man.

35. You decide to become a pediatric dentist. On the first day of your residency you are asked to see a female infant who has a pinkish red, polyplike mass on her maxillary alveolar ridge. Having read and memorized this book, you are ready to dazzle your attending with a diagnosis of _____.
Congenital epulis

36. Brilliant diagnosis, but what is a congenital epulis?
A congenital epulis is a rare benign tumor of newborns. The lesions are almost exclusively seen in females and most often on the maxillary anterior alveolar ridge. The tumors are benign and are treated by surgical excision.

37. Vascular tumors of the oral mucosa are probably developmental anomalies rather than true tumors. What are the two major categories of these lesions?
1. Hemangiomas
2. Lymphangiomas

38. List the types of hemangiomas.
• Capillary hemangiomas
• Juvenile hemangiomas
• Cavernous hemangiomas
• Arteriovenous hemangiomas

39. Describe the clinical features of the most common type of hemangioma to occur in the mouth.
Capillary hemangiomas appear as raised pedunculated, purple-red masses with a pebbly surface, giving them a berrylike appearance. Since these tumors are probably developmental anomalies, they are usually present at birth, although initially they tend to be less raised and discrete. Capillary hemangiomas are most commonly found on the tongue but can occur in other locations. They are relatively firm and blanch on pressure.

40. What is the normal course of most capillary hemangiomas?
They usually peak in size by the end of the first year of life and then may spontaneously regress by age 7.

41. What is the gender predilection for capillary hemangiomas?
Five times more common in females than males.

42. What condition is associated with facial lesions called port-wine stain or nevus flammeus?
Sturge-Weber syndrome includes a dermovenous malformation that involves the brain and the skin, innervated by one or more branches of the trigeminal nerve. Usually the involvement is unilateral. Intraoral involvement is common, with the gingiva being the primary target tissue. Gingival changes range from hyperplasia to dramatic hemangiomatous proliferation typically on the same side as the facial lesions.

43. What neurologic conditions can be seen in patients with Sturge-Weber syndrome?
• Seizures
• Mental retardation
• Hemiparesis

43. DISEASES OF THE SALIVARY GLANDS

Stephen T. Sonis, D.M.D., D.M.Sc.

1. Name the three pairs of major salivary glands.
1. Parotid
2. Submandibular
3. Sublingual

2. According to Fox and Eversole what are the major functions of saliva?
- Hydration
- Cleansing
- Lubrication
- Digestion
- Remineralization of dentition
- Maintenance of mucosal integrity
- Antimicrobial

3. What are the two types of saliva produced by the major salivary glands?
Serous saliva and mucous saliva are produced by the major salivary glands. The parotid glands produce purely serous saliva, the submandibular glands produce both, and the sublingual glands are wholly mucus in their production.

4. What is Wharton's duct and where does it drain?
Wharton's duct is the duct of the submandibular glands and enters the mouth just behind the mandibular incisors.

5. What is Stenson's duct and where does it drain?
Stenson's duct drains the parotid glands. The duct opens on the buccal mucosa opposite the maxillary second molar.

6. As in most conditions, the patient's history reveals a great deal about his or her salivary gland status. What questions can you ask to help elicit this information?
- Does the patient feel like her or his mouth is dry?
- Is the amount of saliva excessive?
- Has the patient's ability to taste changed?
- Does the patient have trouble swallowing solid food?
- Does the patient have salivary gland pain prior to eating?
- Is the patient taking medications known to modify salivary function?
- Does the patient have any systemic illnesses that are associated with salivary gland dysfunction?

7. What elements of the clinical examination are helpful in diagnosing salivary gland dysfunction?
- The patient's facial symmetry should be examined to determine any salivary gland enlargement.
- The quality and quantity of saliva should be observed. Normal saliva is clear, free-flowing, and easily milked from the parotid and submandibular glands. The presence of particulate matter in saliva might represent early sialolith formation. Thickened, discolored saliva could be from a suppuration.
- The mucosa should be observed for signs of dryness, atrophy, and erythema.
- Each of the major salivary glands should be palpated to determine the presence of masses and gland consistency.
- Salivary output can be measured.

239

8. Radiographic and imaging techniques may be useful in the diagnosis of salivary gland disease. What techniques are most commonly available for this purpose?
- Sialography
- Scintigraphy
- Computerized tomography
- Magnetic resonance imaging

9. What is sialography?
Sialography involves the injection of a radio-opaque dye into a salivary duct, followed by taking a radiograph. It is particularly useful to identify blockages of ductal flow.

10. What is scintigraphy and when is it used?
Scintigraphy is generally used to detect suspected glandular inflammatory or neoplastic disease. The procedure relies on the ability of salivary glands to concentrate certain isotopes before they are secreted. Technetium 99m pertechnetate is injected intravenously and then is taken up by the major salivary glands, which are imaged sequentially using a gamma scintillation camera to make a visual recording of isotope uptake and secretion.

11. A patient presents with a firm, expanding mass of one of her parotid glands. You suspect a tumor. What imaging test would be most appropriate?
Computed tomography (CT) is probably the best imaging technique to diagnose a tumor of a salivary gland.

12. Magnetic resonance imaging (MRI) distinguishes the water content of tissue. It is not a radiographic technique but is effective in diagnosing soft-tissue lesions. For what type of salivary gland disease is MRI particularly effective?
MRI is especially good at differentiating between cystic and solid masses.

13. What do you call inflammatory conditions of salivary glands? What are the most common causes of salivary gland inflammation?
Inflammation of the salivary glands is called sialadenitis and is most commonly caused by bacterial or viral infection.

14. What is sialolithiasis?
An acute bacterial infection of the major salivary glands that is caused by the presence of salivary stones or sialoliths in the ducts.

15. What is the composition of a sialolith?
Sialoliths are laminated calcified structures composed of a mineralized matrix of proteins and lipopolysaccharides calcified with calcium phosphate.

16. What symptoms are associated with sialolithiasis?
- Pain in the affected gland, particularly prior to eating.
- Unilateral swelling of the affected gland, especially prior to eating.
- When the duct milked, flow may be intermittent and cloudy.
- If complete obstruction occurs, infection may develop. The gland becomes swollen, tender, and erythematous, and the patient may have signs of infection.

17. How would you diagnose a suspected case of sialolithiasis?
Diagnosis of sialolithiasis is based on history, physical examination, and radiographic examination. See question 17 for history features. Clinical examination may demonstrate tender swelling of the salivary gland. If there is a large stone, it may sometimes be palpated or partially poke out through the duct. An occusal radiograph is often diagnostic for stones in the submandibular ducts. Sialography might also be useful diagnostically.

18. How is sialolithiasis treated?

Treatment varies with the size of the sialoliths. Small stones may pass spontaneously following stimulation of the gland by keeping the patient hydrated and then using sugar-free lemon drops. Larger stones may be removed following dilation of the duct. In some cases, surgical exposure of the stone may be required. If stasis is suspected that results in inflammatory changes in the gland, antibiotic therapy should also be considered.

19. What is acute bacterial sialadenitis?

Acute bacterial sialadenitis is an acute infection of the parotid gland. It is seen almost exclusively in debilitated, elderly patients who become dehydrated. It may also occur in patients who have drug- or disease-induced xerostomia.

20. What appears to be the cause of bacterial sialadenitis?

Salivary stasis within the salivary duct results in a retrograde infection of the gland.

21. What are the clinical characteristics of acute bacterial parotitis?
- Sudden onset (80% of the time)
- Unilateral
- Erythematous swelling
- Initially localized pain and tenderness at the angle of the mandible, then spreads to involve the gland
- Enlargement of the gland
- Overlying skin tense and shiny
- Purulent discharge can be expressed from duct
- Patient may have systemic signs of infection, including fever, chills, leukocytosis, and malaise

22. What organism is most commonly isolated from the infected glands of patients with bacterial parotitis?

Penicillin-resistant *Staphylococcus aureus*

23. How would you manage a patient with acute bacterial parotitis?
- Culture the discharge from parotid duct
- Empirically place the patient on an antistaphylococcal antibiotic such as dicloxacillin. Clindamycin can be used for penicillin-allergic patients.
- Generally, patients should be hospitalized so that antibiotic therapy can be administered intravenously.
- Provide supportive care such as pain medication, fluid support, and bed rest and apply moist heat to the area.
- Discontinue any medication known to cause xerostomia.
- Use surgical drainage if appropriate.

24. What is chronic bacterial parotitis?

Chronic bacterial parotitis is typically the result of an obstructed duct. The condition may occur in patients following acute bacterial parotitis or as a consequence of Sjögren's disease. Because of the chronic nature of the condition, degeneration of the gland may occur.

25. What are the clinical features of chronic bacterial parotitis?
- Recurrent unilateral swelling of one of the parotid glands. Each episode of swelling is rapid in onset, but pain may be intermittent.
- Swelling may last for periods ranging from days to months.
- Pus may be present but is not a constant feature.
- If pus is present, cultures usually show streptococci in children and mixed streptococci-staphylococci in adults.

• Occurs in nondebilitated children and adults.
• Sialography demonstrates multiple cystic cavities of the parenchyma.

26. What is the treatment of chronic bacterial parotitis?
• Elimination of obstruction by careful dilatation of duct.
• Irrigation of duct with antibiotic solution for a week.
• Systemic antibiotics.
• Parotidectomy for persistent cases.

27. Name three viruses that can cause sialadenitis.
1. Mumps
2. Group A Coxsackievirus
3. Cytomegalovirus

28. What is mumps?
Mumps is a very communicable viral disease that used to be extremely common. Since the availability of immunization for the disease, mumps is rare. It was typically seen in children as a part of a springtime endemic. Following a 3- to 5-week incubation period, patients develop a viral prodrome followed by fever, malaise, headache, chills, and swelling of both or either parotid gland. Typically, the infection is self-limiting and resolves in a week or so. Treatment is confined to supportive care.

29. Group A Coxsackievirus occurs primarily in children in the summer and fall. It may cause parotitis in some patients, but the usual oral manifestations are vesicular lesions of the posterior oropharynx. What is the name of the infection caused by this virus?
Herpangina

30. Cytomegalovirus-induced parotitis is commonly associated with what disease?
Acquired immunodeficiency syndrome

31. What are the three major causes of non-inflammatory non-neoplastic swellings of the salivary glands?
1. Drugs
2. Endocrine disturbances
3. Nutritional deficiencies

32. What class of drugs is associated with salivary gland enlargement?
Sympathomimetic drugs such as isoproterenol, and drugs that interfere with autonomic nerve function, such as guanethidine and imidazolamine, may cause salivary gland enlargement.

33. What endocrine disease is most often associated with salivary gland enlargement?
Diabetes mellitus is most often associated with parotid changes. Less frequent salivary gland changes have been reported with hypothyroidism and gonadal disturbances.

34. How can vitamin A deficiency cause salivary gland inflammation?
It has been speculated that vitamin A deficiency results in squamous metaplasia of the specialized epithelium found in salivary glands. As a result, salivary retention occurs, which results in inflammation of the gland.

35. Niacin deficiency has been associated with salivary gland changes. What is the clinical condition that results from deficiency of this vitamin?
Pellegra

36. Which salivary gland may be infected by tuberculosis?
The parotid gland is most often involved, usually secondary to pulmonary involvement.

37. How often is the parotid gland involved in patients with sarcoidosis?
The extent of parotid involvement is unresolved, with reported frequencies ranging from 5 to 60%.

38. What is the clinical presentation of the parotid glands when they are affected by sarcoidosis?
Typically, there is bilateral asymptomatic enlargement of the parotid glands.

39. What is Sjögren's syndrome?
Sjögren's syndrome is a chronic autoimmune disorder that affects the salivary and lacrimal glands and results in xerostomia and dryness of the eyes.

40. How prevalent is Sjögren's syndrome?
Sjögren's syndrome affects about 1% of the population.

41. What is the difference between primary and secondary Sjögren's syndrome?
Sjögren's syndrome may occur in the absence of connective tissue disease (primary Sjögren's) or in association with it (secondary Sjögren's). The distribution of patients is about 50:50 between the two.

42. Xerostomia is a consistent and prominent feature of Sjögren's syndrome. How often is there bilateral enlargement of the parotid glands?
About 50% of the time.

43. What is sicca complex?
Sicca complex consists of dry mouth, dry eyes, and symptoms of an associated connective tissue disease.

44. If you biopsied the parotid gland of a patient with Sjögren's syndrome, what would you expect to see?
Replacement of the normal acinar of the glands by a lymphocytic infiltration.

45. Connective tissue diseases are associated with Sjögren's syndrome in a significant number of cases. Name specific connective tissue diseases that are associated with the syndrome.
- Most common is rheumatoid arthritis
- Systemic lupus erythematosus
- Polyarteritis
- Dermatomyocytis
- Scleroderma

46. Describe the demographics of patients with Sjögren's syndrome.
- More common in women than in men.
- Age of onset typically in the 50s.
- Although rare, has been reported in children and young adults.

47. In patients with secondary Sjögren's syndrome, which comes first, the connective tissue disease or salivary gland involvement?
In the majority (90%) of cases, the connective tissue disease precedes salivary gland involvement.

48. Although the etiology of Sjögren's syndrome is unresolved, all patients with the condition develop antibodies to what antigens?
SSA/Ro antigens

49. What other diseases should you be especially concerned about in patients with Sjögren's syndrome?
Patients with Sjögren's syndrome have a sharply increased risk of developing lymphoreticular malignancies, including lymphoma, reticulum cell sarcoma, and Waldenström's macroglobulinemia.

50. About half of patients with Sjögren's syndrome have skin involvement. What are the most common cutaneous manifestations of the condition?

Xerosis and pruritus

51. How is Sjögren's diagnosed?

• Clinical findings
• Salivary gland biopsy in which the extent of lymphocytic infiltration is evaluated, or immunofluoresence in which antisalivary duct antibody is evaluated.
• Salivary flow rate to demonstrate xerostomia.
• Imaging studies, including secretory sialography and scintigraphy.
• Studies of serologic markers of autoimmunity, including antinuclear antibodies (ANAs), and autoantibodies specific for the condition, anti-SS-A/Ro and anti-SS-BLa.

52. How predictive are serologic tests in diagnosing Sjögren's syndrome?

The ANA test is positive about 80% of the time, whereas the specific autoantibodies are only detectable in 40 to 60% of cases.

53. What are the treatment objectives in treating a patient with dry mouth?

• Establishing a diagnosis.
• Hydration of the oral tissues.
• Caries prevention.

54. What are the major factors that can cause dry mouth?

• Local conditions that produce drying of the oral mucosa.
• Inherent diseases of the salivary glands.
• Systemic conditions that affect salivary gland function

55. What local conditions are associated with dry mouth?

• Mouth breathing
• Smoking, especially pipe, but occasionally cigar or cigarette

56. Many medications may cause xerostomia. Name some classes that can cause dry mouth.

• Antihistamines	• Tricyclic antidepressants
• Antihypertensives	• Antiparkinsonian drugs
• Sympathomimetics	• Antianxiety medications

There are over 300 drugs that can cause xerostomia.

57. What can you do for a patient who has a dry mouth?

• Be sure that the patient drinks plenty of water.
• Have the patient avoid caffeine and carbonated beverages.
• Suggest a mouth moisturizing product such as Biotene rinse or gum.
• Recommend supplemental topical fluoride through the use of a stannous fluoride gel.
• In significant cases consider prescribing a sialagogue such as pilocarpine (Salagen) or cevimeline (Evoxac).

58. Are salivary gland tumors common?

No; tumors of the major salivary glands are rare. Most occur (80%) within the parotid glands. Of parotid tumors, the majority are benign (70%). However, submandibular and sublingual gland tumors have a greater tendency toward malignancy.

59. Many of the symptoms associated with malignant salivary gland tumors are a consequence of local invasion. What are some of the presenting symptoms of malignant salivary gland tumors?

• Pain	• Tongue weakness	• Paresthesia
• Facial paralysis	• Lymphadenopathy	

60. What are the clinical features of a salivary gland containing a malignant tumor?
The gland typically manifests a very firm, unilateral, nontender, fixed swelling.

61. Compare the clinical features of benign and malignant salivary gland tumors:

FEATURE	BENIGN	MALIGNANT
Growth	Slow, steady	Rapid
Pain	Rare	May be present
Facial nerve paralysis	None	May be present
Consistency	Rubbery	Firm
Attachment	None, mobile	Fixed
Trismus	None	May be present
Lymphadenopathy	None	May be present

Adapted from Bales and Norante. Head and Neck Tumors.

62. How are salivary gland tumors diagnosed?
Diagnosis is made by histologic examination of a specimen from a fine-needle aspiration or biopsy. Supplemental imaging studies with CT or nuclear magnetic resonance may be helpful.

63. How are salivary gland tumors treated?
The primary treatment for parotid malignancies is surgical resection. Radiation therapy is often used as an adjunctive therapy.

64. What are the most common types of malignant salivary gland tumors?
• Mucoepidermoid carcinoma
• Cylindroma
• Adenoid cystic carcinoma
• Squamous cell carcinoma of salivary gland origin
• Adenocarcinoma

65. What is the most common benign salivary gland tumor?
Pleomorphic adenoma is the most common salivary gland tumor, accounting for more than 50% of all observed tumors and 90% of benign tumors.

66. What is a mucocele?
Mucoceles are retention cysts that result, typically, from trauma to the ducts of the minor salivary glands. They are common on the mandibular labial mucosa, where they appear as raised, smooth, mucus-filled, and sometimes tender swellings.

44. DISEASES OF BONE

Stephen T. Sonis, D.M.D., D.M.Sc.

1. What hormones influence calcium metabolism?
• Parathyroid hormone
• Calcitonin
• Vitamin D

2. How many parathyroid glands are normally present?
Four.

3. Parathyroid hormone (PTH) is produced in response to what?
Low levels of serum calcium.

4. What are the actions of PTH?
• Increases intestinal absorption of calcium
• Increases renal absorption of calcium
• Stimulates bone resorption

5. Where is calcitonin produced?
Calcitonin is produced in the C cells of the thyroid gland.

6. Vitamin D undergoes a series of steps to become biologically active. Where do they take place?
• Skin
• Liver
• Kidney

7. What functions are associated with Vitamin D?
• Increases intestinal calcium absorption.
• Increases intestinal phosphate absorption.
• Increases renal reabsorption of calcium and phosphate.

8. What is the precursor of prostaglandin?
Arachidonic acid.

9. Name nine regulators of bone metabolism.
1. Glucocorticoids
2. Insulin
3. PTH
4. Prostaglandins
5. Vitamin D
6. Osteoclast-activating factor
7. Bone morphogenic protein
8. Ions
9. Androgens and estrogens

10. Describe the function of each of the above regulators of bone metabolism.
   1. Glucocorticoids: excessive amounts adversely affect skeletal growth and decrease bone mass and bone formation.
   2. Insulin: diabetes mellitus is associated with osteoporosis.

3. PTH is the most important regulator of extracellular calcium concentration.

4. Vitamin D increases mineral supply by stimulating calcium and phosphate intestinal transport systems.

5. Prostaglandins stimulate bone resorption.

6. Osteoclast-activating factor is a lymphocyte-derived cytokine that stimulates bone resorption and bone-collagen synthesis.

7. Bone-derived regulators have a stimulatory effect on bone cell replication and matrix synthesis.

8. Ions: calcium may affect bone formation by controlling secretion of calcium-regulating hormones.

9. Estrogens may reduce the risk of osteoporosis.

11. Define osteoporosis.

Osteoporosis is a common disease of bone metabolism in which the quantity of normally mineralized bone is reduced so that spontaneous fractures or fractures may result from minimal trauma.

12. Exactly how common is osteoporosis?

Very common. The disease affects more than 25 million people in the U.S. and is responsible for more than a million fractures of the spine and 300,000 fractures of the hip each year.

13. What is the most common site for manifestation of osteoporosis?

The most frequent manifestation of osteoporosis occurs in the vertebrae, which undergo spontaneous fracture. The fractures produce lower back pain, the symptom that typically leads the patient to seek medical attention.

14. Can osteoporosis affect long bones?

Yes. Osteoporosis may result in the fracture of long bones after minimal trauma. Although healing occurs, the bone typically does not regain its original strength.

15. What mechanisms that account for osteoporosis-induced fractures?

Low peak bone mass and accelerated bone loss.

16. How is osteoporosis diagnosed?

• Routine radiographic studies for symptoms or a fracture
• Bone density tests using a scanner
• In rare cases, bone biopsy from the iliac crest

17. What causes osteoporosis?

There is no one specific cause of osteoporosis. It has been associated with a variety of factors, including sedentary lifestyle, reduced estrogen production, endocrine abnormalities (e.g., hyperparathyroidism), hematologic malignancies that affect the bone marrow, drugs, arthritis, and, in rare cases, connective tissue diseases such as scurvey and osteogenesis imperfecta.

18. What treatments are available to prevent the progression of osteoporosis?

• Exercise (especially weight-bearing exercise)
• Calcium supplements
• Hormone replacement therapy (estrogen)
• Selective estrogen receptor modulators (SERMs)
• Biphosphonates
• Calcitonin

Rosen CJ: Treatment of postmenopausal osteoporosis: An evidence-based approach. Rev Endocrinol Metab Disord 2:35–43, 2001.

19. What happens to the following laboratory values in patients with osteoporosis: calcium, phosphorous, alkaline phosphatase, and PTH?
Calcium: normal or elevated
Phosphorus: decreased
Alkaline phosphatase: increased
PTH: increased

20. What are some of the possible oral manifestations of osteoporosis?
• Thinning of the cortical plate
• Loss of trabeculation
• Edentulous patients may be at risk for increased ridge resorption
• Delayed healing of extraction sites
• Referred pain to teeth from thinned maxillary sinuses

21. What disorders does vitamin D deficiency produce?
Rickets in children and osteomalacia in adults.

22. What are the major causes of osteomalacia? What populations are at potential risk?
The major causes of osteomalacia are dietary vitamin D deficiency and lack of exposure to sunlight. Consequently, two groups at potential risk are homebound, elderly patients who rarely get into the sun and strict vegetarians.

23. Can any drugs interfere with vitamin D metabolism and lead to osteomalacia?
Yes. Antiseizure medications, particularly phenylhydantoin and phenobarbital, have been reported to be commonly associated with osteomalacia.

24. What systemic conditions have been associated with osteomalacia?
• Gastrointestinal malabsorption syndromes including sprue, regional enteritis, prolonged biliary obstruction, and pancreatic insufficiency
• Chronic renal failure
• Renal transplantation

25. Describe the typical clinical presentation of rickets.
• Bowed legs
• Retarded skeletal growth
• Hypoplastic enamel

26. What are the symptoms of osteomalcia?
• Weakness
• Ataxia
• Skeletal pain

27. If you ordered a blood test on a patient with osteomalacia, what would you expect to find in respect to alkaline phosphatase and PTH?
Both would be elevated.

28. What oral findings are associated with vitamin D deficiency?
The oral findings are neither specific nor, in most cases, dramatic. In children, rickets has been associated with enamel hypoplasia, delayed tooth eruption, and abnormal dentin. Trabecular patterns of bone may be widened, and an indistinct lamina dura may be present in either rickets or osteomalacia. There are reports of increased periodontal disease in patients with osteomalacia.

29. What is the difference between primary and secondary hyperparathyroidism?

Primary hyperparathyroidism is the result of excessive PTH secretion from the gland and in most cases is attributable to a single parathyroid adenoma. It also may be caused by hyperplasia or carcinoma.

Secondary hyperparathyroidism is caused by hypocalcemia, usually secondary to renal disease.

30. What laboratory values are associated with hyperparathyroidism?

Increased serum calcium, decreased serum phosphorus, and increased alkaline phosphatase.

31. What are the clinical manifestations of hyperparathyroidism?

The clinical manifestations of the disease vary depending on its severity and may include any or all of the following:

- Renal colic
- Bone pain
- Debility
- Weight loss
- Weakness
- Bone, renal, and gastric disturbances

32. What oral changes are associated with hyperparathyroidism?

Usually oral changes appear only when the disease is advanced. The most reported oral manifestation is radiographic loss of the lamina dura. Intrabony and extrabony giant cell tumors may be seen.

33. Define fibrous dysplasia.

Fibrous dysplasia is a condition in which normal bone is replaced by fibrous tissue, probably by a developmental process, although the exact cause is undefined. The disease may affect a single bone (monostotic fibrous dysplasia) or multiple bones (polyostotic fibrous dysplasia).

34. Which is more common—monostotic or polyostotic fibrous dysplasia?

Monostotic by a ratio of 4:1.

35. What is the gender predilection for fibrous dysplasia?

Females more than males by a ratio of 2:1.

36. Summarize the clinical course of monostotic fibrous dysplasia.

1. Age of onset: 20s or 30s.
2. Any bone may be affected.
3. Jaws are involved in 20% of cases (the maxilla is involved twice as often as the mandible).
4. Jaw involvement begins as painless swelling with expansion of the buccal or labial plate.
5. Patients may note positional changes of teeth within the jaw.
6. Occasionally bone sensitivity develops.
7. Malocclusions or facial deformities may occur in children.

37. Which occurs at an earlier age, monostotic or polyostotic fibrous dysplasia?

Polyostotic fibrous dysplasia usually occurs at an earlier age, typically in children or adolescents.

38. What are the radiographic manifestations of monostotic fibrous dysplasia?

Although variable, the radiographic manifestations usually fall into one of three patterns:

1. Unilocular radiolucency
2. Multilocular radiolucencies
3. Ground glass

39. What changes in root anatomy may be seen in patients with unilocular fibrous dysplasia?
Roots may be displaced.

40. Describe the typical clinical presentation of fibrous dysplasia in the head and neck.
Fibrous dysplasia presents as a painless, hard swelling of either jaw. Changes in bone may affect the position of teeth and cause tipping or drifting.

41. Can any blood test confirm the diagnosis of fibrous dysplasia?
No. No abnormalities are detectable in blood.

42. How is fibrous dysplasia best diagnosed?
Biopsy.

43. How is monostotic fibrous dysplasia treated?
Localized lesions are treated by surgical resection of involved tissue.

44. Describe the two types of polyostotic fibrous dysplasia.
The first type involves more than one bone, but the majority of bones are normal. Café-au-lait pigmentation of the skin often accompanies this form. Because of the bony involvement, patients are prone to fractures.

The second type of polyostotic fibrous dysplasia affects virtually all bones. Patients also demonstrate disturbances of skin pigmentation and endocrine function. The triad of fibrous dysplasia, endocrine dysfunction, and altered skin pigmentation defines McCune-Albright syndrome.

45. What are the orofacial features of McCune-Albright syndrome?
- Deformity of facial bones
- Café-au-lait pigmentation
- Expansion and deformity of the mandible (in one-third of cases)
- Altered eruption pattern of teeth
- Multilocular cystic mandibular lesions

46. Define cherubism.
Cherubism (familial fibrous dysplasia) is a rare autosomal dominant hereditary disorder that causes expansion of the mandible and maxilla, beginning in childhood. The condition progresses through puberty but may regress spontaneously during early adulthood. The mandible is often more involved than the maxilla, giving affected children a chipmunk-like appearance.

47. List the clinical features of cherubism.
- Onset usually by ages 3 or 4 years
- Progressive symmetric, painless, rockhard swelling of the mandible and/or maxilla
- Bilateral symptoms
- Possible lymphadenopathy due to reticuloendothelial hyperplasia and fibrosis
- Premature loss of the deciduous teeth
- Possible defects in the permanent dentition, including agenesis of the second and third molars in affected areas
- Severe destruction of the jaws with extensive radiolucencies and thinning and expansion of the cortical plates on radiographic examination

48. How should you treat a child with cherubism (assuming that you completed an appropriate specialty training program)?
Since the condition is typically self-limiting, no treatment is required.

49. What is Paget's disease?

Paget's disease, or osteitis derformans, is a chronic, slowly progressing condition characterizeds by remodeling of the bone due to both osteoblastic and osteolytic activity. The condition results in enlargement of bones. The cause of Paget's disease is unknown, although circulatory disturbances have been suggested. Paget's disease typically occurs in people over the age of 40 years and is slightly more common in men.

50. What signs and symptoms are associated with Paget's disease?

• Bone pain
• Blindness
• Bell's palsy
• Dizziness
• Changes in mental status
• Joint pain
• Postural changes
• Changes in gait
• Bowing of the legs
• Spontaneous fractures

51. Is involvement of the jaws common in patients with Paget's disease?

Yes. About 20% of patients have jaw involvement. The maxilla is more often involved than the mandible. The mandible enlarges, resulting in an increase in the size of the ridge, diastema formation, flattening of the palate, and tooth mobility. Because of the changes in the ridges and palate, patients with removable prostheses may first be aware of the disease because the fit of their dentures changes.

52. What laboratory tests may help with a diagnosis of Paget's disease?

The serum alkaline phosphatase level is markedly elevated.

53. What radiographic findings are associated with Paget's disease?

The most consistent radiographic finding is a ground-glass appearance.

54. How is Paget's disease treated?

There is no specific treatment for the condition.

55. Does the presence of Paget's disease predispose to any other condition?

Yes. Patients with Paget's disease are at increased risk for developing osteosarcoma.

56. What is histiocytosis X?

Histiocytosis is a collective term that describes three nonneoplastic, proliferative, nonlipid reticuloendothelioses:

1. Eosinophilic granuloma (localized form)
2. Hand-Schüller-Christian syndrome (chronic disseminated form)
3. Letterer-Siwe disease (acute disseminated form)

57. What causes histiocytosis?

Although the origin of histiocytosis is thought to be the Langherhan's cell, it is not clear what happens to the cells to result in the condition. Some investigators have suggested that the disease is a reactive rather than a neoplastic process. Among the causes or associations are a virally induced hypersensitivity reaction, autoimmune process, intestinal malabsorption, smoking, and pituitary dysfunction.

58. Is there a gender or genetic predilection for histiocytosis X?

No.

59. What are the clinical and radiographic features of eosinophilic granuloma?
- Eosinophilic granuloma is the mildest form of histiocytosis.
- Patients may have single (monostotic) or multiple (polyostotic) bone lesions.
- The skull, ribs, pelvis, and flat bones are most commonly involved.
- The condition affects primarily children and young adults.
- Mandibular (posterior) involvement is common.
- Patients may present with a tender intraoral swelling or mass associated with the mandible.
- Tooth mobility, gingival inflammation, oral ulceration, and halitosis may occur.
- Radiographs indicate bone destruction that may affect tooth roots; teeth may have floating appearance in radiolucent area.

60. How is eosinophilic granuloma diagnosed?
Biopsy. The specimen demonstrates large numbers of reticuloendothelial and eosinophilic cells.

61. How is eosinophilic granuloma treated?
Treatment usually consists of surgical curettage of bony defects. Radiation has been used to treat disseminated forms. Healing is typically complete, and the prognosis is good.

62. Hand-Schüller-Christian syndrome also affects children over 3 years of age and young adults. It is the chronic disseminated form of histiocytosis X. What triad characterizes the syndrome?
1. Bony lesions of the skull
2. Exophthalamos
3. Diabetes insipidus
Patients rarely have all three of the above.

63. What oral findings are most commonly associated with Hand-Schüller-Christian syndrome?
The most common oral lesions are gingival ulcers. Patients also may complain of soreness and halitosis. Precocious exfoliation of teeth, tooth mobility, or an enlarged painful mass may be seen.

64. How is Hand-Schüller-Christian syndrome diagnosed?
Biopsy is the diagnostic procedure of choice. The specimens demonstrate sheets of foamy reticuloendothelial cells. Radiographic examination shows destructive bony lesions, particularly of the mandible.

65. Describe the treatment and prognosis of Hand-Schüller-Christian syndrome.
Treatment consists of surgical excision or curettage of accessible lesions. Chemotherapy is also used. The overall prognosis depends on the extent of involvement, but the extraskeletal nature of the condition and its early onset are negative factors. Usually the disease is progressive, chronic, and of increasing severity.

66. Define Letterer-Siwe disease. What clinical findings are associated with it?
Letterer-Siwe disease is the most severe form of histiocytosis X. The disease often begins in infancy, and the prognosis is terrible. Clinical findings include the following:
- Fever
- Otitis media
- Hepatomegaly
- Anemia
- Lymphadenopathy
- Bleeding
- Seborrhea
- Eczema

The symptoms vary from patient to patient. Involvement of the jaws is less frequent than with the other forms of histiocytosis.

67. Define multiple myeloma. What is the radiographic appearance of the disease in the skull and jaws?

Multiple myeloma is a plasma cell neoplasm that originates in bone marrow and causes destructive bony lesions. Radiographs show a characteristic pattern of punched-out lesions in bone. About 80% of patients with multiple myeloma present with radiolucent ovoid lesions of the mandible or maxilla.

68. What oral symptoms or signs may be seen in patients with multiple myeloma?

The oral signs and symptoms of multiple myeloma are similar to those of other malignancies and include the following:
• Paresthesia
• Swelling
• Tooth mobility
• Tooth movement
• Gingival masses

69. What laboratory findings are unique to patients with multiple myeloma?

Because multiple myeloma is a malignancy of plasma cells, laboratory findings are associated with plasma cell function. Light chains manifested as Bence-Jones proteins are found in the urine of 70% of patients. Anemia also may be seen.

70. How is multiple myeloma treated?

Chemotherapy, radiation, and bone marrow transplant are used to treat multiple myeloma. Thalidomide has been used with some success.

45. ANALGESICS

Robert C. Fazio, D.M.D., and Leslie S.T. Fang, M.D., Ph.D.

1. What are the basic choices for analgesics in dentistry?

There are two basic categories of drugs that the dentist must consider. The peripherally active drugs act at the site of injury. Centrally acting drugs change the perception of pain at the cerebral level.

2. What are examples of peripherally acting drugs?

Aspirin, acetaminophen, and all the drugs in the category of nonsteroidal anti-inflammatory drugs (NSAIDs) and the COX-2 inhibitors.

3. What are the centrally acting analgesics?

All narcotics are centrally acting drugs.

4. How should the dentist deal with mild pain?

Generally, the peripherally acting drugs—aspirin, acetaminophen, or over-the-counter nonsteroidal anti-inflammatory drugs—are chosen.

5. What are the relative potencies?

Acetaminophen and aspirin are relatively interchangeable with regard to analgesia. Aspirin has an anti-inflammatory effect, which acetaminophen does not. Over-the-counter nonsteroidal anti-inflammatory drugs are generally more effective analgesics than full doses of aspirin or acetaminophen, and some have analgesic effects equal to those of oral narcotic combination products (e.g., acetaminophen No. 3).

6. Are there differences in risk among these over-the-counter drugs?

The maximum allowable daily dose of acetaminophen is 4 g (two 500-mg tablets) four times a day. Overdose with acetaminophen can cause serious hepatic injury. There is a growing concern over the potential risk for hepatic injury from acetaminophen in the medical community. Patients who use alcohol on a regular basis appear to be at increased risk of hepatic injury even at lower than maximum doses. This may also be true for patients taking zidovudine (AZT) or a barbiturate concurrently.

7. What are the risks with aspirin?

Aspirin irreversibly inhibits platelet function for the lifetime of the platelet (8–10 days). This interferes with hemostasis and causes a prolonged bleeding time. In the surgical setting, aspirin taken within an 8- to 10-day time frame of surgery and aspirin taken postoperatively can be associated with significant bleeding. This phenomenon is not dose-dependent: the risk for abnormal hemostasis in a patient receiving "baby" aspirin in an 81-mg dose per day may be the same as that for a patient receiving over 1000 mg of aspirin a day for rheumatoid arthritis.

8. Are there other concerns with aspirin?

Yes, gastric toxicity is a significant concern for patients receiving aspirin. Patients on prednisone, patients with a previous history of peptic ulcer disease, and elderly patients are particularly at risk for gastrointestinal bleeding.

Aspirin can also precipitate an acute asthmatic attack in a subgroup of asthmatic patients with aspirin sensitivity. These patients often have the clinical triad of asthma, nasal polyps, and aspirin sensitivity.

9. What are the commonly used NSAIDs for analgesia in dental pain?
A large number of NSAIDs have been shown to be effective in the control of dental pain. These drugs have both an analgesic and an anti-inflammatory effect and are therefore excellent drugs to use for pain control. The following are the commonly prescribed NSAIDs.

GENERIC	BRAND NAME	DOSING	MAXIMUM DAILY DOSE
Ibuprofen	Motrin	po 400 mg q4h 600 mg q6h 800 mg tid	2400 mg
Over-the-counter ibuprofen	Advil, Nuprin, others	po 200 mg q4–6h	1200 mg
Etodolac	Lodine	200–400 mg q6–8h	1200 mg
Naproxen	Naprosyn, others	500 mg q12h	1000 mg
Naproxen sodium	Anaprox	po 550 mg q12h	1100 mg
Over-the-counter naproxen sodium	Aleve	220 mg q8–12h	660 mg
Flurbiprofen	Ansaid	100 mg q8–12h	300 mg
Diflunisal	Dolobid	500 mg q8–12h	1500 mg
Ketoprofen	Orudis	25–75 mg q6–8h	300 mg

10. Is the analgesic effect of the drugs in the above table generally similar?
Yes, in large population studies, there is not a significant difference in analgesic effect among maximum daily doses of any of the above-mentioned drugs.

11. Why therefore do some patients say one agent works better than another? Is this attributable either to a placebo effect or to brand name recognition?
No. Some patients have better analgesic effect from one nonsteroidal drug than from many others. The effect is different for different patients and appears to be quite individualized.

12. How would this affect the prescription of NSAIDs?
Generally, the dentist should inquire if the patient has had success taking NSAIDs in the past. All other considerations being equal, the dentist should choose the agent that the patient has had previous success with.

13. What are the risks of NSAIDS?
The adverse effects of NSAIDs are generally qualitatively similar to those of aspirin. Exacerbations of asthma, gastric toxicity and gastrointestinal bleeding are concerns, particularly in patients on corticosteroid therapy, with a history of peptic ulcer disease, or in elderly patients.
NSAIDs cause reversible inhibition of platelet aggregation. The mechanism for compromising platelet function and, therefore, a prolonged bleeding time are different than those for aspirin. This effect is reversible, and platelet function returns to normal when the drug has been eliminated.

14. Are there other adverse effects of NSAIDs?
Yes, NSAIDs interfere with the synthesis of renal prostaglandins. These are important hormones regulating renal blood flow. In the susceptible patient, even a short course of NSAIDs can precipitate acute renal failure and hyperkalemia. Susceptible patients include elderly patients, those with diabetic renal disease, those with compromised renal function and those with marginal cardiac output and compromised renal perfusion. NSAIDs should be avoided in these patients.

15. Are there significant drug-drug interactions with NSAIDs?

Coumadin dosing can be influenced by NSAIDs. Bleeding complications can result. It is therefore important for patients taking coumadin to avoid NSAIDs.

Lithium used in the management of bipolar disorders and depression interacts with non-steroidals and can cause lithium toxicity. Therefore, NSAIDs have relative contraindications with lithium.

16. What do the terms "nonselective" and "selective" NSAIDs mean?

NSAIDs are currently divided into nonselective and selective categories. It refers to the inhibition of an enzyme called cyclo-oxygenase (COX), which is responsible for the breakdown of arachidonic acid into the various prostaglandin derivatives. In the 1990s, it was discovered that there are two separate cyclo-oxygenase enzymes (COX-1 and COX-2). COX-1 appears to be a constitutive enzyme and is active all of the time. Most important, this enzyme appears to confer protection on the gastric mucosa and is responsible for platelet aggregation. COX-2, on the other hand, is an inducible enzyme and is stimulated at times of tissue injury and inflammation. This enzyme is responsible for mounting an inflammatory response.

Traditional NSAIDs inhibit both COX-1 and COX-2 enzymes and therefore would have not only an analgesic and anti-inflammatory response associated with COX-2 inhibition but also the adverse effects on the gastric mucosa and platelet function associated with COX-1 inhibition. Selective COX-2 inhibitors, however, would primarily have an anti-inflammatory and analgesic effect.

17. What are the selective COX inhibitors (COX-2 inhibitors)?

The selective COX inhibitors are those that in theory have dominant COX-2 inhibition. These drugs, therefore, produce analgesia and an anti-inflammatory response without interfering with COX-1 function.

COX-2 inhibitors are very popular anti-inflammatory agents that inhibit only the COX-2 enzymes. As such, they are potent anti-inflammatory agents and analgesics.

In contrast to NSAIDs that inhibit both COX-1 and COX 2 enzymes, the COX-2 inhibitors have a reduced risk of adverse effects on the gastric mucosa and do not have any effect on platelet aggregation.

These properties make them ideal analgesics in the postoperative arena.

18. What are the COX-2 inhibitors currently available?

Celecoxib (Celebrex) and rofecoxib (Vioxx) are the two COX-2 inhibitors on the market. Both have been approved by the Federal Drug Administration for pain control.

Celecoxib is prescribed as a 400-mg initial dose followed by 200 mg bid. Rofecoxib is prescribed in doses of 50 mg once a day when the primary goal is that of analgesia.

Both have superb anti-inflammatory effects as well. When these drugs are used for arthritis, a reduced dose is used daily.

The efficacy of these agents in the control of pain associated with dental procedures has been amply demonstrated. When Celebrex was first introduced, the drug was not approved for use as an analgesic. Some studies testing 200-mg doses demonstrated superior results to placebo but inferior results to ibuprofen and rofecoxib. Other studies demonstrated equal analgesic effects when compared to Anaprox. It was not until 2001 that celecoxib received approval as an indication for pain control.

Both agents have been shown to be considerably less toxic to the gastric mucosa than traditional NSAIDs. Neither drug interferes with platelet function.

These unique features make celecoxib and rofecoxib ideal agents to use for the control of moderate and moderately severe pain associated with dental therapy.

These agents should generally not be used for more than 5 days in the doses recommended.

19. Which medication do you prefer?

Currently because of the once a day dosing for rofecoxib compared with the dosing for celecoxib, we prefer the former and its 24-hour effects.

20. What concerns have recently been raised about COX-2 inhibitors?

There have been some concerns raised about the possibility that long-term use of COX-2 inhibitors for arthritis may increase cardiovascular risks because of a possible prothrombotic effect of these agents. These concerns are probably not applicable to the very short course of these agents used by dentists for analgesia.

21. Do these two drugs have purely COX-2 inhibition effects?

No, but both drugs have a predominant COX-2 inhibitory effect with very minor influence on the COX-1 enzyme.

22. Are there drug-drug interactions with COX-2 inhibitors?

Yes, the most important one is for patients receiving coumadin. All NSAIDs, both selective and nonselective, increase the International Normalized Ratio (INR, prothrombin time) for patients on coumadin treatment. This could precipitate significant bleeding complications. Celecoxib appears to have less of an effect than rofecoxib.

23. But I thought that the COX-2 inhibitors do not affect platelet function.

Neither rofecoxib nor celecoxib interfere with platelet function. However, the other arm of coagulation relating to the clotting factor production of fibrin from fibrinogen is influenced by both drugs. Both rofecoxib and celecoxib can therefore raise the prothrombin time and INR and can precipitate bleeding complications from excessive anticoagulation.

24. What medication choices do dentists have for moderate pain?

Generally, dentists choose between prescription NSAIDs, COX-2 inhibitors, and codeine or synthetic codeine derivatives compounded with peripherally acting drugs.

25. What are the commonly prescribed codeine derivatives?

Codeine compounds (Tylenol with codeine, Tylenol No. 3), oxycodone compounds (Percocet, Percodan), and hydrocodone compounds (the Vicodin series, the Lortab series, the Lorcet series).

26. What are the differences in potency of these codeine derivatives?

Generally speaking, a dose of 45 mg of codeine is therapeutically equivalent to 5 mg of oxycodone and 7.5 mg of hydrocodone.

Codeine, 45 mg, compounded with Tylenol has a relatively equal analgesic effect to that of Percocet 5/325 (5 mg of oxycodone) or to Vicodin ES, which contains 7.5 mg of hydrocodone. Generally this dose of codeine would be inferior to that of Vicodin HP, which contains 10 mg of hydrocodone, roughly equivalent to 60 mg of codeine compounded with the peripherally acting drug.

27. What are some common examples of codeine derivatives prescribed?

Codeine/Acetaminophen Combinations

NAME	DOSING	MAXIMUM 24-HR DOSE*
Tylenol with codeine No. 2 (15mg) No. 3 (30mg) No. 4 (60 mg)	1 or 2 q4–6h	12

Hydrocodone/Acetaminophen Combinations

NAME	DOSING	MAXIMUM 24-HR DOSE*
Vicodin (5/500)	1 or 2 q4–6h	8
Vicodin ES (7.5/750)	1 q4–6h	5
Vicodin HP (10/600)	1 q4h	6

Cont'd. on next page

Hydrocodone/Acetaminophen Combinations (Continued)

NAME	DOSING	MAXIMUM 24-HR DOSE*
Lortab (2.5/500)	1 q4h	8
Lortab (5/500)	1 or 2 q4–6h	8
Lortab (7.5/500)	1 q4h	8
Lortab (10/500)	1 q4h	8
Lorcet (5/500)	1 q4h	8
Lorcet Plus (7.5/650)	1 q4h	6
Zydone (5/500)	1 q4h	8

Maximum 24-hr Dosing Limited by 4000 mg/24hr Maximum Acetaminophen Dose

Oxycodone/Acetaminophen Combinations

NAME	DOSING	MAXIMUM 24-HR DOSE*
Percocet (2.5/325)	1 q4–6h*	12
Percocet (5/325)	1 q6h	12
Percocet (7.5/500)	1 q4–6h	8
Percocet (7.5/325)	1 q4–6h	8
Percocet (10/650)	1 q4–6h	6
Percocet (10/325)	1 q4–6h	6
Tylox 1	q6h	8
Roxicet (5/500)		

Oxycodone/Aspirin Combinations

NAME	DOSING	MAXIMUM 24-HR DOSE*
Percodan (5/325)	1q4h	12

28. Is there a problem with prescribing narcotic preparations?

There is much confusion over the maximum dose allowable based on the differing contents of acetaminophen and narcotic.

29. Why is this confusion a problem?

The drug Vicodin ES is composed of 7.5 mg of hydrocodone and 750 mg of acetaminophen. Because acetaminophen toxicity occurs over 4000 mg/day, the maximum dose of Vicodin ES in a 24-hour period is five pills (750 mg of acetaminophen times five pills equals 3750 mg of acetaminophen). This provides the patient with a 24-hour dose of 37.5 mg of narcotic.

On the other hand, Vicodin HP has a maximum dose of six pills in a 24-hour period. This is driven again by the content of acetaminophen. Vicodin HP contains 10 mg of the hydrocodone narcotic but only 660 mg of acetaminophen. At six pills in a 24-hour period, this yields a total dose of acetaminophen of 3960 mg (less than the 4000 mg maximum dose). Yet, at six pills in a 24-hour period of Vicodin HP, the patient has been provided with 60 mg of the narcotic. In the setting of more severe pain, therefore, the Vicodin HP may be the better choice of medication.

30. Is there a similar problem with potential acetaminophen toxicity's limiting the dose of oxycodone?

Yes, Percocet 5/325 is 5 mg of oxycodone combined with 325 mg of acetaminophen. The maximum 24-hour dose, therefore, is 12 tablets or the equivalent of 60 mg of oxycodone and 4000 mg of acetaminophen. There are, however, preparations of oxycodone that contain 5 mg of oxycodone compounded with 500 mg of acetaminophen (Tylox, Roxicet/500). For these preparations the maximum 24-hour dose becomes eight tablets. An eight tablet 24-hour prescription of

Tylox yields only 40 mg of oxycodone and 4000 mg of acetaminophen. As with Vicodin ES and Vicodin HP, therefore, Percocet 5/325 is the superior drug in the setting of more severe pain when compared with Tylox.

31. What about comparisons among the different categories?
With regard to the maximum available narcotic for a patient with severe pain in a 24-hour period, Percocet 5/325 appears to be superior to Vicodin HP. Both yield 60 mg of narcotic and roughly 4000 mg of acetaminophen in a 24-hour period. However, the oxycodone to hydrocodone relative potency is 5:7.5. Therefore, the 60 mg of oxycodone available in a 24-hour dosing of Percocet 5/325 has greater analgesic potency than the equivalent Vicodin HP maximum dose.

32. Why are most codeine preparations compounded with either acetaminophen or aspirin?
Peripherally acting medications are synergistic with centrally acting medications. Therefore, the effect of a combination drug is greater than the sum of two individual analgesic drugs.

33. Previously the pharmacy would the a prescription for just Percocet. Now they will not. Why is that?
The oxycodone/acetaminophen combination formerly referred to as Percocet is now Percocet 5/325, denoting 5 mg of oxycodone and 325 mg of acetaminophen. Percocet, however, now has five other formulations: a 2.5/325 (a reduced narcotic dose), a 10/650 preparation, a 10/325 preparation, a 7.5/500 preparation, and a 7.5/325 preparation.

34. What oxycodone preparation is most commonly used?
Percocet 5/325 is by far the most commonly prescribed formulation.

35. As a dentist, what should my strategy be for prescribing analgesics?
For most patients in the absence of contraindications, NSAIDs would generally be first-choice drugs. Pain studies have generally shown nonsteroidals to have equal analgesic as the codeine and codeine-derivative compounds. Opioids commonly cause problems with drowsiness, nausea, constipation, and vomiting. The drowsiness issue prohibits patients from returning to work while using opioid analgesics and therefore may significantly compromise their lifestyles. Patients using NSAIDs do not have this limitation.

36. What are the considerations in choosing among the nonsteroids?
Timing of the drug is important. In general, the fewer the doses the patient has to take, the more likely he or she is to have continuous analgesia and anti-inflammatory effects. Therefore, drugs that are given once a day (e.g., rofecoxib [Vioxx], 50 mg) or two to three times a day (flur-biprofen [Ansaid] 100 mg bid to tid), or three times a day dose (etodolac [Lodine] 400 mg tid or ibuprofen [Motrin] 800 mg tid) would seem to be superior choices. Compare these clinical situations to the patient taking ibuprofen, 400 mg, every 4 hours. The latter patient will more often be exposed to less effective analgesia as the dose wears off. A recurrent pain relief, pain-relief cycle can be psychologically detrimental to the patient. Also, with the short acting NSAIDs, the patient is more likely to wake up in pain during the night.

37. When should shorter acting nonsteroidals such as ibuprofen 400-mg or 600-mg tablets be used?
If the dentist was limiting himself or herself to nonselective nonsteroidals, ideally it is prefer-able to have the patient taking a longer acting nonsteroidal at bedtime. This allows the patient to sleep through the night with therapeutic, analgesic, and anti-inflammatory effects. Few dentists want to have a patient waking up in the middle of the night in pain needing another dose of anal-gesic. Chairside, therefore, many dentists administer short-acting NSAIDs such as 400 mg or 600 mg of ibuprofen in order to allow the patient a full therapeutic dose of the analgesic up until bed-time and then to remedicate at that time. The drug chosen, therefore, depends on the time of day of the procedure. A patient undergoing surgical care in the late afternoon would best receive a

400- to 600-mg dose of ibuprofen chairside. Theoretically, this analgesic would wear off and require remediation at approximately the time the patient goes to bed. A longer acting nonselective NSAID could then be administered by prescription at bedtime, and the patient would now be on a cycle of every 8 to 12 hour dosing, minimizing the risk of his or her awakening at night in pain. The advantage of the selective COX-2 inhibitor rofecoxib (Vioxx) is that this drug can be administered once every 24 hours and give full therapeutic effect.

38. Why not use rofecoxib (Vioxx) or celecoxib (Celebrex) all the time?

The cost of the drug per pill is relatively expensive and some insurance companies will not pay for the drug as a prescription benefit in the setting of acute analgesia.

In the setting of a dental surgical procedure, a case can be made for the exclusive use of selective COX-2 inhibitors because of the lack of interaction with platelet function.

39. Are there other criteria for choosing among the nonselective NSAIDs?

Yes, generally these relate to the gastrointestinal bleeding risk. Etolodac (Lodine) under 1000 mg/day dosing and ibuprofen (Motrin) in under 1600 mg/day dosing seem to have the lowest risk of gastrointestinal complications among the nonselective NSAIDs. These drugs, therefore, are the drugs of choice for the elderly population, with its significantly higher risk of complications. Of course, with the advent of selective COX-2 inhibitors such as rofecoxib and celecoxib, these former drugs are generally being replaced by rofecoxib as the drug of choice even for short-term analgesic care. Other nonselective NSAIDs like naproxen sodium (Anaprox) and flurbiprofen (Ansaid) have moderate or higher gastointestinal complication risks and are relatively contraindicated in the aged and at risk population.

40. If the dentist starts with a NSAID and the patient has more pain, can he or she switch to or add on a narcotic?

There is an intermediate step of analgesic enhancement. Nonsteroidals plus acetaminophen are superior to nonsteroidals alone. In addition, the analgesic efficacy of this combination appeared to be equivalent to that of adding a pure narcotic to an NSAID.

41. What should the patient be told about pain relief?

The dentist will often prescribe an NSAID to the patients and advise them that if this is not sufficient as a pain reliever, over-the-counter acetaminophen can be added to the NSAID following the dosing instructions on the bottle. If, for example, the patient is given rofecoxib, 50 mg once daily, the dentist would advise the patient to continue taking that drug once daily and add, for example, 1000 mg of acetaminophen four times a day as needed for enhanced analgesic effects.

42. Why not just add an oxycodone or hydrocodone preparation to the NSAIDs?

This is an acceptable strategy with one advantage and one disadvantage. The disadvantage is that once a narcotic has been introduced, the patient must be told not to drive a car and not to do anything that requires good reflexes, and this often means not going to work or caring for children. The intermediate step of adding acetaminophen alone to the nonsteroidal may be sufficient to give the patient relief.

The advantage, however, is that the combination of a nonsteroidal, acetaminophen, and a narcotic has been shown by Breivak et al. to be superior to a nonsteroidal and acetaminophen alone or even to a nonsteroidal and a narcotic alone without the addition of acetaminophen. Therefore, for more severe pain, the dentist would choose, for example, rofecoxib, 50 mg, once daily as a baseline analgesic, with Percocet 5/325 every 4 to 6 hours added as an enhancement.

43. What is the mechanism of action of this combination?

The efficacy of NSAIDs is enhanced by acetaminophen. Opioids, when added to non-steroidals alone, have an additive analgesic effect even when the nonsteroidals are insufficient by themselves. Acetaminophen also enhances the effects of the opioids.

44. Are there any add-ons to the hierarchy of analgesics prescribed by the dentist?

In order, dentists prescribe over-the-counter nonsteroidals, prescription nonsteroidals, prescription nonsteroidals plus acetaminophen, and prescription nonsteroidals plus acetaminophen and codeine derivative. Beyond this hierarchy, generally the dentist turns to a sedative drug. Promethazine (Phenergan) in a 25-mg dose, or hydroxyzine (Vistaril), when added to the other analgesics and analgesic compounds, further enhances the analgesic effect. Some preparations incorporate a combination of acetaminophen or aspirin, codeine, and a barbiturate in one pill. Fiorinal (aspirin, caffeine, butalbital with codeine) or Fioricet (acetaminophen, codeine, caffeine, butalbital) can be prescribed as two tablets tid as needed for pain.

45. Are there any other routine adjuncts that can be utilized?

Yes: caffeine enhances the analgesic effect of codeine. Therefore, taking the analgesic pills with coffee or a caffeine-containing soft drink may help the patient.

46. We have established that codeine and codeine derivatives do not work as well as analgesics unless they are mixed with peripherally acting drugs such as aspirin or acetaminophen. Are there any medications that can be used effectively without being combined with peripherally acting drugs like acetaminophen and aspirin?

Yes, there are two that are commonly used. Meperidine (Demerol) is a narcotic that is effective when not used in combination with aspirin or acetaminophen. It is often prescribed as 50 mg every 4 hours as needed for pain. It is often simultaneously prescribed with the drug promethazine (Phenergan) in 25–50 mg doses every 4 hours. The promethazine is a sedative and enhances the effect of the meperidine. Therefore, less meperidine yields more analgesia when in combination with promethazine. In addition, the promethazine is an anti-emetic, which helps negate some of the side effects of meperidine, namely, nausea. Meperidine should be used cautiously in the elderly. It should never be given to patients on monoamine oxidase inhibitors for psychiatric disease and is generally contraindicated in patients receiving phenytoin (Dilantin) for seizure disorders. There is a decreased effectiveness of meperidine in the presence of phenytoin. As an aside, promethazine is also generally not recommended in patients receiving seizure disorder medication.

47. Are there any other medications that work well without peripherally acting drugs?

The drug tramadol (Ultram) is one. It is prescribed in 50 mg tablets. The general prescription is two tablets stat and one tablet every 4 hours as needed for pain, with a maximum daily dose of 400 mg It is a mild oral opioid. It is not scheduled as a controlled substance, but an opioid type dependency can occur. Tramadol is generally contraindicated in patients with a previous history of seizure disorder or for those patients concomitantly receiving a monoamine oxidase inhibitor, an antidepressant, or antipsychotic medication. There is a seizure risk as a side effect to this medication that is exacerbated in these clinical settings. Typically then patients on selective serotonin reuptake inhibitors (fluoxetine [Prozac], sertraline [Zoloft]) tricyclic antidepressants (amitriptyline [Elavil], imipramine [Tofranil]) and monoamine oxidase inhibitors (phenelzine [Nardil], tranylcypromine [Parnate]) should not receive tramadol as an analgesic.

48. Suggest a clinical setting in which a dentist may prefer analgesic drugs that are efficacious in the absence of peripherally acting medication.

A common clinical situation is the patient who is a regular alcohol user. When combined with NSAIDs, or aspirin, alcohol has an increased risk of gastrointestinal toxicity and bleeding. Alcohol, in combination with acetaminophen, increases the risk of hepatotoxicity. Therefore, for patients who regularly consume alcohol, the analgesic strategy may include the following:

• Short-term cessation of the alcohol.
• The use of rofecoxib or celecoxib.
• The prescription of the relatively short-acting drugs meperidine and promethazine or tramadol for analgesia as needed.

Often the dentist is aware that at best the patient will have only short-term cessation of alcohol consumption. Therefore, a drug that is short acting in duration may be advisable.

49. Are there other clinical settings in which peripherally acting drugs may not be desirable?

Warfarin (coumadin) therapy is commonly used in medical practice. Coumadin contraindicates the use of aspirin and NSAIDs, since both markedly enhance the anticoagulation effect of coumadin and will artificially increase the INR (prothrombin time. In the past, dentists were taught to use codeine and acetaminophen combinations for analgesia in patients on coumadin therapy.

50. Is there now a problem with acetaminophen?

Bell, in a 1998 JAMA article, and Hylek, in a separate 1998 JAMA article, suggested that acetaminophen may increase the prothrombin time and, therefore, the bleeding risk in selected patients on coumadin therapy. They demonstrated a statistically significant increase in prothrombin time 18 to 48 hours after multiple doses of acetaminophen and noted that the risk of a spike in prothrombin time was greater if weekly doses of acetaminophen were higher than seven to fourteen standard tablets.

51. What does that mean for the dentist?

Although no one would criticize the prescription of an acetaminophen-codeine compound, in the setting of a high-risk postoperative bleeding situation (extensive intraoral surgical therapy), the dentist may choose an analgesic effective without any peripherally acting medications.

52. Does this mean a meperidine (Demerol) and promethazine (Phenergan) regimen or the tramadol (Ultram) regimen?

Yes and no; meperidine and promethazine are appropriate choices because they have no impact on coumadin activity. It is not clear what influence tramadol has on coumadin therapy. There are some reports that show that tramadol can adversely effect coumadin therapy. Others have reported that tramadol does not influence prothrombin time/INR. Caution is therefore advisable when using tramadol in the patient on coumadin therapy, and prothrombin/INR should be closely monitored.

53. Where does propoxyphene fit in the dentist's analgesic armamentarium?

Propoxyphene compounded with Tylenol as Darvocet-N 100 or compounded with aspirin as Darvon is sometimes chosen as an analgesic. It is prescribed as one tablet every 4 hours as needed for pain. This synthetic opioid agonist drug, however, adversely interacts with coumadin, potentiating the latter's effect. It is, therefore, contraindicated for patients receiving coumadin therapy.

The drug is also contraindicated for patients receiving carbamazepine (Tegretol) for seizure disorders and the anti-anxiety drug alprazolam (Xanax). Toxicity of these drugs is a problem in the presence of propoxyphene.

54. What about analgesics and pregnancy?

The reader is referred to the pregnancy chapter. However, aspirin is a category D risk analgesic with strict contraindication. Tylenol alone carries a category B risk and is generally acceptable in the pregnant patient. The brand names Motrin, Ansaid, and Anaprox generally carry a category B risk acceptable analgesic for the first two trimesters only for pregnant patients.

Other drugs, brand names Lodine (etodolac), Dolobid (diflunisol), and Vioxx (rofecoxib), carry a category C risk analgesic category, and consultation with the obstetrician/gynecologist is advisable. All NSAIDs are a category D risk in the third trimester. A pregnant patient receiving nonsteroidals in the third trimester can have a premature closure of the fetal circulation as a complication. Codeine and the codeine derivatives are generally category C risk drugs requiring obstetrician clearance.

46. ILLUSTRATED CASES

Stephen T. Sonis, D.M.D., D.M.Sc.

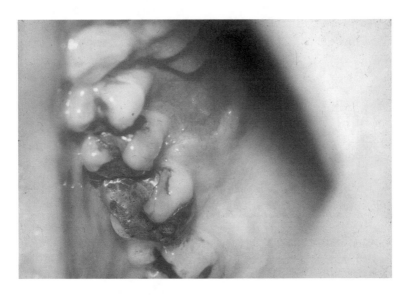

Patient 1. Mr. Jones is a 42-year-old lawyer who comes to see you as a new patient. As you examine his mouth you notice a lesion on his palate. When you question Mr. Jones about the lesion, he tells you that he has been aware of "something up there" for a couple of months, but since it hasn't been symptomatic, he hasn't bothered to see anyone. What kind of lesion is present on the palate?

    Ulceration

What is your next step?
A. Prescribe a topical steroid ointment and check the lesion again in 2 months.
B. No treatment, but have Mr. Jones return in a month to be sure that the lesion has disappeared.
C. Since the lesion might be traumatic, fabricate a nightguard and have Mr. Jones return after it has been in place for at least 6 weeks.
D. Biopsy the lesion immediately.

    Mr. Jones has a non-healing ulcer. The lesion has a noninflammatory look, is asymptomatic, and has caused loss of bone (take a look at the amount of root exposed on the premolars). You should have a high index of suspicion that this may be a malignancy. The answer is **D**.

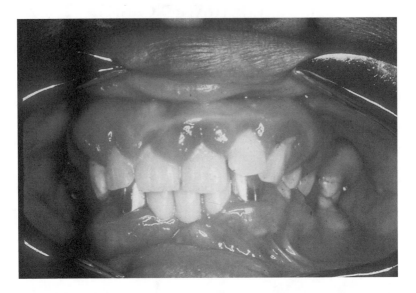

Patient 2. Name three medications that could cause this condition.
    This patient presents with gingival hyperplasia. Phenytoin, cyclosporin, or nifedipine could all cause this condition.

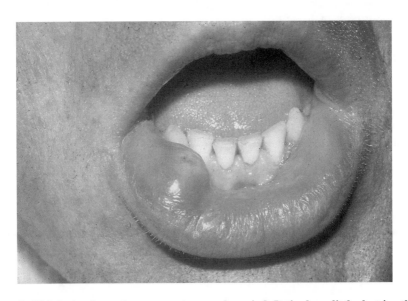

Patient 3. This lesion has arisen over a two-week period. It tingles a little, but is otherwise asymptomatic. What is the most likely diagnosis and what treatment would you recommend?
    This cyst-like lesion is a mucocele and is best treated by surgical removal.

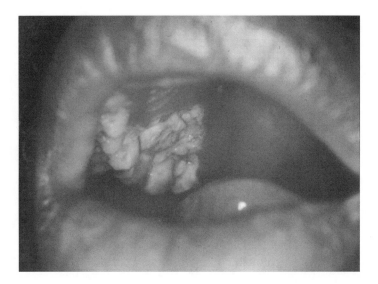

Patient 4. What is the most likely etiology of this firm, white lesion of the palate?
This is a squamous cell carcinoma. The most likely etiology is tobacco use (cigarette smoking).

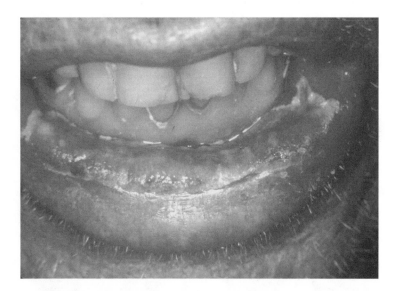

Patient 5. Mr. Smith is a 62-year-old gentleman who is being treated with chemotherapy for lymphoma. He comes to see you 14 days after receiving his last dose of treatment with this painful lesion of his lower lip. He is scheduled for a prophylaxis. What is your diagnosis of the lip lesion? If the lip lesion wasn't present, would you feel comfortable having the hygienist clean his teeth?
The lesion is most likely mucositis caused by his cancer drugs. It is highly likely that Mr. Smith is myelosuppressed because of his treatment and so is both neutropenic and thrombocytopenic. A dental prophylaxis would not be a good move as he is at high risk for both infection and postoperative bleeding.

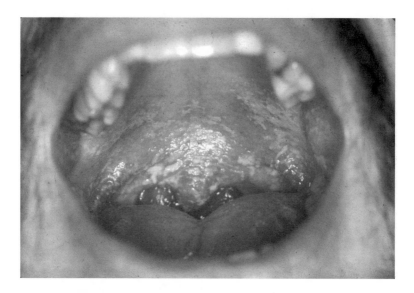

Patient 6. What's the white stuff on the soft palate of this patient who just completed a course of doxycycline? How would you treat it?
    Candidiasis. You could treat this with nystatin oral suspension, clotrimazole, or fluconazole.

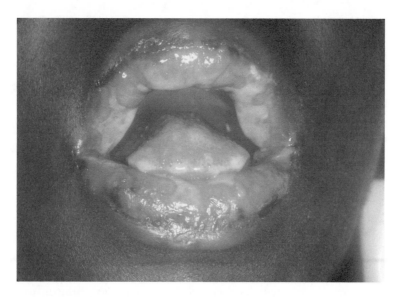

Patient 7. Six weeks after you diagnosed a case of primary herpetic gingivostomatitis, the hysterical mother of this 14-year-old calls you to say that her son awoke with his mouth looking like this. What is it and what would you do?
    The most likely diagnosis for this lesion is erythema multiforme. Although it looks and feels terrible, it should resolve on its own. The major concerns for this patient are adequate palliation and hydration.

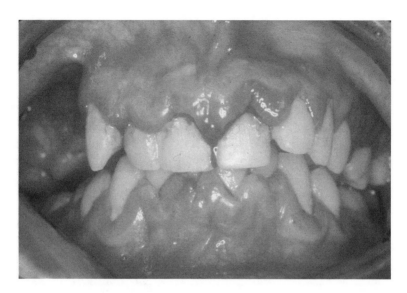

Patient 8. This is a new patient for you. Although she hasn't had routine dental care, she hasn't had gingival bleeding until last week. Now she complains that her gums bleed spontaneously—she found blood on her pillow—and that they are swollen. On questioning, she tells you that she has been dragging around for the last few days. What would you do?

A. Immediately perform scaling and root planing and emphasize oral hygiene.

B. Put the patient on antibiotics (a penicillin) for 10 days and then re-evaluate.

C. Biopsy the gingiva.

D. After determining through radiographs that there is no appreciable bone loss, plan a gingivectomy.

E. Send the patient for a CBC.

   Spontaneous gingival bleeding is indicative of profound thrombocytopenia and usually occurs with platelet counts of under 30,000 cells/mm³. Accompanied by gingival enlargement, spontaneous bleeding should raise a red flag. This patient has acute leukemia. The appropriate course would be to refer her for a complete blood count (CBC). So the answer is **E**.

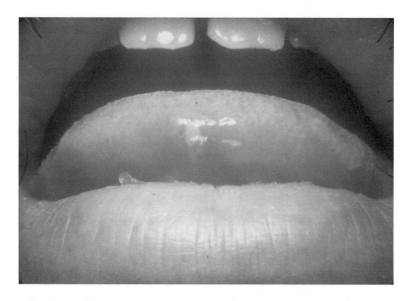

Patient 9. A 19-year-old comes to see you because of this painful lesion on the tip of his tongue. It has only been present for two days, but is driving the patient crazy. There is no history of trauma, but this is the second time the patient has had a painful oral lesion in the last 6 months. What is your diagnosis? How long would you predict the lesion would remain?

The clinical presentation and recurrent history are consistent with a diagnosis of aphthous stomatitis (aphthous minor based on the size of the lesion and the recurrence frequency). Typically these lesions resolve on their own in about 7 to 10 days. In the meantime, treatment options would include amLexanox, triamcinalone acetonide in Orabase, or a topical anesthetic.

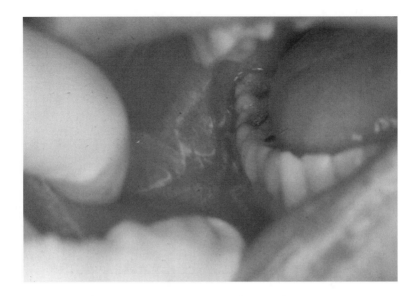

Patient 10. This 54-year-old woman presents to you with a complaint of localized areas of mucosal burning and a feeling of roughness on her cheeks. She has been aware of the cheek roughness for about 3 months. She used to smoke one pack of cigarettes per day, but stopped 7 years ago. How would you describe the lesions on her buccal mucosa? What is your diagnosis? What is the natural history of this disease?

She has white, keratotic, reticulated lesions on her buccal mucosa with areas of surrounding erythema. The lesions are lichenoid in appearance (Wickham's striae) and are consistent with a clinical diagnosis of lichen planus. This condition tends to be chronic and goes through periods of exacerbation and remission. The literature is not clear on the relationship between lichen planus and squamous cell carcinoma. Nonetheless, given her smoking history, a biopsy to establish a baseline and confirm the diagnosis and regular follow-up examinations would be prudent.

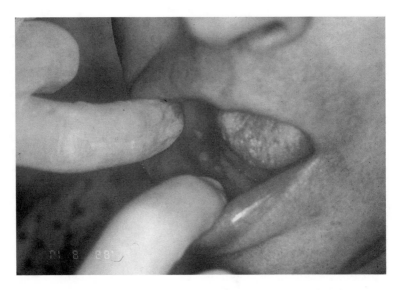

Patient 11. Mr. Butler presents to you complaining of these burning lesions on the right side of his mouth. He is a 62-year-old renal transplant recipient, but is otherwise healthy. What is your diagnosis?

Mr. Butler presents with a linear pattern of vesicular lesions on the right side of his mouth. As a transplant recipient, it is likely that he has been taking immunosuppressive drugs to prevent rejection. The diagnosis is herpes zoster.

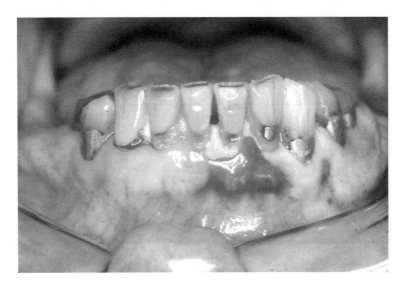

Patient 12. How would you describe the lesion on this woman's mandibular attached gingiva? How would you make a definitive diagnosis?

This patient presents with an intact bullous lesion of the attached gingiva. The differential diagnosis for blistering lesions would include pemphigus vulgaris, pemphigoid, and bullous lichen planus. Diagnosis is made by histologic and immunohistologic criteria, so a biopsy is mandatory.

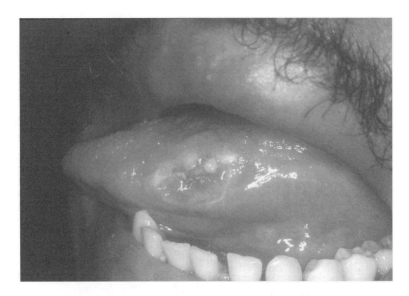

Patient 13. Your neurologist friend refers this patient to you shortly after she saw him immediately following a seizure. During her examination she noted this tongue lesion. The patient uses snuff on a regular basis. What would you do for this patient?

A. Reassure the patient that the lesion is probably benign and have him return in 2 weeks.

B. Biopsy the lesion immediately.

C. After consulting with the neurologist, place the patient on prednisone for 2 weeks and then reevaluate.

D. Place the patient on antibiotics and have him return if the lesion had not resolved in 2 to 4 weeks.

This nasty looking tongue ulcer was induced by the patient biting himself during his seizure. The location of the ulcer and its appearance are consistent with a diagnosis of traumatic ulcer. Consequently, the answer is **A**. The patient should be reassured, but asked to return in two weeks to confirm that the lesion has healed. It would also be reasonable to discuss the carcinogenic effects of snuff use.

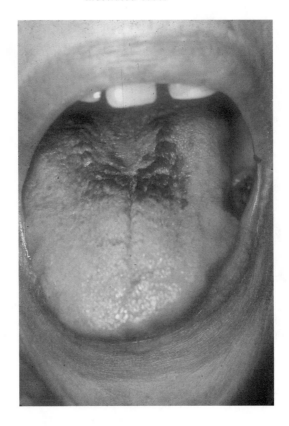

Patient 14. Name three agents that could cause the pigmented lesion noted on this patient's dorsal tongue.

Bismuth-containing compounds such as Pepto Bismol, pipe smoking, and tetracycline use all may cause dark, superficial pigmentation of the tongue.

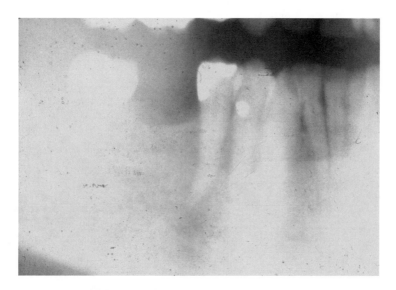

Patient 15. **A 57-year-old woman presents to you complaining of progressive numbness of her right lower lip and tongue. She has no trouble smiling, frowning, or squinting. Her medical history is significant for hypercholesterolemia, borderline hypertension, and mastectomy followed by radiation and chemotherapy. What would be your number 1 concern?**

The periapical radiograph reveals radiolucent areas in the mandible. Your first concern in this case would be metastatic breast cancer to the mandible.

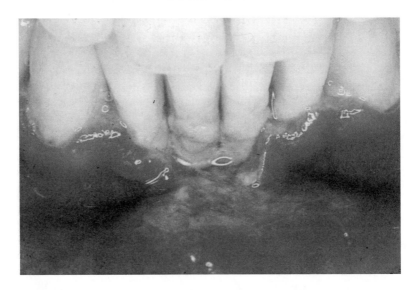

Patient 16.   This 22-year-old healthy student is in the midst of final exams and woke up this morning with this painful gum condition.   He feels a "little sick" and is really concerned that he won't be able to take his scheduled examination the day after tomorrow. What is your diagnosis? How would you treat him? Do you think he'll be feeling better for his examination?

The acute onset, mild systemic symptoms, and clinical appearance (modification of gingival architecture with loss of papillae and necrosis) are consistent with a diagnosis of acute necrotizing ulcerative gingivitis. The disease is caused by a fusospirochetal bacterial complex that is very sensitive to penicillin. Probably best to prescribe penicillin (1 gm loading dose followed by 500 mg q6h for a week) immediately, plus some local irrigation with saline or chlorhexidine gluconate. After 24 hours, have the patient return for local debridement. Typically, this condition responds quickly—he should be good to go for his exam.

BIBLIOGRAPHY

ATHEROSCLEROSIS

1. Chobanian AV: Pathophysiology of atherosclerosis. Am J Cardiol 70:3G, 1992.
2. Collins R, et al: Blood pressure, stroke and coronary artery disease. Part 2: Short-term reductions in blood pressure: Overview of randomized drug trials in their epidemiological context. Lancet 333:827, 1990.
3. Eagle KA, et al: Guidelines for perioperative cardiovascular evaluation for noncardiac surgery. J Am Coll Cardiol 27:910, 1996.
4. Lakier JB: Smoking and cardiovascular disease. Am J Med 93:8S, 1992.
5. Matsuura H: The systemic management of cardiovascular risk patients in dental practice. Anesth Pain Contr Dent 3:49, 1999.
6. Ross R: The pathogenesis of atherosclerosis: A perspective for the 1990s. Nature 362:801, 1993.
7. Schwartz CJ, et al: A modern view of atherogenesis. Am J Cardiol 71:9B, 1993.
8. Sixth Report of the Joint National Committee on Prevention, Detection, Evaluation, and Treatment of High Blood Pressure. Arch Intern Med 157:2413, 1997.

HYPERTENSION

1. Abraham-Inpijn L, et al: Changes in blood pressure, heart rate and electrocardiogram during dental treatment with use of local anesthesia. J Am Dent Assoc 116:531, 1988.
2. Becker D: The autonomic nervous system and related drugs in dental practice: Part II: Adrenergic agonists and antagonists. Compend Contin Educ Dent 9:772, 1997.
3. Chernow B, et al: Local dental anesthesia with epinephrine: Minimal effects in the sympathetic nervous system or on hemodynamic variables. Arch Intern Med 143:2141, 1983.
4. Foster CA, et al: Propranolol-epinephrine interaction: A potential disaster. Plast Reconstr Surg 72:74, 1983.
5. Frohlich ED, et al: Report of a special task force appointed by the Steering Committee, American Heart Association: Recommendations for human blood pressure determinations by sphygmomanometers. Hypertension 11:209A, 1998.
6. Goulet JP, et al: Contraindications to vasoconstrictors in dentistry, part III. Oral Surg Oral Med Oral Pathol Oral Radiol Endod 74:682, 1992.
7. Hanssbrough JF, et al: Propranolol-epinephrine antagonism with hypertension and stroke. Ann Intern Med 92:717, 1980.
8. Hastak JT, et al: Vasoconstrictors and local anesthesia: A review and rationale for use. J Am Dent Assoc 107:623, 1983.
9. Joint National Committee on Preventions, Detection, Evaluation of Treatment of High Blood Pressure: Sixth Report of the Joint National Committee on Detection, Evaluation, and Treatment of High Blood Pressure. Arch Intern Med 127:2412, 1997.
10. MacMahon S, et al: Blood pressure, stroke, and coronary heart disease. Part I: Prolonged differences in blood pressure: Prospective observational studies corrected for regression dilution basis. Lancet 225:765, 1990.
11. Perusse R, et al: Contraindications to vasoconstrictors in dentistry, part I. Oral Surg Oral Med Oral Pathol Oral Radiol Endod 74:679, 1992.
12. Perusse R, et al: Contraindications to vasoconstrictors in dentistry, part II. Oral Surg Oral Med Oral Pathol Oral Radiol Endod 74:687, 1992.
13. Quock RM: Clinical complications in the psychiatric dental patient. Compend Contin Educ Dent 6:333, 1985.
14. Steele RM, et al: Calcium antagonist-induced gingival hyperplasia. Ann Intern Med 120:663, 1994.
15. van Herwaarden CL, Binkhorst RA, Fennis JF, van t'Laar A: Effects of adrenaline during treatment with propranolol and metoprolol. Br Med J 1(6067):1029, 1977.
16. Westbrook P, Bednarczyk EM, Carlson M, et al: Regression of nifedipine-induced gingival hyperplasia following switch to same class calcium channel blocker, isradipine. J Periodontol 68:645-650, 1997.
17. Wynn RL: Epinephrine interactions with beta blockers. Gen Dent 42:16, 1994.
18. Wynn RL: Recent research on mechanisms of local anesthetics. Gen Dent 43:316, 1994.
19. Yagiela J: Adverse drug interactions in dental practice: Interactions associated with vasoconstrictors. Part V of a series. J Am Dent Assoc 130:701, 1999.

ANGINA PECTORIS

1. Cutler LS: Evaluation and management of the dental patient with cardiovascular disease. III. Angina and myocardial infarction. J Conn State Med Assoc 61:21, 1987.
2. Eagle KA, et al: Guidelines for perioperative cardiovascular evaluation for noncardiac surgery. J Am Coll Cardiol 27:910, 1996.
3. Findler M, et al: Dental treatment in very high risk patients with active ischemic heart disease. Oral Surg Oral Med Oral Pathol Oral Radiol Endod 76:298, 1993.
4. Kotler TS, et al: Exercise thallium-201 scintigraphy in the diagnosis and prognosis of coronary artery disease. Ann Intern Med 113:684, 1990.
5. Matsuura H: The systemic management of cardiovascular risk patients in dental practice. Anesth Pain Contr Dent 3:49, 1999.
6. Perusse R, et al: Contraindications to vasoconstrictors in dentistry, part I. Oral Surg Oral Med Oral Pathol Oral Radiol Endod 74:679, 1992.
7. Perusse R, et al: Contraindications to vasoconstrictors in dentistry, part II. Oral Surg Oral Med Oral Pathol Oral Radiol Endod 74:687, 1992.
8. Solomon AJ, et al: Management of chronic stable angina: Medical therapy, percutaneous transluminal coronary angioplasty, and coronary artery bypass graft surgery. Lessons from the randomized trials. Ann Intern Med 128:216, 1998.
9. Willard JE, et al: Use of aspirin in ischemic heart disease. N Engl J Med 327:175, 1992.

MYOCARDIAL INFARCTION

1. Abraham-Inpijn L, et al: Changes in blood pressure, heart rate and electrocardiogram during dental treatment with use of local anesthesia. J Am Dent Assoc 116:531, 1988.
2. Becker D: The autonomic nervous system and related drugs in dental practice: Part II: Adrenergic agonists and antagonists. Compend Contin Educ Dent 9:772, 1997.
3. Clintron G, et al: Cardiovascular effects and safety of dental anesthesia and dental interventions in patients with recent uncomplicated myocardial infarction. Arch Intern Med 146:2203, 1986.
4. Cutler LS: Evaluation and management of the dental patient with cardiovascular disease. III. Angina and myocardial infarction. J Conn State Med Assoc 61:21, 1987.
5. Eagle KA, et al: Guidelines for perioperative cardiovascular evaluation for noncardiac surgery. J Am Coll Cardiol 27:910, 1996.
6. Findler M, et al: Dental treatment in very high risk patients with active ischemic heart disease. Oral Surg Oral Med Oral Pathol Oral Radiol Endod 76:298, 1993.
7. Goulet JP, et al: Contraindications to vasoconstrictors in dentistry, part III. Oral Surg Oral Med Oral Pathol Oral Radiol Endod 74:682, 1992.
8. Matsuura H: The systemic management of cardiovascular risk patients in dental practice. Anesth Pain Contr Dent 3:49, 1999.
9. McCarthy FM: Safety treatment of the post-heart-attack patient. Compend Contin Educ Dent 10:598, 1989.
10. Hastak JT, et al: Vasoconstrictors and local anesthesia: A review and rationale for use. J Am Dent Assoc 107:623, 1983.
11. Perusse R, et al: Contraindications to vasoconstrictors in dentistry, part I. Oral Surg Oral Med Oral Pathol Oral Radiol Endod 74:679, 1992.
12. Perusse R, et al: Contraindications to vasoconstrictors in dentistry, part II. Oral Surg Oral Med Oral Pathol Oral Radiol Endod 74:687, 1992.

CONGESTIVE HEART FAILURE

1. Baker DW, et al: Management of heart failure. I. Pharmacologic treatment. JAMA 272:1361, 1994.
2. Braunwald E: ACE inhibitors: A cornerstone of the treatment of heart failure. N Engl J Med 325:351, 1991.
3. The CONSENSUS Trial Study Group: Effects of enalapril on mortality in severe congestive heart failure. N Engl J Med 23:1429, 1987.
4. Eagle KA, et al: Guidelines for perioperative cardiovascular evaluation for noncardiac surgery. J Am Coll Cardiol 27:910, 1996.
5. Mulligan R: Pretreatment for the cardiovascularly compromised geriatric dental patient. Special Care Dentist 5:116, 1985.
6. Smith TW: Digoxin in heart failure. N Engl J Med 329:51, 1993.

ARRHYTHMIAS

1. el Hakim M: Cardiac dysrhythmias during dental surgery: Comparison of hyoscine, glycopyrrolate and placebo premedication. Anesthesiol Reanim 16:393–398, 1991.
2. Feinberg WM, et al: Prevalence, age distribution and gender of patients with atrial fibrillation: Analysis and implications. Arch Intern Med 155:469, 1995.
3. Frabetti L, et al: Cardiovascular effects of local anesthesia with epinephrine in periodontal treatment. Quintessence Int 23:19, 1992.
4. Kannel WB, et al: Epidemiologic features of chronic atrial fibrillation: The Framingham Study. N Engl J Med 306:1018, 1982.
5. Matsuura H: The systemic management of cardiovascular risk patients in dental practice. Anesth Pain Contr Dent 3:49, 1999.
6. Rashad A, et al: Cardiac dysrhythmias during oral surgery: Effect of combined local and general anesthesia. Br J Oral Maxillofac Surg 28:102, 1990.
7. Rodrigo CR: Cardiac dysrhythmias with general anesthesia during dental surgery. Anesth Prog 35:102, 1988.
8. Roelofes JA, et al: Cardiac dysrhythmias associated with intravenous lorazepam, diazepam and midazolam during oral surgery. J Oral Maxillafac Surg 52:247, 1994.

BACTERIAL ENDOCARDITIS AND MANAGEMENT OF THE CARDIAC SURGICAL PATIENT

1. Burket LW, et al: Bacteremias following dental extraction. Demonstration of source of bacteria by means of a non-pathogen (*Serratia marcescens*). J Dent Res 16:521, 1937.
2. Clemens JD, et al: A controlled evaluation of the risk of bacterial endocarditis in persons with mitral valve prolapse. N Engl J Med 307:776, 1982.
3. Dajani AS, et al: Prevention of bacterial endocarditis: Recommendations by the American Heart Association. Clin Infect Dis 25:1445–1458, 1997.
4. DeMoor CE, et al: The occurrence of *Streptococcus mutans* and *Streptococcus sanguis* in the blood of endocarditis patients. Abstracts of paper presented at the Eighteenth ORGA Congress, 1968.
5. Durack DT: Prevention of infective endocarditis. N Engl J Med 332:38, 1995.
6. Durac DT: Antibiotics for prevention of endocarditis during dentistry: Time to scale back? Ann Intern Med 129:829, 1998.
7. Iver TS, et al: Prosthetic valve endocarditis. Circulation 69:223, 1984.
8. Nelso CI, et al: Physicians' and dentists' compliance with AHA guidelines for prevention of bacterial endocarditis. J Am Dent Assoc 118:169, 1989.
9. Sadowsk D, et al: Recommendations for prevention of bacterial endocarditis: Clinician non-compliance. J Am Dent Assoc 1181:175, 1989.
10. Simmon NA, et al: Antibiotic prophylaxis and infective endocarditis. Lancet 339:1252, 1992.
11. Stro BL, et al: Dental and cardiac risk factors for infective endocarditis. Ann Intern Med 129:761, 1998.
12. Van der Meer JT, Van Wijk W, Thompson J, et al: Efficacy of antibiotic for prevention of native valve endocarditis. Lancet 339:135–139, 1992.
13. Van der Meer JT, et al: Awareness of need and actual use of prophylaxis: Lack of patient compliance in the prevention of bacterial endocarditis. J Antimic Chemother 29:187, 1992.

DIABETES MELLITUS

1. Albrecht M, et al: Dental and oral symptoms of diabetes mellitus. Community Dental Oral Epidemiol 16:378, 1988.
2. Centers for Disease Control and Prevention: The status of diabetes mellitus in the U.S.: Surveillance report. MWWR 50:101, 2001.
3. Clark CM, et al: Prevention of complications of diabetes mellitus. N Engl J Med 332:1210, 1995.
4. Collin H, et al: Periodontal finding in elderly patients with non-insulin dependent diabetes mellitus. J Periodontol 69:962, 1998.
5. Diabetes Control and Complications Trial Research Group: The effect of intensive treatment of diabetes on the development and progression of long-term complications in insulin-dependent diabetes mellitus. N Engl J Med 329:977, 1993.
6. Ervastis T, et al: Relationship between control of diabetes and gingival bleeding. J Periodontol (March):154, 1985.
7. Firatli E: The relationship between clinical periodontal status and insulin-dependent diabetes mellitus. Results after 5 years. J Periodontol 68:136, 1997.
8. Golden EA: Preventing complications of diabetes by controlling hyperglycemia. Diabetes Care 22:1408, 1999.

9. Grossi S, et al: Periodontal disease and diabetes mellitus: A two-way relationship. Ann Periodontol 3:51, 1998.
10. Guggeneheimer J, et al: Insulin-dependent diabetes mellitus and oral soft tissue pathologies. Oral Surg Oral Med Oral Pathol Oral Radiol Endod 89:563, 2000.
11. Harris MI, et al: Prevalence of diabetes and impaired glucose tolerance and plasma glucose levels in U.S. population ages 20 to 74 years. Diabetes 36:523, 1987.
12. Kannell WB, et al: Diabetes and cardiovascular disease: The Framingham Study. JAMA 241:2035, 1979.
13. Kinane DF, et al: Relationship of diabetes to periodontal disease. Curr Opin Periodontol 4:29, 1997.
14. Mealey B: Impact of advances in diabetes care on dental treatment of the diabetic patient. Compend Cont Educ Dentistry 19:41, 1998.
15. Nathan DM: Long-term complication of diabetes mellitus. N Engl J Med 328:1676, 1995.
16. Perusse R, et al: Contraindications to vasoconstrictors in dentistry: Part II. Hyperthyroidism, diabetes, sulfite sensitivity, corticosteroid-dependent asthma and pheochromocytoma. Oral Surg Oral Med Oral Pathol Oral Radiol Endod 62:687, 1992.
17. Piche J: The glycosylated hemoglobin assay for diabetes: Its value to the periodontist. J Periodontol 60:640-642, 1989.
18. Rosenthal IM, et al: The relationship of inflammatory periodontal disease to diabetic status in insulin-dependent diabetes mellitus patients. J Clin Periodontol 15:425, 1988.
19. Satrowijoto SH, et al: Relationship between bleeding/plaque ratio, family history of diabetes mellitus and impaired glucose tolerance. J Clin Periodontol 17:55, 1990.
20. Sastrowijoto SH, et al: Improved metabolic control, clinical periodontal status and subgingival microbiology in insulin-dependent diabetes mellitus. A prospective study. J Clin Periodontol 17:233, 1990.
21. Scheen AJ, et al: Antihyperglycemia agents. Drug interactions of clinical importance. Drug Safety 12:32, 1995.
22. Sholssman M, et al: Type 2 diabetes mellitus and periodontal disease. J Am Dent Assoc 121:532, 1990.
23. Taylor G, et al: Non-insulin dependent diabetes mellitus and alveolar bone loss progressive over two years. J Periodontol 16:76, 1998.
24. Taylor G, et al: Glycemic control and alveolar bone loss progression in type 2 diabetes. Ann Periodontol 3:29–30, 1998.
25. Tervonen T, et al: Long term control of diabetes mellitus and periodontitis. J Clin Periodontol 20:431, 1993.
26. Tervonen T, et al: Relation of diabetes control to periodontal pocketing and alveolar bone level. Oral Surg Oral Med Oral Pathol Oral Radiol Endod 61:346, 1986.
27. Van Dis ML, et al: Prevalence of oral lichen planus in patients with diabetes mellitus. Oral Surg Oral Med Oral Pathol Oral Radiol Endod 79:696, 1995.

ADRENAL DISORDERS AND STEROID THERAPY

1. Boumpas DT, et al: Glucocorticoid therapy for immune-mediated diseases: Basic and clinical correlates. Ann Intern Med 119:1198, 1993.
2. Gersema L, et al: Use of corticosteroids in oral surgery. J Oral Maxillofac Surg 50:270, 1992.
3. Glowniak JV, et al: A double-blind study of peri-operative steroid requirements in secondary adrenal insufficiency. Surgery 121:123, 1997.
4. Hempenstall PD, et al: Cardiovascular, biochemical and hormonal responses to intravenous sedation with local analgesia versus general anesthesia in patients undergoing oral surgery. J Oral Maxillofac Surg 44:441, 1986.
5. Krasner AS: Glucocorticoid-induced adrenal insufficiency. JAMA 282:671, 1999.
6. Parnell AG: Adrenal crisis and the dental surgeon. Br Dent J 116:294, 1964.
7. Perusse R, et al: Contraindications to vasoconstrictors in dentistry: Part II. Hyperthyroidism, diabetes, sulfite sensitivity, corticosteroid-dependent asthma and pheochromocytoma. Oral Surg Oral Med Oral Pathol Oral Radiol Endod 62:687, 1992.

THYROID DISORDERS

1. Helfand M, et al: Screening for thyroid disease: An update. Ann Intern Med 129:144, 1998.
2. Hurley DL, et al: Detection and treatment of hypothyroidism and Graves' disease. Geriatrics 50:41, 1995.
3. Mandel SJ, et al: Levothyroxine therapy in patients with thyroid disease. Ann Intern Med 119:492, 1993.
4. Perusse R, et al: Contraindications to vasoconstrictors in dentistry: Part II. Hyperthyroidism, diabetes, sulfite sensitivity, corticosteroid-dependent asthma and pheochromocytoma. Oral Surg Oral Med Oral Pathol Oral Radiol Endod 62:687, 1992.
5. Singer PA, et al: Treatment guidelines for patients with hyperthyroidism and hypothyroidism. Standards of Care Committee, American Thyroid Association. JAMA 273:808, 1995.

6. Surks MI, et al: Drugs and thyroid function. N Engl J Med 333:1688, 1995.
7. Weetman AP: Graves' disease. N Engl J Med 343:1236, 2000.

PREGNANCY
1. Balligan FJ, et al: Analgesic and antibiotic administration during pregnancy. Gen Dent 41:220, 1993.
2. Chiodo GT, et al: Dental treatment during pregnancy: A preventive approach. J Am Dent Assoc 110:365, 1985.
3. Loe H: Periodontal changes in pregnancy. J Periodontol 36:209, 1965.
4. Moore P: Selecting drugs for the pregnant dental patient. J Am Dent Assoc 129:1281, 1998.
5. Schwartz M, et al: Care of the pregnant patient. J Can Dent Assoc 55:299, 1987.
6. Schrout MK, et al: Treating the pregnant dental patient: Four basic rules addressed. J Am Dent Assoc 123:75, 1992.
7. Tarsitano BF, Rollings RE: The pregnant dental patient: Evaluation and management. Gen Dent 41:226–234, 1993.

ASTHMA
1. Abramowicz M (ed): Drugs for Asthma. Med Lett Drugs Ther 37:1, 1996.
2. Babu KS, Salvi SS: Aspirin and asthma. Chest 118:1470–1476, 2000.
3. Barnes PJ, et al: Asthma: Basic Mechanisms and Clinical Management, 2nd ed. New York, Academic Press, 1992.
4. Suissa S, et al: Albuterol in mild asthma. N Engl J Med 336:129, 1997.

CHRONIC OBSTRUCTIVE PULMONARY DISEASE
1. Bellamy D: Progress in the management of chronic obstructive pulmonary disease. Practitioner 244:24, 2000.
2. Burrows B: Physiologic variants of chronic obstructive pulmonary disease. Chest 58(suppl):415, 1979.
3. Ferguson G: Recommendations for the management of chronic obstructive pulmonary disease. Chest 117:23S, 2000.
4. Fletcher CM: Chronic bronchitis: Its prevalence, nature, and pathogenesis. Am Rev Resp Dis 111:719, 1975.
5. Hugh-Jones P, et al: The etiology and management of disabling emphysema. Am Rev Resp Dis 117:343, 1978.

TUBERCULOSIS
1. Bleed DM: Worldwide epidemiology of tuberculosis. Pediatr Pulmonol Suppl 23:60, 2000.
2. Laskaris G: Oral manifestation of infectious diseases. Dent Clin North Am 40:395–423, 1996.
3. Mignogna MD, Zuzioll, Favia G, et al: Oral tuberculosis: A clinical evaluation of 42 cases. Oral Dis 6:25–30, 2000.
4. Reichler MR, Reves P, Bur S, et al: Evaluation of investigations conducted to detect and prevent transmission of tuberculosis. JAMA 287:991–995, 2002.

PEPTIC ULCER DISEASE
1. Fendick AM, et al: Alternative management strategies for patients with suspected peptic ulcer disease. Ann Intern Med 123:260, 1995.
2. Graham D, et al: Effect of triple therapy (antibiotics plus bismuth) on duodenal ulcer healing: A randomized controlled trial. Ann Intern Med 115:266, 1991.
3. Lam S: Aetiological factors of peptic ulcer: Perspectives of epidemiological observation this century. J Gastroenterol Hepatol 9:S93, 1994.
4. Manton PN: Omeprazole. N Engl J Med 324:965, 1991.
5. McCarthy D: Non-steroidal anti-inflammatory drug related gastrointestinal toxicity: Definitions and epidemiology. Am J Med 105:3S, 1998.
6. Walsh J, et al: The treatment of *Helicobacter pylori* infection in the management of peptic ulcer disease. N Engl J Med 333:984, 1995.
7. Wolfe M, et al: Gastrointestinal toxicity of non-steroidal anti-inflammatory drugs. N Engl J Med 340:1720, 2000.

INFLAMMATORY BOWEL DISEASE

1. Becker J: Surgical therapy for ulcerative colitis and Crohn's disease. Gastroenterol Clin North Am 28:371, 1999.
2. Ghosh S, et al: A regular review: Ulcerative colitis. BMJ 320:1119, 2000.
3. Glotzer DJ, et al: Comparative features and course of ulcerative and granulomatous colitis. N Engl J Med 282:582, 1970.
4. Halme L, Meurman JH, Laine P, et al: Oral findings in patients with active or inactive Crohn's disease. Oral Surg Oral Med Oral Pathol Oral Radiol Endod 76:175–181, 1993.
5. Kornbluth A, et al: Ulcerative colitis practice guidelines. American College of Gastroenterology Practice Parameters Committee. Am J Gastroenterol 92:204, 1997.
6. Peppercorn MA: Advances in drug therapy for inflammatory bowel disease. Ann Intern Med 112:59, 1990.
7. Tremaine WJ, et al: Practice guidelines for inflammatory bowel disease: An instrument for assessment. Mayo Clinic Proc 74:495, 1999.
8. Williams AJ, et al: The clinical entity of orofacial Crohn's disease. Q J Med 79:451, 1991.

HEPATITIS

1. ADA Council on Scientific Affairs, ADA Council on Dental Practice: Infection control recommendations for the dental office and the dental laboratory. J Am Dent Assoc 127:672, 1996.
2. Advisory Committee on Immunization Practices (ACIP) and the Hospital Infection Control Practices Advisory Committee: Immunization of health-care workers: Recommendations of the Advisory Committee on Immunization Practices and the Hospital Infection Control Practices Advisory Committee. MMWR 46:1, 1997.
3. Center for Disease Control and Prevention: Recommended infection-control practices for dentistry. MMWR 41:1, 1993.
4. Center for Disease Control and Prevention: Update towards the elimination of hepatitis B virus-United States. MMWR 44:574, 1995.
5. Center for Disease Control and Prevention: recommendations for prevention and control of hepatitis C virus infection and HCV-related chronic disease. MMWR 47:1, 1998.
6. Cleveland JL, et al: Risk and prevention of hepatitis C virus infection: Implications for dentistry. J Am Dent Assoc 130:641, 1999.
7. Davis GL, et al: Treatment of chronic hepatitis C with recombinant interferon alfa: A multicenter randomized controlled trial. N Engl J Med 321:1501, 1989.
8. Demas PN, et al: Hepatitis: Implications for dental care. Oral Surg Oral Med Oral Pathol Oral Radiol Endod 88:2, 1999.
9. Gerberding J: Management of occupational exposures to blood-borne viruses. N Engl J Med 332:444, 1995.
10. Klein RS, et al: Occupational risk for hepatitis C virus infection among New York City dentists. Lancet 338:1539, 1991.
11. London TW, Evans AA: The epidemiology of hepatitis viruses B, C and D. Clin Lab Med 16:251–271, 1996.
12. Pianko S: Treatment of hepatitis C with interferon and ribavirin. J Gastroenterol Hepatol 15:581, 2000.
13. Rosenberg PM, et al: Therapy with nucleoside analogues for hepatitis B virus infection. Clin Liver Dis 3:349, 1999.
14. Sywasssink JM, et al: Risk of hepatitis B in dental care providers: A contact study. J Am Dent Assoc 106:182, 1983.
15. Thomas DL, et al: Occupational risk of hepatitis C infections among general dentists and oral surgeons in North America. Am J Med 100:41, 1996.

CIRRHOSIS

1. Epstein M: Treatment of refractory ascites. N Engl J Med 321:1675, 1989.
2. Friedlander AH, et al: Alcoholism and dental management. Oral Surg 62:42, 1987.
3. Galili D, et al: A modern approach to prevention and treatment of oral bleeding in patients with hepatocellular disease. Oral Surg 54:277, 1982.
4. Glassman P, Wong C, Gish R: A review of liver transplantation for the dentist and guidelines for dental management. Special Care Dentist 13:74–80, 1993.
5. Glick M: Medical considerations for dental care of patients with alcohol-related liver disease. J Am Dent Assoc 128:61, 1997.
6. Powell WJ Jr, et al: Duration of survival in patients with Laennec's cirrhosis. Am J Med 33:406, 1968.
7. Riordan SM, et al: Treatment of hepatic encephalopathy. N Engl J Med 337:473, 1997.
8. Seeff LB, et al: Acetaminophen hepatotoxicity in alcoholics: A therapeutic misadventure. Ann Intern Med 104:399, 1986.

ANEMIA

1. Carr MM: Dental management of patients with sickle cell anemia. J Can Dent Assoc 59:180, 1993.
2. Cash JM, et al: The anemia of chronic diseae: Spectrum of associated diseases in a series of unselected hospitalized patients. Am J Med 87:638, 1989.
3. Clarke GM, et al: The laboratory investigation of hemoglobinopathies and thalassemias: Review and update. Clin Chem 46:1284, 2000.
4. Drummond JF, et al: Megaloblastic anemia with oral lesions. A consequence of gastric bypass surgery. Oral Surg Oral Med Oral Pathol Oral Radiol Endod 59:149, 1985.
5. Imbery TA: Dental management of a patient with aplastic anemia. Gen Dent 40:316, 1992.
6. May DA: Dental management of sickle cell anemia patients. Gen Dent 39:182, 1991.
7. Thacker JM, et al: Oral epithelial dysplasia in vitamin B12 deficiency. Oral Surg Oral Med Oral Pathol Oral Radiol Endod 67:81, 1989.
8. Wood M, et al: Symptoms of iron deficiency anemia: A community survey. Br J Prev Soc Med 20:117, 1966.

BLEEDING DISORDERS

1. Carr MM, et al: Dental management of anticogaulated patients. J Can Dent Assoc 58:838, 1992.
2. Gill FM: Congenital bleeding disorders: Hemophilia and von Willebrand's disease. Med Clin North Am 68:601, 1984.
3. Herman WW, Konzelman JL Jr, Sutley SH: Current perspectives on dental patients receiving coumarin anticoagulation therapy. J Am Dent Assoc 128:327–335, 1997.
4. Johnson WT, et al: Management of dental patients with bleeding disorders: Review and update. Oral Surg Oral Med Oral Pathol Oral Radiol Endod 66:297, 1988.
5. Katz JO, et al: Dental management of the patient with hemophilia. Oral Surg Oral Med Oral Pathol Oral Radiol Endod 66:139, 1988.
6. Litin SC, et al: Current concepts in anticoagulation therapy. Mayo Clin Proc 70:266, 1995.
7. McNeil Consumer Product Company: Acetaminophen and other risk factors for excessive warfarin anti-coagulation. JAMA 279:9, 1998.
8. O'Grady J, et al: Aspirin: A paradoxical effect on bleeding time [letter]. Lancet 2:780, 1978.
9. Rakoca M, et al: Dental extractions in patients with bleeding disorders. The use of fibrin glue. Oral Surg Oral Med Oral Pathol Oral Radiol Endod 75:280, 1993.
10. Ramstrom G, et al: Prevention of postsurgical bleeding in oral surgery using tranexamic acid without dose modification of oral anticoagulants. J Oral Maxillofac Surg 51:1211, 1993.
11. Rossman J, et al: The use of hemostatic agents in dentistry. Postgrad Dentistry 3:3, 1996.
12. Santo J, et al: Oral surgery in anticoagulated patients without reducing the dose of oral anticoagulant: A prospective randomized study. J Oral Maxillofac Surg 54:27, 1996.
13. Schafer A: Effects of non-steroidal anti-inflammatory drugs on platelet function and systemic hemostasis. J Clin Pharam 35:209, 1995.
14. Staffileno H Jr, Ciancio S: Bleeding disorders in the dental patient: Causative factors and management. Compendium 8:501, 504–507, 1987.
15. Troulis M, et al: Dental extractions in patients on oral anticoagulants: A survey of practices in North America. J Oral Maxillofac Surg 56:914, 1998.
16. Weibert R: Oral anticoagulant therapy in patients undergoing dental surgery. Clin Pharm 11:851, 1992.

ANTICOAGULATION

1. Carr MM, et al: Dental management of anticogaulated patients. J Can Dent Assoc 58:838, 1992.
2. Herman WW, Konzelman JL Jr, Sutley SH: Current perspectives on dental patients receiving coumarin anticoagulation therapy. J Am Dent Assoc 128:327–335, 1997.
3. Litin SC, et al: Current concepts in anticoagulation therapy. Mayo Clin Proc 70:266, 1995.
4. McNeil Consumer Product Company: Acetaminophen and other risk factors for excessive warfarin anti-coagulation. JAMA 279:9, 1998.
5. Rakoca M, et al: Dental extractions in patients with bleeding disorders. The use of fibrin glue. Oral Surg Oral Med Oral Pathol Oral Radiol Endod 75:280, 1993.
6. Ramstrom G, et al: Prevention of postsurgical bleeding in oral surgery using tranexamic acid without dose modification of oral anticoagulants. J Oral Maxillofac Surg 51:1211, 1993.
7. Rossman J, et al: The use of hemostatic agents in dentistry. Postgrad Dentistry 3:3, 1996.
8. Santo J, et al: Oral surgery in anticoagulated patients without reducing the dose of oral anticoagulant: A prospective randomized study. J Oral Maxillofac Surg 54:27, 1996.
9. Troulis M, et al: Dental extractions in patients on oral anticoagulants: A survey of practices in North America. J Oral Maxillofac Surg 56:914, 1998.
10. Weibert R: Oral anticoagulant therapy in patients undergoing dental surgery. Clin Pharm 11:851–864, 1992.

HEMATOLOGIC MALIGNANCIES

1. Epstein JB, Epstein JD, Len D, et al: Characteristics of oral and paraoral malignant lymphoma: A population-based review of 361 cases. Oral Surg Oral Med Oral Pathol Oral Radiol Endod 92:519–525, 2001.
2. Estey EH: Therapeutic options for acute myelogenous leukemia. Cancer 92:1059–1073, 2001.
3. Fowler CB: Benign and malignant neoplasms of the periodontium. Periodontol 1999:33–85, 2000.
4. O'Dwyer ME, Mauro MJ, Druker BJ: Recent advancements in the treatment of chronic myelogenous leukemia. Annu Rev Med 53:369–381, 2002.
5. Stafford P, Sonis S, Lockhart P, et al: Oral pathoses as diagnostic indicators in leukemia. Oral Surg Oral Med Oral Pathol Oral Radiol Endod 50:1349, 1980.

ARTHRITIS

1. American College of Rheumatology: Guidelines for monitoring drug therapy in rheumatoid arthritis. Arthritis Rheum 39:723, 1996.
2. American Dental Association, American Academy of Orthopedic Surgeons Advisory Statement: Antibiotic prophylaxis for dental patients with total joint replacement. J Am Dent Assoc 128:1004, 1997.
3. Amrein PC, et al: Aspirin-induced prolongation of bleeding time and peri-operative blood loss. JAMA 245:1825, 1981.
4. Arnett FC, et al: The American Rheumatism Association 1987 revised criteria for the classification of rheumatoid arthritis. Arthritis Rheum 31:315, 1988.
5. Fries JF, et al: Reduction in long-term disability in patients with rheumatoid arthritis by disease-modifying anti-rheumatic drug-based treatment strategies. Arthritis Rheum 39:616, 1996.
6. Hochberg MC, et al: Guidelines for the medical management of osteoarthritis. Part 1. Osteoarthritis of the hip. Part 2. Osteoarthritis of the knee. American College of Rheumatology. Arthritis Rheum 38:1535, 1995.
7. Jeurissen MEC, et al: Influence of methotrexate and azathioprine on radiologic progression in rheumatoid arthritis: A randomized, double blind study. Ann Intern Med 114:999, 1991.
8. Liang MH, et al: Management of osteoarthritis of the hip and knee. N Engl J Med 325:125, 1991.
9. Little JW: Patients with prosthetic joints. Are they at risk when receiving invasive dental procedures? Special Care Dentist 17:153, 1997.
10. Moreland LW, et al: Treatment of rheumatoid arthritis with a recombinant human tumor necrosis factor reception (p75)-Fc fusion protein. N Engl J Med 337:141, 1997.

CEREBROVASCULAR DISORDERS

1. Almog DM, Illig KA, Khin M, et al: Unrecognized carotid artery stenosis discovered by calcification on panoramic radiograph. J Am Dent Assoc 131:1593–1597, 2000.
2. August M: Cerebrovascular and carotid artery disease. Oral Surg Oral Med Oral Pathol Oral Radiol Endod 92:253–256, 2001.
3. Bendisen BH, Ocava L: Evaluation and management of acute ischemic stroke. Cur Cardiol Rep 4:149–157, 2002.
4. Carter LC, Heller AD, Nadarjah V, et al: Use of panoramic radiography among an ambulatory dental population to detect patients at risk of stroke. J Am Dent Assoc 128:977–984, 1997.
5. Nuva H, Sugimusa M, Satdr Y, et al: Cardiovascular response to epinephrine-containing local anesthesia in patients with cardiovascular disease. Oral Surg Oral Med Oral Pathol Oral Radiol Endod 92:610–616, 2001.
6. Weinberger J: Stroke and TIA prevention and management of cerebrovascular events in primary care. Geriatrics 57:38–43, 2002.

CRANIOFACIAL NEUROLOGIC DISORDERS

1. Cady R, Dodick DW: Diagnosis and treatment of migraine. Mayo Clin Proc 77:255–261, 2002.
2. Dionne RA: Pharmacologic advances on orofacial pain from molecules to medicine. J Dent Edu 65:1393–1403, 2001.
3. Loeser JD: Tic douloureux. Pain Res Manag 6:156–165, 2001.
4. MacFarlane TV, Glenny AM, Worthington HV: Systemic review of population-based epidemiological studies of orofacial pain. J Dent 29:451–467, 2001.
5. Madland G, Feinmann C: Chronic facial pain: A multidisciplinary problem. J Neurol Neurosurg Psychiatry 71:716–719, 2001.
6. Wiiebe S, Nicolle UW: Recent developments in neurology. BMJ 324:656–660, 2002.
7. Zakrzewska JM: Diagnosis and differential diagnosis of trigeminal neuralgia. Clin J Pain 18:14–21, 2002.

SEXUALLY TRANSMITTED DISEASES INCLUDING HIV
1. Greenspan D, Greenspan JS: Oral manifestations of HIV infection. AIDS Clin Care 11:18–24, 1997.
2. Laskaris G: Oral manifestations of infectious diseases. Dent Clin North Am 40:395–423, 1996.
3. Ryder MI: Periodontal management of HIV-infected patients. Periodontol 23:85–93, 2000.
4. Tapprini AR, Fleming GJ: The effect of antiretroviral therapy on the prevalence of oral manifestations of HIV-infected patients: A UK study. Oral Surg Oral Med Oral Pathol Oral Radiol Endod 92:625–628, 2001.

VIRAL INFECTIONS
1. Holbrook WP, Gudmandsson GT, Ragnarsson KT: Herpetic gingivostomatitis in otherwise healthy adolescents and young adults. Acta Odontol Scand 59:113–115, 2001.
2. Naesens L, DeCheug E: Recent developments in herpesvirus therapy. Herpes 8:12–16, 2001.
3. Roizman B, Whitley RJ: The nine ages of herpes simplex virus. Herpes 8:23–27, 2001.
4. Villarreal EC: Current and potential therapies for the treatment of herpes virus infections. Prog Drug Res (spec no.):185–228, 2001.

FUNGAL INFECTIONS
1. Farah CS, Ashman RB, Challacombe SJ: Oral candidiasis. Clin Dermatol 18:553–562, 2000.
2. Glick M, Siegel MA: Viral and fungal infections of the oral cavity in immunocompetent patients. Infect Dis Clin North Am 13:817–831, 1999.
3. Redding SW: The role of yeasts other than *Candida albicans* in oropharyngeal candidiasis. Curr Opin Infect Dis 14:673–677, 2001.
4. Reichart PA, Samaranayake LP, Philipsen HP: Pathology and clinical correlates in oral candidiasis and its variants: A review. Oral Dis 6:85–91, 2000.
5. Scully C, deAlmeida OP, Sposto MR: The deep mucoses in HIV infection. Oral Dis 3(suppl 1):2200–2207, 1997.

ULCERS
1. Kinane DF: Periodontal disease in children and adolescents: Introduction and classification. Periodontol 26:7–15, 2000.
2. Porter SR, Hegarty A, Kaliatson F, et al: Recurrent aphthous stomatitis. Clin Dermatol 18:569–578, 2000.
3. Ship JA, Chavez EM, Doerr PA, et al: Recurrent aphthous stomatitis. Quintessence Int 31:95–112, 2000.
4. Sykes LM, Sukha A: Potential risk of serious oral infections in the diabetic patient: A clinical report. J Prosthet Dent 86:569–573, 2001.
5. Von Arx DP, Husain A: Oral tuberculosis. Br Dent J 190:420–422, 2001.

WHITE LESIONS
1. Callen P: Oral manifestations of collagen vascular disease. Semin Cutan Med Surg 16:323–327, 1997.
2. Grbic JT, Lamster IB: Oral manifestations of HIV infection. AIDS Patient Care 11:18–24, 1997.
3. Kupper R, Lombardi T: Premalignant lesions of the oral mucosa. A discussion about the place of oral intraepithelial neoplasia (OIN). Oral Oncol 38:125–130, 2002.
4. Reichart PA, Samaranaylke LP, Philipsen HP: Pathology and clinical correlates in oral candidiasis and its variants: A review. Oral Dis 6:85–91, 2000.
5. Sugarman PB, Savage NW, Zhou X, et al: Oral lichen planus. Clin Dermatol 18:533–539, 2000.

VESICULOBULLOUS DISEASES AND AUTOIMMUNITY
1. Casiglia J, Woo SB, Ahmed AP: Oral involvement in autoimmune blistering diseases. Dermatol Clin 19:637–648, 2001.
2. Chan LS, Ahmed AR, Anhalt GJ, et al: The first international consensus on mucous membrane pemphigoid: Definition, diagnostic criteria, pathogenic factors, medical treatment, and prognostic indicators. Arch Dermatol 138:370–379, 2002.
3. Dabelsteen E: Molecular biological aspects of acquired bullous diseases. Crit Rev Oral Biol Med 9:162–178, 1998.
4. Robinson JC, Lozada-Nur F, Frieden I: Oral pemphigus vulgaris: A review of the literature and a report on the management of 12 cases. Oral Surg Oral Med Oral Pathol Oral Radiol Endod 84:349–355, 1997.

5. Scully C: The mouth in dermatological disorders. Practitioner 245:942–944, 946, 949–952, 2001.
6. Scully C, Carrozzo M, Gandolfo S, et al: Update on mucous membrane pemphigoid: A heterogenous immune-mediated subepithelial blistering entity. Oral Surg Oral Med Oral Pathol Oral Radiol Endod 88:56–68, 1999.

PIGMENTAL LESIONS
1. Eisen D, Voorhees JJ: Oral melanoma and other pigmented lesions of the oral cavity. J Am Acad Dermatol 24:527–537, 1991.
2. Scully C, Porter S: AMC of oral health. Swellings and red, white, and pigmented lesions. BMJ 321:225–228, 2000.
3. Seoane Leston JM, Vazquez Garcia J, Agreado Santos A, et al: Dark oral lesions: Differential diagnosis with oral melanoma. Curtis 61:279–282, 1998.

ORAL CANCER
1. Brown JS, Lowe D, Kalavrezon V, et al: Patterns of invasion and routes of tumor entry into the mandible by oral squamous cell carcinoma. Head Neck 24:370–383, 2002.
2. Casiglia J, Woo SB: A comprehensive review of oral cancer. Gen Dent 49:72–82, 2001.
3. Frenk GF, Karnell LH, Robinson RA, et al: Presentation, treatment, and outcome of oral cavity cancer: A National Cancer Data report. Head Neck 24:165–180, 2002.
4. Reichart PA: Identification of risk groups for oral precancer and cancer and preventive measures. Clin Oral Investig 5:207–213, 2001.
5. Sciubba JJ: Oral precancer and cancer etiology, clinical presentation, diagnosis, and management. Compend Contin Educ Dent 21:8400–8402, 2000.
6. Silverman SJ: Demographics and occurrence of oral and pharyngeal cancers. The outcomes, the trends, the challenge. J Am Dent Assoc 132(suppl):7S–11S, 2001.
7. Weinberg MA, Estefan DJ: Assessing oral malignancies. Am Fam Physician 651:379–384, 2002.
8. Yellowitz JA, Horowitz AM, Drury TF, et al: Survey of VS dentists' knowledge and opinions about oral pharyngeal cancer. J Am Dent Assoc 131:653–661, 2000.

BENIGN TUMORS
1. Alawi F, Stratton D, Freedman PD: Solitary fibrous tumors of the oral soft tissues: A clinicopathologic and immunohistochemical study of 16 cases. Am J Surg Pathol 25:900–910, 2000.
2. Epivatianos A, Markopoulos AK, Papanayotou P: Benign tumors of adipose tissue of the oral cavity: A clinicopathologic study of 13 cases. J Oral Maxillofac Surg 58:1113–1117, 2000.
3. Maita JK: Oral tumors in children: A review. J Clin Pediatr Dent 24:133–135, 2000.
4. Practorius F: HPV-associated diseases of oral mucosa. Cliln Dermatol 15:399–413, 1997.

SALIVARY GLANDS
1. Brennan MT, Sandar V, Lenkan RA, et al: Risk factors for positive minor salivary gland biopsy findings in Sjögren's syndrome and dry mouth patients. Arthritis Rheum 47:189–195, 2002.
2. Bull PD: Salivary gland stones: Diagnosis and treatment. Hosp Med 62:396–399, 2001.
3. Carsons S: A review and update of Sjögren's syndrome: Manifestations, diagnosis, and treatment. Am J Manag Care 7:5433–5443, 2001.
4. Grisius MM: Salivary gland dysfunction: A review of systemic therapies. Oral Surg Oral Med Oral Pathol Oral Radiol Endod 92:156–162, 2001.
5. Nederfors T: Xerostomia and hyposalivation. Adv Dent Res 14:48–56, 2000.
6. Pedersen AM, Nauntofte B: Primary Sjögren's syndrome: Oral aspects on pathogenesis, diagnostic criteria, clinical features and approaches for therapy. Expert Opin Pharmacother 2:1415–1436, 2001.
7. Zbaren P, Schar C, Hotz MA, et al: Value of fine-needle aspiration cytology of parotid gland masses. Laryngoscope 111:1989–1992, 2001.

DISEASES OF BONE
1. Ardekian L, Peled M, Rosen D, et al: Clinical and radiographic features of eosinophilic granuloma in the jaws: Review of 41 lesions treated by surgery and low-dose radiotherapy. Oral Surg Oral Med Oral Pathol Oral Radiol Endod 87:238–242, 1999.
2. Christiansen P: The skeleton in primary hyperplasia thyroidism: A review focusing on bone remodeling, structure, mass, and fracture. APMIS Suppl (102):1–52, 2001.

3. Faire MP: Dietary factors related to preservation of oral and skeletal bone mass in women. J Prosthet Dent 73:65–72, 1995.
4. Jeffcoat MK: Osteoporosis: A possible modifying factor in oral bone loss. Ann Periodontal 3:312–321, 1998.
5. Rose LF, Steinberg B, Minsk L: The relationship between periodontal disease and systemic conditions. Compend Contin Educ Dent 21:870–877, 2000.
6. Waldron CA: Fibro-osseous lesion of the jaw. J Oral Maxillofac Surg 51:825–835, 1993.

CHRONIC RENAL FAILURE

1. Aradhye S: Clinical management of early progressive renal failure. Dis Mon 44:178–195, 1998.
2. Bennett WM, Aronoff GR, Morrison G, et al: Drug prescribing in renal failure: Dosing guidelines for adults. Am J Kidney Dis 3:155–193, 1983.
3. Eschbach JW: The anemia of chronic renal failure: Pathophysiology and the effects of recombinant erythropoietin. Kidney Int 35:134–148, 1989.
4. Ifudu O: Care of patients undergoing hemodialysis. N Engl J Med 339:1054–1062, 1998.
5. MacKenzie HS, Brenner BM: Current strategies for retarding progression of renal disease. Am J Kidney Dis 31:161–170, 1998.
6. Mooradian AD, Morley JE: Endocrine dysfunction in chronic renal insufficiency. Arch Intern Med 144:351–353, 1984.
7. Pastan S, Bailey J: Dialysis therapy. N Engl J Med 338:1428–1437, 1998.
8. Rahman M, Smith MC: Chronic renal insufficiency: A diagnostic and therapeutic approach. Arch Intern Med 158:1743–1752, 1998.
9. Ziccardi VB, Saini J, Demas PN, Braun TW: Management of the oral and maxillofacial surgery patient with end-stage renal disease. J Oral Maxillofac Surg 50:1207–1212, 1992.

TRANSPLANTATION

1. Daly CG: Resolution of cyclosporin A (CsA)-induced gingival enlargement following reduction in CsA dosage. J Clin Periodontol 19:143–145, 1992.
2. Eigner TL, Jastak JT, Bennett WM: Achieving oral health in patients with renal failure and renal transplants. J Am Dent Assoc 113:612–616, 1986.
3. First MR: Long-term complications after transplantation. Am J Kidney Dis 22:477–486, 1993.
4. Funakoshi Y, Ohshita C, Moritani Y, Hieda T: Dental findings of patients who underwent liver transplantation. J Clin Pediatr Dent 16:259–262, 1992.
5. Hayes JM: The immunobiology and clinical use of current immunosuppressive therapy for renal transplantation. J Urol 149:437–438, 1993.
6. King GN, Fullinfaw R, Higgins TJ, et al: Gingival hyperplasia in renal allograft recipients receiving cyclosporin A and calcium antagonists. J Clin Periodontol 20:286–293, 1993.
7. Little JW, Rhodus NL: Dental management of the liver transplant patient. Oral Surg 73:419–426, 1992.
8. Rhodus NL, Little JW: Dental management of the renal transplantation patient. Compendium 14:518–524, 526, 528, 1993.
9. Seymour RA, Jacobs DJ: Cyclosporin and the gingival tissues. J Clin Periodontol 19:1–11, 1992.

PSYCHIATRIC DISEASES

1. Black JL, Richelson E, Richardson JW: Antipsychotic agents: A clinical update. Mayo Clin Proc 60:777–789, 1985.
2. Friedlander AH, Brill NQ: Dental management of patients with schizophrenia. Spec Care Dentist 6:217–218, 1986.
3. Friedlander AH, West LJ: Dental management of patients with major depression. Oral Surg Oral Med Oral Pathol Oral Radiol Endod 71:573–578, 1991.
4. Mulchahey JJ, Malik MS, Sabai M, Kasckow JW: Serotonin-selective reuptake inhibitors in the treatment of geriatric depression and related disorders. Int J Neuropsychopharmacol 2:121–127, 1999.

ANTIBIOTICS

1. Barnett ML: Inhibition of oral contraceptive effectiveness by concurrent antibiotic administraton: A review. J Periodontol 56:18–20, 1985.
2. Greenberg RN: Overview of patient compliance with medication dosing: A literature review. Clin Ther 6:592–599, 1984.
3. Harrison JW, Svec TA: The beginning of the end of the antibiotic era. Part 1: The problem: Abuse of the "miracle drugs." Quintessence Int 29:151–162, 1998.

4. Kivisto KT, Lamberg TS, Kantola T, Neuvonen PJ: Plasma buspirone concentrations are greatly increased by erythromycin and itraconazole. Clin Pharmacol Ther 62:348–354, 1997.
5. Malizia T, Tejada MR, Ghelardi E, et al: Periodontal tissue disposition of azithromycin. J Periodontol 68:1206–1209, 1997.
6. Sefton AM, Maskell JP, Beighton D, et al: Azithromycin in the treatment of periodontal disease: Effect on microflora. J Clin Periodontol 23:998–1003, 1996.
7. Seppala H, Klaukka T, Vuopio-Varkila J, et al: The effect of changes in the consumption of macrolide antibiotics on erythromycin resistance in group A streptococci in Finland. Finnish Study Group for Antimicrobial Resistance. N Engl J Med 337:441–446, 1997.

ANALGESICS

1. Acetaminophen, NSAIDs, and alcohol. Med Letter Drugs Ther 38(977):55–56, 1996.
2. Beaver WT: Aspirin and acetaminophen as constituents of analgesic combinations. Arch Intern Med 141:293–300, 1981.
3. Bell WR: Acetaminophen and warfarin: Undesirable synergy [editorial]. JAMA 279:702, 1998.
4. Breivik EK, Barkvoll P, Skovlund E: Combining diclofenac with acetaminophen or acetaminophen-codeine after oral surgery: A randomized double-blind single dose study. Clin Pharmacol Ther 66:625–635, 1999.
5. Deykin D, Janson P, McMahon L: Ethanol potentiation of aspirin-induced prolongation of bleeding time. N Engl J Med 306:852–854, 1982.
6. Dionne R: Additive analgesic effects of oxycodone and ibuprofen in the oral surgery model. J Oral Maxillofac Surg 57:673–678, 1999.
7. Dionne R: Additive analgesia without opioid side effects. Compendium 26:572, 2000.
8. Ehrich DG, Lundgren JP, Dionne RA, et al: Comparison of triazolam, diazepam, and placebo as outpatient oral premedication for endodontic patients. J Endod 23:181–184, 1997.
9. Hylek EM, Heiman H, Skates SJ, et al: Acetaminophen and other risk factors for excessive warfarin anticoagulation. JAMA 279:657–662, 1998.
10. Slattery JT, Nelson SD, Thummel KE: The complex interaction between ethanol and acetaminophen. Clin Pharmacol Ther 60:241–246, 1996.
11. Zimmerman HJ, Maddrey WC: Acetaminophen (paracetamol) hepatotoxicity with regular intake of alcohol: Analysis of instances of therapeutic misadventure. Hepatology 22:767–773, 1995.

SEIZURE DISORDERS

1. Consensus statements: Medical management of epilepsy. Neurology 51(suppl 4):S39–S43, 1998.
2. Mattson RH: Medical management of epilepsy in adults. Neurology 51(5 suppl 4):S15–S20, 1998.
3. Thomason JM, Seymour RA, Rawlins MD: Incidence and severity of phenytoin-induced gingival overgrowth in epileptic patients in general medical practice. Community Dent Oral Epidemiol 20:288–291, 1992.

INDEX

Page numbers in **boldface type** indicate complete chapters.